Symptomatic Subjects

ALEMBICS: PENN STUDIES IN LITERATURE AND SCIENCE

Mary Thomas Crane and Henry S. Turner, Series Editors

Symptomatic Subjects

Bodies, Medicine, and Causation
in the Literature of Late Medieval England

Julie Orlemanski

PENN

UNIVERSITY OF PENNSYLVANIA PRESS

PHILADELPHIA

Published by
University of Pennsylvania Press
Philadelphia, Pennsylvania 19104-4112
www.upenn.edu/pennpress

Printed in the United States of America on acid-free paper
10 9 8 7 6 5 4 3 2 1

Library of Congress Cataloging-in-Publication Data

Names: Orlemanski, Julie, author.
Title: Symptomatic subjects : bodies, medicine, and causation in the literature of
    late medieval England / Julie Orlemanski.
Other titles: Alembics.
Description: Philadelphia : University of Pennsylvania Press, [2019] | Series:
    Alembics : Penn studies in literature and science | Includes bibliographical
    references and index.
Identifiers: LCCN 2018045209| ISBN 9780812250909 (hardcover : alk. paper) |
    ISBN 0812250907 (hardcover : alk. paper)
Subjects: LCSH: Literature and medicine—England—History—To 1500. |
    Diseases—England—Causes and theories of causation—History—To 1500. |
    English literature—Middle English, 1100–1500—History and criticism. |
    Human body in literature. | Causation in literature.
Classification: LCC R702 .O75 2019 | DDC 610.942—dc23
LC record available at https://lccn.loc.gov/2018045209

For my family

Contents

PART IV. PERSONALIZING *PHISIK*

Abbreviations

DMLBS *Dictionary of Medieval Latin from British Sources.* 3 vols.
Ed. Richard Ashdowne, David Howlett, and Ronald Latham.
Oxford: British Academy, 2018. Online edition:
http://www.brepolis.net.

DOST *A Dictionary of the Older Scottish Tongue.* Oxford: Oxford
University Press, 2001. Online edition, 2004:
http://www.dsl.ac.uk/.

Du Cange *Glossarium mediae et infimae latinitatis.* 10 vols. Ed. Charles
du Fresne, sieur du Cange. Niort : L. Favre, 1883–1887.
Online edition: http://ducange.enc.sorbonne.fr/.

EETS Early English Text Society (o.s., Original Series, e.s., Extra Series,
s.s., Supplementary Series).

Godefroy *Dictionnaire de l'ancienne langue française et de tous ses dialectes
du IXe au XVe siècle.* 10 vols. Ed. Frédéric Godefroy. Paris:
F. Vieweg, 1881–1902. Online edition:
http://micmap.org/dicfro/search/dictionnaire-godefroy/.

MED *Middle English Dictionary.* Ed. Hans Kurath, Sherman M. Kuth,
and Robert E. Lewis. Ann Arbor: University of Michigan Press,
1954–2001. Online edition: http://quod.lib.umich.edu/m/med/.

ODNB *Oxford Dictionary of National Biography.* Oxford: Oxford
University Press, 2004. Online edition:
http://www.oxforddnb.com/.

OED *Oxford English Dictionary.* Oxford: Oxford University Press,
2014. Online edition: http://www.oed.com/.

Introduction

Early in Geoffrey Chaucer's romance *Troilus and Criseyde*, the officious match-maker Pandarus advises Troilus on how to write a love letter. He warns against jumbling "discordant thyng yfeere [together], / As thus, to usen termes of phisik / In loves termes [for example, to use terms of medicine among love's terms]."[1] Mixing medicine's lexicon with lovespeak, he admonishes, would make Troilus comparable to a painter who depicts a fish "With asses feet, and hedde[s] it as an ape [with donkey's feet, and gives it the head of an ape]."[2] Different conceptual idioms, Pandarus seems to think, have different bodies that go with them; combining them "cordeth naught [does not accord]."[3] And yet, in spite of Pandarus's advice, Chaucer and many other late medieval writers show themselves to have been great jumblers of "termes of phisik." Their writings mingle medical vocabulary with the generic stylings of romance, consolation, satire, exemplum, miracle story, and devotional meditation, among others. The physiological descriptions of lovesickness woven through *Troilus and Criseyde* are enough to suggest that Pandarus's poetics are not, in fact, Chaucer's own.[4] But Pandarus's stylistic injunction nevertheless does imply that the distinction of "termes of phisik" from their putative others—the terms' at least imaginary cordoning off from other conceptual vocabularies—was a comprehensible one, perhaps as clear as the difference between a fish and an ape.

This study investigates what late medieval writers were up to in using "termes of phisik" in their compositions, which is to say, what notions of embodiment, subjectivity, and causality medicine made available and what writers did with them. *Phisik* in fourteenth- and fifteenth-century England was a discourse in ascent. In this era just prior to what we think of as medicine's dawning modernity—before Renaissance anatomy, before the centralized regulation of medical professions, before the rise of empiricism or the rationalist division of mental from physical substance—England was the scene of a remarkable upsurge in medical writing. Between the arrival of the Black

Death in 1348 and the start of English printing in 1476, thousands of discrete medical texts were copied, translated, or composed, the large majority for readers without university degrees.[5] These sundry texts shared a model of the universe crisscrossed with physical forces and a picture of the human body as a changeable, composite thing, tuned materially to the world's vicissitudes. This book tells the story of how embodied subjectivity was narrated in its entangled relation to the world in the era of medicine's unprecedented textual vitality. In that, it offers one approach to the phenomenology of medieval selfhood, or what it was like, within the era's mix of discourses, to reflect on both having and being a body.

The period was one of intellectual ferment for lay and vernacular readers. By the later fourteenth century, it had been more than two hundred years since new Latin translations of Galenic medicine, Aristotelian natural philosophy, and their Arabic commentators began circulating in western Christendom, offering distinctive accounts of why the physical world was as it was. Medicine was where the inquiry into nature scaled itself to the human form, and one effect of its widespread textualization was to render the material body, it seemed, less human. *Phisik* showed persons strafed with the impersonal systems of life—elements, mixtures of qualities, humors, members, powers, faculties, and spirits.[6] They were vulnerable to a volatile economy of physical forces. Such ideas reached new audiences in formats like encyclopedias, mirrors for princes, plague tracts, physiognomies, surgical compendia, gynecological treatises, sermons, devotional literature, and many others. The play of unsystematized authorities and the wrangling over explanations without a solidified framework to order them characterized intellectual inquiry outside university walls, where *scientia* and skill, Latin and Middle English, and speculation and pragmatics each had its part to play.

Medicine's model of the strange and symptomatic body tangled in skeins of cause and effect called forth answering paradigms. Personal agency and its theological counterpart, free will, remained crucial to medieval conceptions of the person. Penitential discipline recoded the body's sufferings; spiritual analogy made medicine the repository of metaphor; and courtly idealization conscripted bodily harm into spectacles of social cohesion. As naturalistic models of causation mingled with penitential, miraculous, and socially symbolic ones, their juxtaposition demanded that a growing number of readers negotiate the divided claims of material forces, willful action, and divine power. Partly as a result, the later Middle Ages became a period of what I will call *etiological imagination*—an era broadly fascinated with projects of explanatory invention and the tasks of envisioning, arbitrating among, and emplotting intricate causal chains. Why did one patient recover and a second worsen? Why did a husband contract leprosy when his wife did not? Was it on account of the man's melancholic disposition, the miasmatic air, or his sinfulness? Case by case, medieval men and women pieced together distinctive causal explanations, often drawing on divergent intellectual traditions, and so acted as bricoleurs of etiology. At the center of this book's investigations is the claim that when we attend to the language of *phisik*, both in the intricacy of its conceptual system and in its promiscuous uptake, we discover previously unremarked experiments in combining causation and selfhood in the texts of late medieval England. These experiments transpire, I will show, in the space of a stubborn phenomenological gap between one's materiality and one's experience, or between having and being a body.

Literary narratives played a distinctive role in the endeavors of etiological imagination. Authors like Geoffrey Chaucer, Robert Henryson, Thomas Hoccleve, Margery Kempe, and the playwright of the *Croxton Play of the Sacrament* adopted the rich terminology of the body and its ailments to depict characters struggling to control their bodies and to control the interpretations that gave their bodies meaning. These writers tell the stories of *symptomatic subjects*, figures marked with leprous pustules, or the pallor of lovesickness, or lunacy's rolling eyes—who try to gloss and construe their own bodily conditions. Such figures inhabit a contentious hermeneutic circle that churns between competing systems of explanation, in the interchange of symptoms and speech acts, flesh and rhetoric.

Because poetic narratives could encompass multiple kinds of causation in their plots and could orchestrate competing discourses within their polyvocal bounds ("termes of phisik," "loves termes," and many more besides), they came to act as *meta*-etiological forms, or arenas for commenting on the relations among causal and explanatory models. Stories like Chaucer's "Knight's Tale" and Henryson's *Testament of Cresseid* gather together and then tangle the etiological categories that determine bodies. They draw into a single plot powers as varied as the pagan gods, the planets, humoral physiology, erotic compulsion, political history, chance, fate, a benevolent monotheistic deity, and metafictional determination. Such a dizzying array renders the ultimate significance of stories like these difficult to decide, and such interpretive resistance, I will argue, acts to thematize the workings of etiological imagination. Extended self-narrations, like the *Book of Margery Kempe* and Thomas Hoccleve's *Series*, give such meta-etiology a further twist. The portrayal of the author's wildly symptomatic body directs readers' etiological scrutiny to the text's narrating voice. As interpreters try to parse the balance of external impingement and narrative design, the text threatens to become itself a symptom—a possibility to which Margery Kempe's *Book* and Hoccleve's *Series* show themselves keenly alert.

The aim of the extended close readings that make up the latter half of *Symptomatic Subjects* is not primarily to contextualize the literary works, for instance by demonstrating which contemporary practices of *phisik* informed them (though some of this will be necessary). It is rather to reveal these works' speaking back to *phisik*, in part by speaking through it. Poetry and imaginative narrative, I will contend, participated in the late medieval project of remapping the self's causal impingements, a project at once broadly shared and fractured into distinctive and sometimes conflicting idioms like medicine, natural philosophy, pastoralia, theology, and mythography. *Symptomatic Subjects* tracks this remapping as it unfolds across several genres and scenes, with an eye to the shifting domains, the mobile and unrationalized patterns of continuity and discontinuity, that characterize the etiological imagination in the later Middle Ages.

The structure of this book follows a trajectory from "termes of phisik" to those terms' reinvention in literary narrative. It arcs from accounting for medicine as a distinctive if heterogeneous discourse in fourteenth- and fifteenth-century England, through medicine's uptake in the registers of satire and exemplum, and onward to the frictional interface of causation and embodied agency in some of the most important works of Middle English writing. These topics constitute a series of overlapping investigations that cumulatively show how and why *phisik* mattered in late medieval England. The book falls into four parts. Part I, "Thinking with *Phisik*," introduces medicine as medieval people practiced and articulated it. The first chapter, "Imagining Etiology," serves as an introduction to the study as a whole. It describes the historical conditions of medicine's textual efflorescence in England and maps out the crucial tensions defining *phisik*'s cultural role—tensions between theory and practice, science and art, generality and particularity, symptom and expression, and causation and agency. Chapter 2, "Cause, Authority, Sign, and Book," explores *phisik* from four angles—how it grappled with causal understanding, how the authority to heal was negotiated, what the semiotics of the medical body looked like, and what bookish forms medicine assumed.

In Part II, "Playing with *Phisik*," I turn to medicine's implication in two literary modes. Chapter 3, "Satire and Medical Materialism," shows how medicine's jargon and its focus on the materiality of the body acted as the stimulus to satirical invective, particularly in Chaucer's "Nun's Priest's Tale," Henryson's "Sum Practysis of Medecyne," and the East Anglican miracle play the *Croxton Play of the Sacrament*. The fourth chapter, "Embodying Causation in Exempla," argues that exemplary stories operated in ways that are parallel to medicine's own modes of understanding: both sought to recognize a more general realm of governing principles in the fate of particular bodies. I trace the growing role of narrative in the medical writings of the later Middle Ages as well as the place of medicine and disease in homiletic literature, including the *Gesta Romanorum* and *Piers Plowman*.

Part III, "Emplotting *Phisik*," tracks how medical terminology, the impingements of the material body, and etiological complexity come to be incorporated into the plots of two vernacular poems. "The Metaphysics of *Phisik* in the 'Knight's Tale'" focuses on the seemingly gratuitous medical language used to describe Arcite shortly before his death. I argue that Theseus's final speech of consolation allows us to recognize *phisik*'s role in the tale's imagination of alternatives to the monotheistic order of the Prime Mover. Chapter 6, "Desire and Defacement in the *Testament of Cresseid*," shows how Henryson's decision to strike Cresseid with leprosy effects a shift from the romance conventions of Chaucer's *Troilus and Criseyde* to those of the exemplum. However, an incoherence in the exemplary plot creates uncertainty about what kind of justice is served. The would-be story of punitive disease is haunted by another tradition of leprosy's medieval representation, that of affective devotion.

In the last part of *Symptomatic Subjects*, "Personalizing *Phisik*," narrative voice, rather than plot, becomes the central object of literary analysis. The seventh chapter, "Symptoms and the Signifying Condition in Hoccleve's *Series*," explores the symptomatic self-loss that Hoccleve's narratorial persona undergoes during his madness. I argue that Hoccleve knits together accounts of symptomatic and textual expression to offer a new embodiment of the signifying condition. Chapter 8, "From Noise to Narration in the *Book of Margery Kempe*," reads Margery's paramystical crying as a symptom. Her involuntary vocalizations, I argue, allow the *Book* to construct its own textual voice through iterative circuits of symptom and explanation, noise and narration. Finally, in the coda, I remark on *Symptomatic Subjects* in light of the scholarly subfield of the history of the body and issues of historical periodization.

PART I

Thinking with *Phisik*

Chapter 1

Imagining Etiology

On the final decorated folio of a fifteenth-century English medical manuscript, a figure gazes out. This is the Wound Man, a conventional surgical diagram that has been rendered here, in what is now London, Wellcome Library MS 290, with extraordinary delicacy (Figure 1).[1] His well-proportioned body stands with a naturalistic grace, left leg slightly bent, even though the outline of his body is punctured with arrows, swords, clubs, and spears, and his skin gapes with open sores. He regards his viewers calmly from this unbearable embodiment, displaying his gashes and lesions. The picture is the last in a series of eight full-page medical illustrations in the manuscript, occupying their own quire after a pair of anatomical treatises in Middle English.[2] The minute strokes of the artist's shading evoke the heft of the Wound Man's limbs and testify to a degree of mimetic craftsmanship in excess of the image's technical purpose. Like the medical diagrams of the Disease Man, the Blood-Letting Man, and the Zodiac Man, the Wound Man is designed for heuristic reference, not verisimilar representation; he gives schematic and mnemonic shape to a long list of cutaneous conditions. But in this manuscript, unusually, the image has little connection to the accompanying medical texts, and the Latin labels that unfurl around him are not linked to further elaborations.[3] He is unmoored from any straightforward purpose. The floating tools and weapons around him suggest the instruments of the *arma Christi*, the oft-depicted instruments of the Passion, and even more closely he echoes warnings against Sabbath breakers found in medieval English wall paintings, where images of the "Sunday Christ" show implements biting into Christ's limbs just as they do into the Wound Man's.[4] Finely detailed features, his closed lips and heavy-lidded eyes, intimate a sense of lucid endurance and, together with this, the impression of inwardness, some self that is the locus of his undergoing.

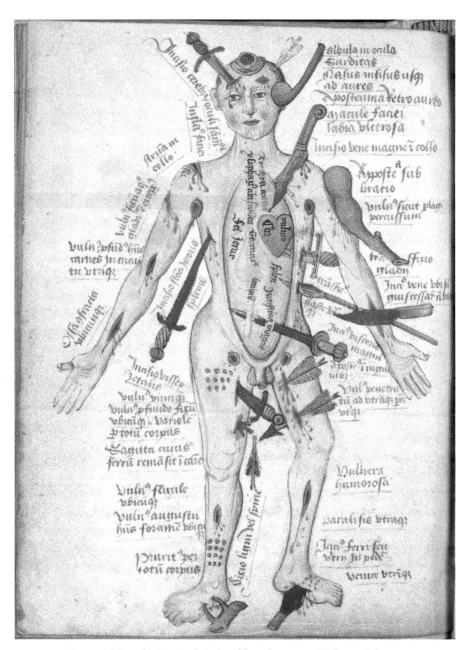

Figure 1. Wound Man. English, late fifteenth century, Wellcome Library
MS 290, fol. 53v. Courtesy of the Wellcome Library, London.

Whatever depths are hinted at, however, recede from the shallow openness of his chest cavity and the Wound Man's bright, bared heart.

Untethered from texts describing treatment for his injuries, then, the Wellcome Wound Man is at least as much about the emotional and aesthetic pull of his injured figure as he is about surgical expertise.[5] Like many of the corporealized figures discussed in the chapters to follow, he conjures a multitude of discourses and associations. The contents of the manuscript bespeak theoretical anatomy; his iconography's origins are in surgical therapeutics; and the parallels with Christian devotional imagery are too obvious to be missed. But he also signifies in terms less bound by discursive context. Insofar as medicine addresses broadly shared conditions like pain, mortality, and physical flourishing, the line between technical expertise and palpable experience is never secure. The Wound Man, with his finely modeled limbs and face, exerts a mimetic and thus a recognitive claim. He is *like us*—and that intuition is perceptible in the minor discomfort of calling him an *it*. At the same time, this is unambiguously a diagram, a pigmented shape. Medical knowledge depends on the abstraction and inscription of corporeality, and the ontological gap between representation and flesh ongoingly qualifies interpretation. Between *him* and *it*, the Wound Man holds viewers' gaze in the image's crosscurrents.

Because the significance of the human body is never strictly scientific—because it attracts multiple schemes of regulation and recognition and calls up notions of experience, consciousness, and self—situations of medical explanation verge constantly into dramas of embodiment and expression, interpretation and feeling. This chapter and those that follow attend to such dramas as they unfolded in the era of medical writing's popularization in England. Wellcome Library MS 290 is a small part of what was a sea change in how men and women in medieval England read and wrote about their bodies. During the later fourteenth century and throughout the fifteenth, medical textuality flourished. English readers demanded and produced an enormous number of manuscripts addressing why bodies thrived and suffered and how they could be healed. The spread of medical literacy called for imagination as well as intellectual and practical skills. It asked audiences to picture their bodies, their world, and the interactions between them differently. Readers experimented with seeing themselves medically and seeing their bodies as the materialization of causes. Optimistically, medical textuality helped to realize a causally labile universe, one in which readers might understand and influence their corporeal conditions. More darkly, medicine articulated the constitutive vulnerability of the microcosm to the macrocosm—a vulnerability figured in the Wound Man's opened flesh.

The Wellcome Wound Man acts as something of a found allegorical figure, embodying dynamics that are at play across the length of *Symptomatic Subjects*. In the simultaneity of his woundable passivity and his upright carriage, he brings to a point of high tension the qualities of determination and agency that recur in medieval depictions of symptomatic expression. By seeming to *show* his wounds, to relate himself to them in the midst of his hyperbolic suffering, he suggests the centripetal pull of the self as an idea that gathers the porous, dissolving body back together. The Wound Man is also a crossroads for narrative. Each of his particular harms—*incisio cerebri* (incision to the brain), *inflatio faciei* (swelling of the face), *sagitta cuius ferrum remansit in carne* (arrowhead stuck in the flesh)—unspools an incipient case history. Finally, what turns out to be his melancholy joke is that he is no one. He portrays no singular body, not even an idealized one. The extravagance of his injuries is a function of his generality: he condenses in one figure what medical practitioners would have encountered across dozens of patients. Medieval theories of knowledge, which were shaped by Aristotelian thought, held that there could be no true science of particulars. Accordingly, the translation from individual patient to general rule and back again was required for the understanding that *phisik* made possible. But it is the Wound Man's wit and pathos that he at once embodies and evades that translation. He sets generality in the teeth of individuation, so that it is hard not to see him, this compendium of maladies, as an ill-fated and piteous fellow.

The present chapter explores some of the dynamics exemplified in the Wellcome Wound Man, which are also endemic to the interpretation of bodies in late medieval England. The Wound Man personifies these dynamics in a decidedly extreme form, on the edge of paradox. However, as will become clear, the strange conditions of the Wound Man's flesh—the polarized interplay of determination and agency, the embodiment of causes, and the flickering between generality and particularity—can be traced through much of medieval medicine and other endeavors of somatic interpretation in the period, as they helped set in motion novel projects of explanation, expression, and imagination.

Symptoms and Selves

Among the pilgrims described in the General Prologue of the *Canterbury Tales*, it is Chaucer's Summoner who is least at home in his own skin. No doubt, the man has his physical pleasures: he loves eating garlic, onions, and leeks, drinking strong red wine, belting out a duet with the Pardoner in his "stif burdoun [strong bass]," and enjoying the company of "his concubyn," not to mention the other "yonge girles of the diocise."[6] But the Summoner's portrait begins with his irritated, abraded, and discomfiting face and all the remedies that fail to change it:

> A Somonour was ther with us in that place,
> That hadde a fyr-reed cherubynnes face,
> For saucefleem he was, with eyen narwe.
> As hoot he was and lecherous as a sparwe,
> With scalled browes blake and piled berd.
> Of his visage children were aferd.
> Ther nas quyk-silver, lytarge, ne brymstoon,
> Boras, ceruce, ne oille of tartre noon,
> Ne oynement that wolde clense and byte,
> That hym myghte helpen of his whelkes white,
> Nor of the knobbes sittynge on his chekes. (623–33)

[A Summoner was with us there, who had a fire-red cherubim's face and narrow eyes, for he was afflicted with saucefleme. He was as hot and lecherous as a sparrow, with scabby brows and a patchy beard. Children were afraid of his appearance. No quicksilver, lead oxide, brimstone, borax, white lead, cream of tartar, nor any ointment that cleans and burns might help him with his white pustules, nor the knobs sitting on his cheeks.]

Saucefleme—*salsum flegma* or "salt phlegm"—was an itchy, scabby inflammation of the face, which entailed swelling, discoloration, and pustules. It could be a symptom of leprosy but was generally regarded as a dermatological ailment in its own right. That the term is unusual in the late fourteenth century is suggested by the fact that the General Prologue is the earliest recorded usage, with nearly all subsequent attestations coming from remedy collections or surgical treatises.[7] The word's technical flavor marks the Summoner's individuating details as notably *medical* phenomena. The diagnostic quality of readers' attention is bolstered by the lines' implication of causal links between the Summoner's intemperate behavior and his pathology. Numerous scholars have catalogued the echoes between the portrait and medieval medical writings.[8] Yet even if some of Chaucer's contemporary readers were unin-formed about the details of *phisik*, the similarity between the Summoner's "fyr-reed" visage and the "strong wyn, reed as blood" and the rhyme between his pimpled "chekes" and diet of "lekes" would insinuate correlations between what the Summoner does and what he physically is (624, 635, 633–34).

By the point that the Summoner appears in the General Prologue, Chau-cer's readers have grown familiar with their hermeneutic task—to glean from details of dress, habit, physiognomy, and diction hints of each pilgrim's moral disposition and style of social inhabitation. The momentary encounter, we are given to understand, is a metonym for the greater life, and each visible exterior ciphers a distinctive personality. So, the Yeoman's "broun visage" reflects his life outdoors, and the Prioress's vast "fair forheed" imports courtly mien (109, 154). That the Monk is "ful fat" is not unrelated to his appetite for "fat swan" (200, 206), and so on. The General Prologue is one of the great documents of characterological implication in medieval literature, and features like the Miller's wart and the Cook's mormal have primed readers to conjecture among behavior, persona, and bodily form. As the audience looks through the narra-tor's eyes, they exercise a symptomizing regard, discovering in each pilgrim's appearance traces of those forces—institutional, natural, and subjective—that shape the life. Diagnosis and etiological imagination mingle with the everyday business of social discernment.

When the narrator reports of the Summoner, "saucefleem he was, with eyen narwe. / As hoot he was and lecherous as a sparwe," the lines' three char-acterizing adjectives (*saucefleem*, *hoot*, and *lecherous*) all point, from different angles, toward the mediating notion of *complexio*. Complexion—the relative calibration of the body's four primary physical qualities (hot, cold, moist, and dry) and its humors (phlegm, blood, black bile, and red or yellow bile)—was perhaps the most widely known idea from Galenic medicine in the Middle Ages. Complexional theory acted as a rational basis for linking together the body's circumstances, its state of health, its appearance, and its unseen material reality. Understood in terms of complexion, *saucefleem* represents an imbal-ance in the humors. Disease in the Middle Ages was conceived not in terms of an underlying invasive entity but as temperamental disequilibrium. The idea that the Summoner's dietary and sexual excess is somehow responsible for his *saucefleem* partakes of the understanding of *complexio* as a proportionality that varies constantly, fluctuating with every change in someone's intake, environs, and behavior.

The adjective *hoot*, by contrast, hints at a more permanent physiological condition. As Nancy Siraisi explains, in medieval medical theory "each person was endowed with his or her own innate complexion; this was an essential identifying characteristic acquired at the moment of conception and in some way persisting throughout life. . . . Thus, a particular person might be characterized as having a hot complexion relative to other human beings, and this characterization would apply to him or her throughout life."[9] Such categories became sweeping social typologies in the later Middle Ages, as their use elsewhere in the General Prologue suggests: the Reeve is "a sclendre colerik man," while the Franklin's "complexioun" is "sangwyn" (587, 333). In these cases, the order of causation partly reverses itself: it may be *because* the Summoner is "hot" that he craves what he craves and does what he does. Complexion produces action, as well as action producing complexion. *Lecherous* shifts the Summoner's description more squarely into the moral realm, though the disposition to lust too could be entailed by humoral disposition. The comparison to a sparrow reinforces the apparent innateness of the Summoner's characteristics. The sparrow "is a ful hoot bridde and lecherous," reads John Trevisa's translation of Bartholomaeus Anglicus's popular encyclopedia *De proprietatibus rerum*.[10] How different are the sparrow's species traits from the Summoner's proclivities? Does the man's complexion determine him, or does he determine it? Would physiological and moral change demand an Archimedean point beyond the confines of the Summoner's own flesh?

In no way does the General Prologue force such questions, which after all were among the most contentious of the Middle Ages and edged swiftly into disputes about inclination and free will.[11] It is part of the narrator's blithe tact not to dwell on matters like these. Tensions between choice and disposition, or between individual and type, are allowed to remain suspended, and in this way Chaucer's General Prologue is similar to the medical discourse that partly undergirds it. Both *phisik* and Chaucer-the-pilgrim leave aside dogmatic pronouncements to concentrate on the intricately particularized individuals at hand. But in the process of doing so they end up instantiating a distinctive way of seeing the world, focused on persons' jointly material and semiotic constitutions and how these constitutions might be read.

The co-implication of natural impulse and human action is raised in no less prominent a place than the first lines of the General Prologue. It is "*Whan* that Aprill" moves the nectar in the flowers and sets the mechanisms of spring into lush operation, "*Thanne* longen folk to goon on pilgrimages."

The temporal coincidence of season and devotion allows nature and religion to share the stage, and the mischievous rhyme between the songbirds' *corages* (where they feel Nature's prick) and the people's *pilgrimages* needles a connection that remains unsettled and unsettling throughout the *Canterbury Tales*, namely, the link between what we are (our longings, our actions, our bodies, our identities) and the forces in which we are enmeshed, like the prickling warmth of April and our answering flesh. These are the relations, between conditions and causes, that medieval medicine addresses as well. The more that readers of the General Prologue wish to pin down a given character—to diagnose the Summoner, interpret the Wife's gapped teeth, determine whether or not the Physician is blameworthy, or know if the Pardoner is "a geldyng or a mare" (691)—the more urgently do uncertainties about causation, agency, and the stability of signs circulate. But the breezy narration, like *complexio*'s manifestly flexible apparatus, keeps radical incoherence out of sight. Both the General Prologue and medieval physiological theory generate a sense of knowing that trails off in the details, leaving room for indeterminacy. In Chaucer's hands, this trailing off nourishes the impression that each pilgrim has a subjectivity in excess of the available grids of explanation.[12] He invites his readers, then, to follow the advice of Galen (d. c. 210 CE), who declares that interiority can be known "if not by means of an absolutely firm kind of knowledge [*disciplinam certam*], then at least by 'artful' conjecture [*secundum coniecturam quandam artificialem*]."[13]

Throughout this book, I use the term *symptom* to name a somatic disturbance that, in its departure from expectations of bodily appearance or function, provokes interpretation. Symptoms appear when we regard bodies as animated systems of signs that refer to the nonconscious or only partly conscious processes in which material selves are entangled. Symptoms need not be medical. Miraculous indices of God's favor appear frequently on medieval bodies, and romances are full of characters whose bodies mutely testify to their noble origins, like the light pouring from the mouth of Havelock the Dane. For their construal, symptoms require not only that interpreters work back from effects to cause but also that they make a decision among explanatory systems. Hermeneutic instructions are not *in* symptoms—not in the body's pallor, excretions, pulse, or pain—but rather in the discursive environment where the body is embedded and becomes legible. The General Prologue pulls readers through a shifting series of discourses—moralistic, satirical, courtly, penitential, exemplary, physiognomic—to interpret the pilgrims' figures. In the Summoner's portrait and the "artful conjectures" it inspires, medicine's primary operations of diagnosis, etiology, and treatment blend seamlessly into the structuring themes of the General Prologue, like the tensions between natural impulse and human action, type and individual, and sign and self.

My broad definition of the symptom, as an involuntary bodily sign, is at odds with the word's narrow use in medieval Latin (*symptoma, sinthoma*) and in Middle English (*sinthome*), where it almost always appears in the context of learned medicine.[14] The ancient Greek term originally meant a mischance, something that happens to or befalls someone, and it is relatively late in the development of Greek medical writing that *sumptōmata* came to denominate those bodily phenomena from which disease is inferred.[15] In the twelfth century a transliterated form of the Greek word made its way into Latin translations of classical medical writings, to denote a quality or condition of the body—as in the *Liber de sinthomatibus mulierum*, or the "Book on the Conditions of Women," as Monica Green translates it.[16] From Latin, the word eventually entered medical writing in Middle English. More often, medical writers and translators employed the terms *accidens* (in Middle English, *accident*) and *significatio* (*signe* or *token*) to name the indices of disease. "Accident" forms a neat etymological counterpart to the Greek *sumptōmata*: from *ad* and *cadere*, it also means a falling to, or something that befalls, which gives it its philosophical sense as a contingent attribute.

Medieval theories of the natural sign (*signa naturalia*) are one framework for understanding the symptom's yoking of causation and signification. According to Augustine's foundational *De doctrina christiana*, the division between natural signs and conventional signs (*signa data*) is a basic distinction of semiotic theory. Whereas words proceed from a desire to communicate via a mutually recognized system of signs, *signa naturalia* make something known "without a wish or any urge to signify [*sine voluntate atque ullo appetitu significandi*]."[17] Augustine's examples are smoke, an animal footprint, and the face of someone angry or sad. Smoke "means" fire because smoke is caused by fire; the face indicates the mind's feelings independently of the will (*etiam nulla ejus voluntate*).[18] Relations of signifier and signified map onto relations of effect and cause. Augustine acknowledges briefly that such signifying is not itself merely natural; it depends on someone's "observation and memory of experience with things [*rerum expertarum animadversione et notatione*]."[19] Roger Bacon, in his 1267 treatise *De signis*, elaborates on this point. Bacon was one of the leading interpreters of the "new" Aristotle and a controversially original thinker in natural philosophy. In *De signis*, he notes that "according to the order of nature [*ordinem naturae*] one thing is the cause of another without having a relation of themselves to a knowing power, but solely from the fact of their relation with one another."[20] In other words, causes produce effects regardless of whether anyone knows about them. But signification works differently: "By contrast, the relations of sign, of signified, and of the one to whom signification occurs are applied through a relation to the mind apprehending [*animam apprehendentem*]."[21] Despite the symptom's natural, causal entailment, its legibility depends on learned systems of signs. For *accidens* to become *significatio*, the "mind apprehending" must track its meaning.

One of the foundational texts of medieval medical study, the *Isagoge* of Joannitius (Hunayn ibn Ishaq, d. 873), illustrates how the gap between causation and signification comes to be charged with social import. In its discussion of different categories of symptoms (*de generibus significationum*), it makes one distinction that depends not on the signs' bodily location or timing but rather on the vantage from which the symptoms are perceived. "There is a distinction between signs and accidents," the treatise states, even though "they have a single physical appearance"—namely, "to the patient [*infirmo*] these are accidents [*accidentia*], while to the doctor [*medico*], they are signs [*significationes*]."[22] The same corporeal phenomena—sweating, racing pulse, trembling lips—are here endowed with two different states of existence, depending on whether they appear to the physician or the sick person. The treatise subtracts the semiotic quality of the symptom insofar as it happens to the patient. By reserving the symptom's signifying power to the *medicus*, the *Isagoge* testifies to its place in a self-consciously learned tradition of healing, where interpretive authority rests with the educated practitioner. The distinction of sign from accident, even though "they have a single physical appearance," also opens on to a much broader issue, namely, what authority (if any) the person bearing a symptom has to interpret it. Does the immediacy of her perspective yield any special insight, or is it disqualifyingly close? How does first-person knowledge rate alongside systematized expertise? Questions like these, about embodied experience and medical authority, are negotiated in many of the texts discussed in the chapters to follow.

It is the symptom's medium, the living body, that gives the semiotic category its distinctiveness.[23] Consciousness has only dim awareness of the biological processes that support its existence—the thickening of mucus membranes, the secretions of glands, the regulation of the heartbeat, and so on—processes that during the Middle Ages were categorized under the body's "natural" and "vital" powers. Usually these processes carry on beneath the level of direct awareness, but in illness they spring to notice. Pain and bodily malfunction exaggerate the felt distinction between one's sense of self and one's corporeality, lending the body a kind of aggression: my stomach hurts; my stomach hurts *me*.[24] In a sermon from the early fifth century, Augustine captures something of this phenomenological insight when he seeks to define illness's opposite, health. "What is health?" he asks and answers, "Sensing, feeling nothing."[25] He continues, clarifying: "It isn't just not to feel, as a stone doesn't feel, as a tree doesn't feel, as a corpse doesn't feel; but to live in the body and to feel nothing of its being a burden, that's what being healthy is."[26] In health, according to Augustine's account, the body fades from concern, in what for him is a faint foretaste of resurrection. By contrast, symptoms, in their disturbance of somatic operation, trouble the body's easy absorption into the self and insist that we feel its burden.

Strikingly, as the sermon continues, Augustine links the body's obtrusion in sickness to the alien quality of medical discourse:

> Indeed, we have many things inside us, in our entrails; would any of us know about them unless we had seen them in butchered bodies? Our guts, our innards, which are called intestines, how do we know about them? And then, precisely, it's good, when we don't feel them. When we don't feel them, after all, when we are unaware of them, is when we are healthy. You say to someone, "Observe the esophagus." He answers you, "What's the esophagus?" Lucky ignorance! He doesn't know where he keeps what is always healthy. If it wasn't healthy, he would feel it; if he could feel it, he would be aware of it, and not for his own good.[27]

Here the very strangeness of medicine's perspective and jargon is made into a premonition of suffering. Physiological vocabulary speaks for parts thrust into awareness by discomfort and breakdown. Augustine's remarks dramatize how illness's felt disjunction between body and self functions as an opening for discourse, when medicine's language and gaze find their way into self-perception. To imagine our insides, according to Augustine, we project the sight of corpses inside ourselves, mingling our most private sensations with the observation of dead flesh. The passage's brief imagined dialogue—*Observe the esophagus. What's the esophagus?*—emphasizes the difference that perspective makes in speaking about the body. The terms of physiology seem alien to the healthy man; they name what he does not even know he has. But if he falls ill, he will need to speak in medicine's idiom. On Augustine's account, then, first-person experiences of sickness estrange us from our bodies and drive us to find new languages to describe them, to come to terms with what he calls the body's burden.

None of this is to imply, however, that the Middle Ages had a dualistic conception of body and self. Christian theology and natural philosophy insisted on the ultimately embodied nature of human identity, albeit from different angles.[28] Scholastic Aristotelianism taught that the soul was the substantial form of the body, and the incarnational theology central to late medieval devotion foregrounded the inextricability of flesh and salvation. But medieval culture, with its many ways of articulating corporeality, simultaneously spoke about what could not be directly identified with the body—self, subject, soul, spirit, person, reason, will. Through myriad explanations and practices, such terms were then re-related to the self's materiality. Embodied subjectivity was negotiated between physical determination and willful agency and among the many historically specific ways of describing that interplay.

Returning to Chaucer's Summoner, we can see that he exemplifies a number of key aspects of what it's like to inhabit and respond to the observable disturbances of the flesh. Symptoms, as the Summoner's portrait shows, are both material and social, taking shape between physiology and the expectations that frame it. His face is symptomatic because it is scabby and *fyr-reed* but also because of the fear that children express when they see it. As readers make their way through his portrait, his anomalous body catalyzes etiological speculation. Details of his life are drawn centripetally around his swollen, carbuncled features. We are called to fit his symptoms into a network of causes running both inside and outside his body and through various moments of biographical time. Etiological inference, it seems, is good at establishing correspondences between body and world but less adept at deciding the priority of cause and effect, or determining the relative fixedness, or fluidity, of embodied identity. And so, symptoms pose riddles of agency. They cannot be controlled merely by someone's intending: the Summoner cannot directly will his skin fair or his complexion balanced. But symptoms respond to altered circumstances, to changed behaviors and habits. *Phisik* offers a backdoor to agency, through the manipulation of bodily causes, though in the case of the Summoner's pharmaceutical self-fashioning, the seven medicines mentioned in the portrait all fall short.

These would-be remedies of quicksilver, lead oxide, brimstone, borax, white lead, and cream of tartar are all topical treatments to be applied to the skin. The superficial nature of the cures is of a piece with the Summoner's preference for shallow pleasures over spiritual depths and for easy fixes over moral labor. But the remedies' topicality may also say something meaningful about how the Summoner addresses himself to his body. It is from the outside that he tries to fix his symptomatic visage—from the same vantage that the gawking children *aferd* of his face look at him and, for that matter, from the position of the appraising narrator and readers. Like Augustine's account of how someone comes to name her own intestines or esophagus, it is by way of others' gaze that the Summoner recognizes his appearance as frightful, symptomatic, and in need of alteration. What could have been a mere accidental quality, a reddened roughness of the skin, assumes the role of stigma. The friction that Chaucer famously evokes between each pilgrim's social role and that role's idiosyncratic performance becomes in the Summoner's case a friction at his own bodily surface, between his materiality and his desires, between what others see and what he wishes them to see. It is a resistance that, one imagines, is perceptible in the medicated abrasion of his skin, raw with borax, mercury, lead, and *brymstoon*—a corroded redness that is finally inextricable from the symptoms he treats.

English *Phisik*

The sense that *saucefleem*'s remedies might be near at hand and bodily infirmity susceptible to medical know-how are hopes that Chaucer's Summoner would have shared with many in late medieval England. Medical discourse was on the rise. In the later fourteenth century, readers began to seek out and produce unprecedented numbers of texts addressed to the tasks of understanding and caring for human bodies. England's growing culture of medical literacy and care was in many ways unique—a bricolaged, miscellaneous, and constantly renegotiated set of practices.

The absence of even incipient structures of regulation and professionalization distinguished England's medical marketplace from the contemporary situation elsewhere in western Europe. The Royal College of Physicians was not founded until 1518, and medieval Oxford and Cambridge had only paltry medical faculties: "At Oxford . . . fewer than 100 men left any record of medical study [before 1500]. This was about one percent of recorded students. Cambridge's body of medical students was about half the size of Oxford's."[29] This differed from the powerful medical faculties in Paris, Montpellier, Bologna, and Padua.[30] England's cities lacked the broadly organized medical guilds of a place like late medieval Florence, and none of them paid salaries to physicians to help the poor and sick, in contrast to France, Italy, and the Crown of Aragon.[31] The lack of opportunities for official employment disincentivized medical credentialing. Instead, patients in England sought health care within a heterogeneous network of physicians, apothecaries, astrologers, members of barber-surgeon guilds, itinerant "leeches" with and without formal education, midwives, tooth-drawers, oculists, parish priests, monastic communities, saints' shrines, and members of their own or local households. While a few shared assumptions about complexion and pharmacopoeia, based upon broadly Galenic foundations, lent consistency to this range of healing authority, there is little else that these several modes of care can be presumed to share.

And yet one finds evidence for marked, punctual growth in medical writing. Thousands of medical texts in Middle English and Anglo-Latin survive from the late fourteenth and fifteenth centuries.[32] While many kinds of informational writing were on the rise in the period, "the greatest growth was seen in the number of medical and surgical texts written in medieval English. The increase was nothing less than explosive," writes historian of medicine Faye Getz.[33] The acceleration of textual production is evident in the calculations of Peter Murray Jones, based on Dorothea Waley Singer's hand-list of scientific manuscripts in the British Isles from before the sixteenth century—which deals with an estimated 30,000 to 40,000 texts across several languages. Jones estimates that six times as many texts survive from the fifteenth century as do from the fourteenth—despite the falling population and the more ephemeral (because more utilitarian) manuscript formats. These numbers "argue sufficiently strongly for dramatic developments in the way medical and scientific books were valued and used."[34] Moreover, Jones's analysis shows the strongly medical orientation of the developing interest in science: the sum of texts and manuscripts dealing with medicine "amounts to more than all those dealing with the remaining subjects."[35]

The database of scientific and medical writings in Old and Middle English, compiled by Linda Voigts and Patricia Deery Kurtz, provides another window onto the remarkable growth of medieval English medical writing. In 1995, when the first iteration of the database was nearly complete, it included "records for approximately 7,700 witnesses to texts, of which two hundred are Old English and the rest Middle English."[36] When the CD-ROM version of the database was issued five years later, it contained entries from 1,200 manuscripts.[37] A search of the updated and revised version, made available online in 2014, turns up 7,048 scientific and medical texts when sixteenth-and seventeenth-century witnesses, as well as Old English texts, are omitted.[38] Not all of this enormous number are medical, but the majority are, falling under such indexed subject categories as medical recipe-collections (1,926 records), herbs and herbal medicine (624), urine and uroscopy (459), bloodletting (408), humors (349), regimens of health (298), diet (274), gynecology and obstetrics (197), plague (174), etiology (146), and surgery (132). Other popular genres—works of alchemy, charms, aids to prognostication, astrological and calendrical texts, and veterinary medicine—often overlapped *phisik*'s concerns, aided in its practice, or shared its ways of perceiving and interacting with the material world.

Chapter 2 continues these reflections of the expansion of Middle English medical writing, but one point bears emphasizing in the meantime. Anglo-Latin medical writing also flourished during the later fourteenth and fifteenth centuries. Though exact figures are wanting, it is clear that England's Latin medical corpus grew in absolute terms, even if it declined as a proportion of all medical and scientific writing.[39] In an earlier study, Voigts examined 117 medical and medical-scientific manuscripts (or discrete booklets) from late medieval England. Of these, only 30, or about a quarter, are entirely in Middle English; the rest are either entirely in Latin (16 manuscripts) or partly so (71 manuscripts).[40] Thus the uptick in scholarly resources devoted to Middle English medicine should not obscure the reality that Latin and especially macaronic medical texts flourished at the same time. Latin works often appeared in the same codices as Middle English ones or in identical textual formats. No straightforward differentiation in audience was indicated solely by the choice of Latin or English.

The best name for this freshly textualized, decentralized discourse of medicine is *phisik*, a Middle English word that became prevalent just as the increase in medical writing was underway. *Phisik* sediments in its etymological history two successive developments in the medieval history of medicine: what might be called healing's *intellectualization* and its subsequent *popularization*. The intellectualization began in the late eleventh century with the Latin term *physica*.[41] In classical Latin *physica* denoted the branch of philosophy concerned with the natural world, deriving from *physis*, the Greek term for (roughly) "nature." As classical natural philosophy, *physica* encompassed all inquiry into the qualities and operations of the mobile universe. During the Middle Ages, however, it took on a new meaning. As new Latin translations of Greco-Arabic medical writings began circulating first in southern Italy and then the rest of Europe, *physica* came to function as an alternative for the Latin term *medicina*, derived from the verb *medeor, mederi*—to heal or cure. To call medicine *physica* was to make claims about the rational character of medical knowledge—that it concerned fundamentally philosophical questions about what causes bodies to be as they are and to change. These are questions concerning the general order of nature, its categories and regularities. *Physica* in its medical sense, then, was inquiry into the human body insofar as the body was part of the orderly, rule-bound cosmos.

This sense of *physica* gained intellectual prominence in western Christendom through projects of translation, commentary, and teaching.[42] Constantine the African (d. c. 1099) was the first major translator of Arabic medical writings into Latin. Working in the Benedictine monastery of Monte Cassino, he translated what would become some of the most widespread texts of medieval rational medicine, including the *Isagoge* of Joannitius, the *Viaticum* (based on a treatise by Ibn al-Jazzar, d. c. 979), and the *Pantegni* (from the compendium by Ali ibn al-Abbas al-Majusi, d. 994). By the 1130s, Constantine's translations are recorded in England. At the nearby "school" of Salerno, the *Isagoge* became a foundational text in the medical curriculum and so part of the *articella*, the collection of texts that would serve as the basis of medical teaching in Europe until the sixteenth century. Meanwhile, the labor of scientific translation picked up steam elsewhere in Europe. Gerard of Cremona (d. 1187), working in Toledo, translated inter alia several works of Galen and the very influential *Canon on Medicine* by Avicenna (Ibn Sina, d. 1037).[43] Burgundio of Pisa (d. 1193) produced perhaps ten translations of Galenic treatises from Greek.[44] As Michael McVaugh observes, the wealth of translations was such that by the latter half of the thirteenth century, "it was no longer possible to assume that a scholar could easily search out whatever text he might happen to want," and ingenious précis and concordances, adapting developments in biblical scholarship, began to be devised, so that (in the words of one of these précis-makers, John de Saint-Amand) "students who pass sleepless nights looking for information among the works of Galen may be relieved of their struggles."[45] *Medicina* was established as one of the three higher faculties at medieval universities, and elite physicians and surgeons across Europe began composing "a newly self-conscious medical literature" of their own.[46] Centers of medical learning took root in Montpellier and Paris in the late twelfth century and in Bologna in the early thirteenth.

The art of healing, then, had become a full-blown intellectual discipline. Thanks to the prominence of Aristotelian philosophy in the thirteenth century, the sense of natural philosophy as a science whose principal end was truth rather than practical action gained ground. But if *medicina* and *scientia naturalis* came to be defined against one another in this way, *physica* could still name their overlap in the newly rational medicine. And that systematic knowledge reached new audiences in formats like encyclopedias, how-to manuals, sermons, vernacular translations, miracle collections, and poetry.

When *phisik* became part of the standard vocabulary of Middle English in the fourteenth century, it did so in tandem with the remarkable upsurge in medical writing. While *phisik* maintained some of the bookish and philosophical associations of its Latin cognate, its semantic range also broadened and loosened. It continued to denote natural philosophy, as *physica* had in classical Latin, as well as medical science, as it had come to do in medieval Latin. Yet it also designated the medical profession, a medicinal substance, a medical treatment, a healthy practice, and a healthful regimen.[47] It was sometimes used in contradistinction to surgery, which was understood to be a manual craft and therefore lower in the hierarchy of arts. Yet the mildness of *phisik*'s academic connotations is clear from its ready exchangeability with the originally Anglo-Saxon (and therefore markedly non-Latinate) term *leechcraft*. For instance, a translation of Guy de Chauliac speaks of the body's role in "alle lechecrafte or phisic," and John Paston complains about the cost of "my lechecrafte and fesyk."[48] The banns advertising a fifteenth-century medical practitioner proclaim, "Here is a man that is a conyng [knowledgeable] man in leche-craftis, bothyn in ffysykke & surgere."[49] Rather than marking a strong distinction between vernacular handicraft and Latinate science, *phisik* was an index of their overlap. If, in the two centuries preceding, *physica* had fitted healing to the systemicity of scholastic education, Middle English *phisik* adapted those academic ambitions to the decidedly unsystematic conditions of learning outside universities—and to the hopes for health that various categories of readers harbored.

The messy, makeshift, and profoundly generative labors of medical writing undertaken in late medieval England answered to two overarching purposes: the organization of information and the social accommodation of suffering. Medicine was simultaneously a system for explaining the entanglement of bodies in the material world and a set of techniques for managing that entanglement. "Iff mens bodies wern of irn [were made of iron]," speculates one work of Middle English medicine, "thei needen no rule of helth."[50] But human bodies were not iron. The remedy books so popular in the later fourteenth and fifteenth centuries were produced in and for communities that faced high levels of illness and infirmity. Nutrition and sanitation conditions contributed to the prevalence of diseases like tuberculosis, influenza, malaria, typhus, smallpox, and dysentery—to say nothing of the plague, which recurred periodically in England from the mid-fourteenth century to the seventeenth.[51] Conditions like toothache, blindness, skin disease, paralysis, gout, kidney stones, and bone fractures further added to what Paul Slack calls the "burden of sickness," or the costs imposed on a society by the poor health of its members.[52] It is in light of such corporeal precarity that practices of vernacular medical learning took on their full significance. And it is against the shadowy background of the period's largely unrecorded habitus of everyday embodiment—the lived varieties of physical care and embodied self-relation that were themselves reflective and imaginative undertakings—that medieval writings about the body should assume their meaning for us now.

The Body's Causes

What models of embodiment did this newly accessible archive of theory-rich medical learning entail? Broadly based on the writings of Galen and his Arabic and Latin heirs, this system of ideas held that human physiology was made from the same components as the rest of the universe—namely, the elements (earth, water, air, and fire) endowed with their respective qualities (hot, cold, wet, and dry). The four bodily humors (black bile, phlegm, blood, and choler) were called the "children" of the elements, and they combined in each person to produce her unique complexion. Elements and humors could not be observed directly but they underlay observable things. Their qualities of heat and moisture did not merely differentiate the natural world but gave it its dynamism, drawing each element toward its proper place and in the process fueling physical change. The Middle Ages did not have an "ontological" concept of disease—that is, there was no entity, like a microorganism, that disease was understood to be—so medieval pathology dealt instead with the patterned conditions of the human body as the result of causal factors. A wide range of influences could affect an individual's physiology—from the planets to daydreams, from the west wind to the scent of flowers, from sexual intercourse to the recitation of prayers. Not germs but the world itself "infected" the permeable microcosm.

The most common medical framework for explaining the hidden dimensions of the body was a triad of categories known as the "naturals," the "contra-naturals," and the "non-naturals" (*res naturales, res contra natura, res non naturales*). Ubiquitous across the medical corpus, this scheme provided countless thinkers with a ready means of thinking about somatic structure and alteration. *Res naturales* encompassed what was intrinsic to the body: "the elements, the mixture [of qualities] [*commixtiones*], the humors [*compositiones*], the members [of the body], the powers [*virtutes*], the faculties [*operationes*], and the spirits."[53] Contra-naturals opposed the health of the body; they were diseases and their symptoms. The non-naturals stood in between, neither good nor bad in themselves. They were the quotidian factors that influenced sickness and health: "The first is the air which surrounds the human body, [then] food and drink, exercise and rest, sleep and waking, fasting and fullness, and incidental conditions of the mind."[54] This widely known system propounded a model of corporeality as an amalgamated composite, knit together by the constant interchange of physical forces and stuffs. Bodily changes could be analyzed into a series of micro-events, each with its own contingencies. Imagining etiology might entail zooming in to the body's constituents or zooming out to trace someone's path through the world.

The Zodiac Man, a diagrammatic aid to bloodletting common in late medieval English manuscripts, offers an image of the body's susceptibility to such a cause-struck world (Figure 2). The man's naked body literally crawls with the symbols of the zodiac, representing the influence on various body parts of the moon's path through the heavens. Painted in lavish color in many of the folded physicians' calendars that were unique to late medieval England, the image was likely intended to be seen by patients and practitioners alike during consultations.[55] Its effect, one imagines, was multivalent: bespeaking bodily vulnerability but also medicine's learned mastery of that vulnerability; diagramming practical information while emblematizing, with strange acuity, the feeling of a body not quite under human control. Like the Wellcome Wound Man, the Zodiac Man is aesthetically arresting as well as informational. It suggests how newly accessible scientific information might have redounded on images of the body in an era when creaturely life was being reconceived within a web of material forces and technical explanations.

One particularly urgent occasion for etiological imagination was the Black Death. The epidemic ravaged Europe between 1348 and 1350, killing perhaps a third of England's population in its course, with mortality rates much higher in some communities. A second massive outbreak hit in the early 1360s, and a total of thirteen epidemics on a national scale occurred in England between 1349 and 1485, along with numerous regional outbreaks.[56] In

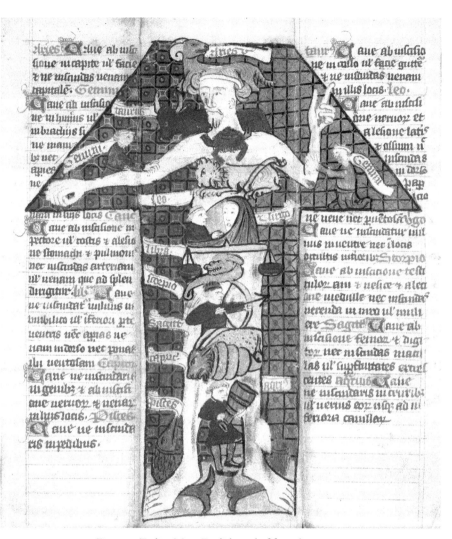

Figure 2. Zodiac Man. English, early fifteenth century.
© The British Library Board, Sloane MS 2250, fol. 12.

the course of its devastation, the plague posed a number of etiological puzzles to medical thought.[57] At least in its bubonic form, it was characterized by unusual and distinctive symptoms, reinforcing authorities' sense that this was something new. Because it occurred in so many places at once, it could not be explained solely with reference to the elements and humors, nor on the basis of local environmental factors. Physicians agreed that it must have its origins in the heavens, in celestial events that could poison the atmosphere on such a vast scale. At the same time, differentiation in the plague's effects also needed to be explained. After witnessing the first outbreak in England, the French physician and astrologer Geoffrey of Meaux announced his intentions "to write something about the cause of this general pestilence, showing its natural cause, and why it affected some countries more than others, and why within those countries it affected some cities and towns more than others, and why in one town it affected one street, and even one house, more than another, and why it affected nobles and gentry less than other people, and how long it will last."[58] To explain the plague, Geoffrey would need to grapple with causes at multiple scales, accounting for the disease's massive reach as well as its variability across regions, between social groups, and even from household to household.

An early and important attempt at explanation was undertaken in the shocking plague year of 1348. Writing at the behest of the French king, the medical faculty at the University of Paris located the disease's "distant and first cause [*remota et primeva causa*]" in the astrological conjunction of three planets in 1345, which led to the poisoning of the atmosphere and to the corruption of susceptible bodies.[59] The doctors enumerated other possible causes as well: winds blown from alien places, earthquakes releasing rotten vapors in the earth, unseasonable weather, and complexions that were especially hot and moist. This causal proliferation reflects the range of factors known to influence human sickness. It also registers the doctors' uncertainty, "for a sure explanation [*certa ratio*] and perfect understanding [*perfecta cognitio*] of these matters is not always to be had."[60] The effort to reckon with an abundance of causes is entirely characteristic of late medieval etiological thought. In the first lines of their prologue, the physicians even pitch their report in terms of an idealized psychology of causal inquiry: "Seeing things which cannot be explained [*effectibus quorum causa latet*], even by the most gifted intellects, initially stirs the human mind to amazement; but after marveling, the prudent soul yields to its desire for understanding and, anxious for its perfection, strives with all its might to discover the causes of the amazing events [*effectuum mirabilium causas*]."[61] This lofty philosophical opening should not, however, obscure the decidedly practical and social concerns motivating the king's charge and the faculty's recommendations for prevention and cure.

Between the mid-fourteenth century and 1500, 281 plague tractates are known to have been composed, typically explaining the causes of the disease and recommending a variety of precautions and treatments.[62] Etiologically, most share the Parisian faculty's tactics; they link the planets' influence to the corruption of the air, while adding information about individual complexions and regimen, occasionally with a nod to God's power.[63] The genre was seized on by English readers. The tract of the otherwise unknown John of Burgundy (also called John of Bordeaux and John de la Barbe) was by far the most popular plague work in late medieval England. Probably compiled in 1365, it circulated in various Latin versions and gave rise to at least six independent Middle English translations.[64] Something like forty-six witnesses to Middle English translations and adaptations survive from before 1500.[65] As one Englishing explains, while the "influence or impressioun of the hevenly or high bodies" makes the air "corrupt" and "pestilencial in effect," this environmental change is "nat al-only [not the only] cause of moreyne [plague]."[66] The treatise cites Galen for the general principle that "the body suffrith no corrupcioun but if [unless] the matier of the body be prompt or redy."[67] So, it is not only the heavens above but flesh "stuffed ful of humours that bien [are] mystempered" that together create the conditions for plague.[68]

John of Burgundy's treatise stresses the importance of the causal understanding it provides. For instance, in the words of the Middle English translation, whoever "han nat drunken of that sweete drynke of astronomy" will not be able to "put to this pestilencial sores no parfit remedy" because those who "knowe nat the cause and the qualite of the sikenes, they may not hele it, as saide the prince of medicyne, Avicen."[69] Averroes is also cited, with the Aristotelian truism that "a man knowith nat a thyng but if he knowe the cause both fer and nygh [distant and proximate]."[70] In this vernacular rendering, such scholastic promotions of causational knowing reached new readers and charged etiological knowledge with the urgency of survival.

John of Burgundy's treatise includes an acknowledgment of God's power: whoever follows its advice may survive "if the helply [merciful] wil of God be with hym."[71] Likewise, the Parisian doctors duly state that "any pestilence proceeds from the divine will [*epidimia aliquando a divina voluntate procedit*]."[72] Indeed, naturalist explanations did not contradict the supernatural etiologies that were ubiquitous in sermons and chronicles, where plague was cast as divine punishment for humankind's sins. However, the intellectual energy of both the Parisian faculty and John of Burgundy was occupied with routing that ultimate divine cause through the intricate etiological apparatus of the physical world.

This emphasis on natural and especially astrological causation sometimes raised hackles, despite (or because of) its evident popularity. For instance, *Dives and Pauper*, a moderately popular Middle English dialogue on the Ten Commandments from the early fifteenth century, pushes back against naturalist presumption.[73] In the section on the First Commandment, Dives mocks those who consider themselves astrological experts. They believe, he declares, "Noon hungyr [famine], noo moreyn [plague], noo tempest, noo sekenesse, noo werre [war] shal falle [befall]" unless caused by the heavenly bodies and predicted by the astrologers' calculations—"for, as they seyn, the bodyis abovyn rewlyn [rule] alle thyngge here benethyn."[74] Such explanatory naturalists, according to Dives, make God "more thral [lowly] and of lesse power than ony kyng or lord is upon erthe."[75] Later, it is the remarkable diversity of natural phenomena that provides a further reason to doubt astrological causes—because, on this account, the planets cannot account for such variation. Ironically, Pauper's description of the plague sounds at first very much like that of Geoffrey of Meaux:

> Sumtyme is moreyn general, sumtyme parcyal, in on contree
> nought in anothir; sumtyme in on toun and nought in the nexte;
> sumtyme in the to syde of the strete and nought in the tothir. Sum
> houshold is takyt up al hool; at the nexte it takyt noon.[76]

> [Sometimes plague is general, and sometimes partial, in one country
> and not in another; sometimes in one town and not in the next;
> sometimes on the near side of the street and not on the other side.
> Some household is completely devastated; at the next, no one is
> struck.]

Rather than pursuing an ever more intricate causal explanation to account for these variations (as Geoffrey of Meaux does), Dives and Pauper reject the utility of any such account and recommend turning to God instead.

Pauper prefers demons to celestial conjunctions as the intermediary explanation for pestilence: devils often "have leve [permission]" from God, for reason of "mannes synne," to "doon [create] wondres, to causen hedows [terrible] tempest, to enfectyn and envenymen the eyr and causen moreyn [plague] and syknesse, hunger and droughte."[77] Strikingly, the dialogue even wades into the murky overlap between causation and semiotics. Pauper is eager to show that natural signs—especially the position of the planets—may *signify* without acting as causes. After all, he reasons, condensation on a stone "is tokene of reyn [rain]" but "nought cause of the reyn."[78] Just so, by means of the planets' positions, someone gains knowledge not "as be [by] causis but as be tokenys, for God made hem to been tokenys to man, beste, bryd, fysh and othere creaturys."[79] Here is a passage of vernacular theory on the semiotics and etiology of the natural world.

As the example of *Dives and Pauper* suggests, medicine (together with natural philosophy) existed in a changeable, sometimes volatile relation with God's omnipotence and the health of the soul. The impulse to regulate medicine's and religion's tangled jurisdictions is nowhere more evident than in the 1215 decree of the Fourth Lateran Council stating that "physicians of the body [*medicis corporum*]" must "warn and persuade" their patients "first of all to call in physicians of the soul [*medicos animarum*]."[80] The statute justifies itself in terms of the well-being of patients: because "sickness of the body may sometimes be the result of sin [*infirmitatis corporalis nonnumquam ex peccato proveniat*]," it follows that once spiritual health (*spirituali salute*) has been seen to, patients "may respond better to medicine for their bodies; for when the cause ceases so does the effect [*cum causa cessante cesset effectus*]." Moreover, the writers explain, some patients, when their physicians advise them "to arrange for the health of their souls, [they] fall into despair and the more readily incur the danger of death."[81] Yet if all physicians did this, there would be no reason for fear. A final sentence dispels any ambiguity about the relative claims of body and soul: "Since the soul is much more precious than the body, we forbid any physician, under pain of anathema, to prescribe anything for the bodily health [*pro corporali salute*] of a sick person that may endanger his soul [*in periculum animae convertatur*]."[82] The Lateran rule was often quoted or paraphrased in later texts, including medical ones.[83]

This decree was issued amid tensions concerning the role of Aristotelian philosophy in scriptural and moral matters. In no uncertain terms, the rule about physician of the soul takes the moralists' side in seeking to subordinate naturalistic concerns to spiritual ones. Importantly, however, it leaves room for debate about causation. Bodily sickness is only sometimes (*nonnumquam*) the result of sin, which means that humoral, astrological, and other natural forces remain explanations circulating uneasily alongside moral and divine ones. This unsettledness necessitates the ongoing work of causal discernment and etiological narration. Given the ceaseless negotiation between medicine and religion throughout the Middle Ages, it is notable that Darrel Amundsen has found a close predecessor for the 1215 decree, in a twelfth-century medical treatise on physicians' etiquette. It advises the physician to send his patient to confession *before* commencing any examination, because if the patient "hears mention of this [confession] after you have examined him and have considered the signs of disease, he will begin to despair of recovery, because he will think you despair of it too."[84] The Lateran decree offers an identical version of patient psychology; a recommendation for confession in the course of treatment makes the patient despair, perhaps fatally. In the overlap of these two documents, one sees *medici* of body and soul worrying, in almost identical terms, over how the sick will navigate the crisscrossing urgencies of physical and sacramental care.

When, in the General Prologue of the *Canterbury Tales*, Chaucer sketches his archetypical member of the medical profession, he makes explicit reference to etiology. The portrait of the "Doctour of Phisik" marks the close relation between medical skill and the knowledge of causes:

> He knew the cause of everich maladye,
> Were it of hoot, or coold, or moyste, or drye,
> And where they engendred, and of what humour.
> He was a verray, parfit praktisour:
> The cause yknowe, and of his harm the roote,
> Anon he yaf the sike man his boote.[85]

> [He knew the cause of every disease, whether it was hot, cold,
> moist, or dry, and where they were engendered, and from what
> humor. He was a true and perfect practitioner: having learned
> the cause and the root of the harm, he soon gave the sick man
> his remedy.]

Etiological know-how is tied directly to the physician's success in healing. According to the verses, identifying the "cause" of every illness means being able to place it within the system of elemental qualities at the foundation of medieval pathology. Although the basis of the Galenic system in the four qualities may seem simple, the portrait emphasizes the elaborate learning that makes such explanation possible. The narrator lists a rather staggering library of medical authorities that the Physician "wel knew" (lines 429–34), and also mentions his expertise in surgery, astrology, and the crafting of measured regimens. It is the fact that his treatments are informed by etiological acumen that makes the Doctour "a verray, parfit praktisour": because he understands the cause and "roote" of the patient's "harm," he is able to give the "sike man" the proper remedy.

Yet the narrator's famously offhand comment that the Doctour of Phisik's "studie was but litel on the Bible" also suggests a limit to the physician's explanatory authority. His current journey to the shrine of the "hooly blisful martir" who "hath holpen [has helped]" pilgrims "whan that they were seeke [sick]" gently qualifies the practical effectiveness of his remedies.[86] The shrine was famous for its curative properties, and many of the *ampullae* that pilgrims used to collect holy water, which was supposedly tinctured with Saint Thomas's blood, bear the words *Optimus egrorum medicus fit Toma Bonorum*, or "Thomas is the best doctor of the worthy sick." The Doctour of Phisik may be a master of some causes but ignorant of others. In the Middle Ages there was no a priori principle to guarantee that a naturalistic explanation for health was more appropriate than a supernatural one, or vice versa.[87] The controversy that the Physician has inspired among modern readers—does Chaucer portray him as laudable or blameworthy?[88]—reflects what was an open question in the later Middle Ages. How legitimate was it to bracket the Bible and concentrate on the intricate technicalities of the medical arts? Chaucer's portrait implies at once the height of the Physician's learned authority and its provisionality within the wider frame of the Canterbury pilgrimage and the Christian cosmos. The narrator's lightness of touch in evoking both medical authority and its limits suggests something of the undecidability of religion's and medicine's claims on the body.

The "Specific Rationality" of Medicine

Medieval medicine's special relation to etiology stemmed not only from the vast number of physical causes it sought to comprehend. It arose as well from the unique position of *phisik* among medieval discourses of knowledge. More than any other, medicine was aware of itself as an amalgam of theoretical and practical expertise and sensitive to the fact that this produced its "specific rationality," or its logic and style of thought.[89] The standard primer in medieval medical education, the *Isagoge*, opens by stating that "Medicine is divided into two parts, namely, the theoretical and the practical [*Medicina dividitur in duas partes, scil. in theoricam et practicam*]."[90] Similarly, Avicenna, at the start of his influential *Canon*, explains medicine's division into theory and practice: "Theory is that which, when mastered, gives us a certain knowledge, apart from any question of treatment. Thus we say there are three forms of fever and nine complexions. The practice of medicine is not the work which the physician carries out, but is that branch of medical knowledge which, when acquired, enables one to form an opinion upon which to base the proper plan of treatment."[91] Almost all systematic treatments of medicine begin by dividing medical learning into theory and practice. In doing so, writers flagged medicine's special responsibility to hold together generality and particularity, philosophy and experience, and universal principles and individual cases.

The epistemological status of medicine was of special concern in the Middle Ages thanks to Aristotelian hierarchies of knowledge. Writing in the early eleventh century, Avicenna was already anxious to synthesize Galenic and Aristotelian systems. That task became urgent for medical thinkers in western Christendom following the ascent of the "new" Aristotle in the thirteenth century. At stake was the standing of *medicina* in the emerging culture of the university. In the hierarchies that structured academic learning, the more that a discipline mixed in the realm of contingent particulars, the lower its status was on the scale of intellectual value. In accord with Aristotle, thinkers tended to doubt that real truths could be based on particular experiences of an ever-changing physical world. Such observations lacked the necessity and universality proper to *scientia*, which depended on a rigorous demonstration through deductive process beginning with first principles and definitions.[92] Medicine sat uneasily astride the definitions of *scientia* and *ars*. It was both a theoretical discipline with its own principles and a practical discipline proceeding by empirical observation and inductive judgment and aiming to affect patients' health.

Uneasiness about medicine's epistemological status is nowhere more visible than in the scholastic prologues, or *accessus*, of medical treatises, which became increasingly elaborate as writers sought to describe medicine in Aristotelian terms.[93] There, medical writers questioned whether medicine was a *scientia* or an *ars*; if a *scientia*, whether it was speculative, practical, operative, active, or mechanical; if an *ars*, whether it was mechanical or "real" (*realis*); whether it was the most perfect art; and so on.[94] Most agreed that to the extent that medical thought moved from causes to effects, it, like natural philosophy, possessed demonstrably true knowledge based on axiomatic principles—and was thus a *scientia*. But to the extent that the physician tried to infer causes from observable effects and to read etiologies from symptoms, medicine was far from a pure science. Among the medieval disciplines of understanding, then, medicine played fretfully between causes and effects.

Such considerations did not remain confined to academic prefaces. The innovative French surgeon Henri de Mondeville (d. 1316) negotiated medicine's double role in his *Chirurgia*.[95] On the one hand, Henri was eager to dismiss mere empiricism. Speaking of the necessity of theory and abstraction, he warns that "particular cases are and always will be infinite in number, and consequently unknown [*quia particularia sunt et erunt infinita et per consequens ignota*]."[96] And yet, he points out soon after, in a warning against overly abstract theory, "medicine is carried out not on mankind in general, but on every individual in particular [*medicina enim non fit homini in universali, sed unicuique individuo*]."[97] Traces of similar oscillation and compromise are evident even in Galen's writings, composed in what was already an Aristotelian age. The Greek physician's disagreements with both sides of his era's polarized medical culture, the medical "rationalists" and "empiricists," show him trying to balance the sure knowledge of natural philosophy against the insights of sensory observation and experience.

A related epistemological point is made in no less prominent a place than the beginning of the *Metaphysics*, where Aristotle states that it is a matter of experience (*experientia*) "to have a judgment that when Callias was ill of this disease, this did him good, and similarly in the case of Socrates, and so in many individual cases." However, it is a matter of *art* (*ars*) to judge that the treatment "has done good to *all persons* of a certain constitution."[98] While art is a higher form of knowledge than experience, the imperatives of clinical treatment appear to upend the hierarchy:

> For the physician [*medicans*] does not cure "man," except in an incidental way [*secundum accidens*]—but rather Callias or Socrates or someone else called by some such individual name, who just happens to be a man [*cui esse hominem accidit*]. If, then, someone has the explanation [*rationem*] without the experience [*sine experimento*], and recognizes the universal [*universale*] but does not know the individual [*singulare*] included in this, he will often fail to cure [*curatione peccabit*]; for it is the individual that is to be cured [*singulare namque magis curabile est*].[99]

This passage should not be taken as a defense of empiricism. Aristotle leaves no doubt that wisdom comes with explaining the causes behind observed facts. But the passage distances such wisdom from practical success. Because healing is a matter of particulars, of *this* embodied individual, experience might prove superior. While treating the patient as "man" may be essential to medicine's scientific project, it is a particularized person, designated here by the proper names Callias and Socrates, who wants healing. The passage captures something of the epistemological pathos of medieval medicine, as it weaves from general knowledge to singular scenes of suffering and care, and back again. The flickering between generality and particularity is what the Wellcome Wound Man (discussed at this chapter's opening) likewise sets in motion—as the image's diagrammatic universality warps but does not subsume the individuality of the man's figure and face.

Joel Kaye's magisterial study of the new "idea of balance" arising between 1250 and 1375 locates medicine at the heart of scholastic intellectual history, despite what would seem to be its problematically practical focus. Kaye's book follows the vicissitudes of a conceptual model, that of "equalization," as it was gradually developed and disseminated in scholastic thought. This wide-ranging paradigm, based partly on Galen's ever self-calibrating body, focuses on the "dynamic interaction" of a system's working parts and the production of balance as the "*aggregate product* of the systematic interaction of multiple moving parts within the whole."[100] This model "made possible a form of naturalistic explanation that did not require the existence or intervention of an intelligence or ordering power existing above or outside the sphere that it governed."[101] In other words, the interaction of causal forces themselves produced the qualitative identity of the system in which they participated. Though Aristotle had an intellectual cachet with which scholastic thinkers were eager to associate themselves, Kaye argues that it was Galenic thought that actually acted as a crucial, if partly disavowed, intellectual model: "While the writings of Aristotle are generally taken as the textual point of departure for scholastic speculation, I have found that the most dynamic and productive texts behind the new model of equilibrium came not from Aristotle but from Galen and his continuators, both Arabic and Latin."[102]

Symptomatic Subjects picks up where Kaye's study concludes. In the later fourteenth century, according to Kaye, the scholastic model of equilibrium broke down. He hazards two speculations as to why. The first is the development of a "plethora of competing models," which dispersed the paradigms's coherence just as "the university ceased to be the center and arbiter of speculation."[103] The phenomenon of explanatory proliferation, which accompanies the diffusion of intellectual authority beyond the university, creates the conditions of etiological imagination to which I have gestured, especially among lay and vernacular audiences. The second reason Kaye hazards for the breakdown of the scholastic model of equilibrium is what he describes as the widespread "failure of faith in the potential of systematic self-ordering and self-equalization: a failure in the assumption that the process of interior self-ordering can, in itself, replace the ordering power of an intervening or over-arching intelligence."[104] Indeed, such distrust in systematic self-balancing is found frequently in the sources discussed in the ensuing chapters of this study, whether in the physician Arnau of Vilanova's worry over medical contingency or in Arcite's corrupting body in Chaucer's "Knight's Tale."

Behind such pessimism, Kaye speculates cautiously, may be all the bad news of the fourteenth and fifteenth centuries—plague, labor unrest, authoritarian politics, heterodoxy and its suppression. Yet, I think, just as important to the pessimism expressed in my sources is these sources' scale. Both practical medicine and imaginative literature tend to think at the scale of the individual. If natural philosophy and avowedly theoretical medicine concentrate on the regularities of the species, medical practice and literary narrative proceed from the exigencies of individuals. It is "the individual that is to be cured," as Aristotle writes, and it is also the individual who perishes, as all eventually do. The model of equilibrium that Kaye so persuasively identifies does, I think, find its way into the late medieval milieu of *phisik*—but as something fragilized and perhaps faulty. The self-equalizing model is the occasion for intellectual experimentation in various texts, as the body's causal determinants are imagined and reimagined. But the numerousness of the factors involved tends to overwhelm powers of comprehension and control. After all, embodiment always turns out to be terminal.

Medicine's position between theory and practice, between universal and particular, draws it into close alignment with two other intellectual procedures, narration and exemplification. As the causal forces understood to structure the physical world became more multifarious in the later Middle Ages, the task of interpreting individual bodies became more delicate.[105] It required picking out the relevant threads of explanation and then charting singular itineraries of implication and consequence. This often happened through narrative, the efficacy of which was increasingly recognized in contemporary trends in academic medical writing.[106] *Experimenta*, or "case histories," and *consilia*, or didactic accounts of cases, became increasingly important genres for late medieval physicians and surgeons, as they responded to the perceived inadequacies of systematic theorization.[107] Moreover, to put medical principles into action, practitioners had to recognize patients as *examples*, by discovering each body under examination as an instance of broader medical categories, and so to bring that individual, here and now, into the medicine's system of interpretation.

Late medieval medicine, then, shares with practices of medieval narrative a vivid interest in the exemplary and explanatory functions of individual bodies. This fascination, with how general principles and overarching laws might (or might not) be legible in the flesh, animates an extraordinary passage from a mid-fourteenth-century devotional work. Henry of Lancaster's (d. 1361) Anglo-Norman *Le Livre de Seyntz Medicines* (*The Book of Holy Medicines*) consistently imagines penitential spirituality through a series of intricately physicalized images of wounds, sickness, treatment, and healing. In this passage, however, his meditations turn to a body marked by learned medicine in particular. Henry prays:

> Most sweet Lord, I entreat you that it please you that I may then be cut up and opened up before you [*defait et overt par devant vous*], my Lord and my master, as certain people are before the surgeons at those schools in Montpellier and elsewhere [*devant ces surgens qe sont a ces escoles de Monpelers et aillours*], to whom is given a man lawfully executed [*mort par le droit de juggement*]; he is given to them to open [*est donee pur overir*], in order to see and understand how and in what fashion the veins, nerves, and other parts are disposed in a man [*a veoir et conoistre coment les veynes, les nerfs et les autres choses gisent dedeinz un homme et la manere*]. Sweet Lord, I should wish to be opened up like this before you, that you might see fully openly how my flesh and my veins and all my limbs are suffused with sin [*tout en apert veoir coment ma char et mes veynes et touz mes menbres sont pleyns de pecchés*]; not at all, Lord, because I do not know full well that there is nothing you do not know; but to be healed of my evil illness [*mes pur estre garry de ma male maladie*]. Furthermore, I am a man condemned to death by law for my crimes, so that you can, Lord, with good reason, open and cut me up rather than another, and make an example of me to others so that they may see and recognize the abscesses in me [*pur ensample doner de moi as autres des enpostumes q'ils purront veoir et conoistre en moi*].[108]

Here, Henry asks to be made an example like the corpses dissected in anatomical demonstrations at Montpellier. The executed criminals turned over to surgeons are cut open to illustrate what is characteristically human, how veins and nerves and other parts are disposed in the body. Medical learning, here, renders the human body illustrative, exemplary of the natural principles according to which it is formed. But this body is also particular. *Les veynes, les nerfs et les autres choses* of the anonymous corpse become Henry's own— *ma char et mes veynes and touz mes menbres*—which, he explains, are riddled with sin. Like the Wellcome Wound Man, this image trades on the unstable interchange between didactic generality and individual embodiment, between inert exemplification and the urgency of a cure. In a rather fantastic imaginative exercise, Henry identifies himself not with someone sick or suffering but with a corpse—perhaps because, as Augustine's sermon claims, we know that "we have many things inside us" only because we have seen such things "in butchered bodies." Here, the dead man, *mort par le droit de juggement*, becomes the paradoxical avatar of a desire for medicalized healing. In this metaphor, the surgeon's cut unites violence and cure in a fantasy that anatomical exposure will make the self whole. Healing is tied not to medical therapeutics but to becoming an *ensample* for *autres*. The circuit between the reifying estrangement of the dissected corpse and the imaginative reclamation of flesh's dead weight shows the power of the medicalized body as a literary resource for medieval writers.

Chapter 2

Cause, Authority, Sign, and Book

Phisik in late medieval England was many things. It was written in university textbooks and in the margins of household manuscripts. Its practitioners were learned and unlearned, men and women, variably Latin- and English-literate. Medical care was sometimes a craft and sometimes a science. In the midst of this heterogeneity, however, *phisik* also fostered a set of ideas and practices peculiar to it. The later Middle Ages saw the dissemination of the medical framework, in which bodies were explained and manipulated as natural things, composite and changeable. Inquiry into the forces that sustained life assumed new relevance as more and more readers came into contact with medical expertise. In order to capture both the widespread tendencies of late medieval medicine and the variability of their expressions, the following chapter examines *phisik* under four different rubrics: *cause*, *authority*, *sign*, and *book*. These four words cut different, twisting paths through the thickets of medical discourse, from the classrooms of Montpellier to the small towns of Nottinghamshire, from leprosy's diagnosis to John Lydgate's most popular poem. The chapter aims to throw light on some of the central concerns of *phisik*, including its interests in why bodies change, the grounds of medical authority, how to interpret symptoms, and the best ways to transmit medical knowledge. Together, these topics yield a portrait of the plural and contentious nature of late medieval medicine.

Cause

One of the central projects of medieval medical inquiry was the investigation of causes. Chaucer's Physician on his way to Canterbury is called a "verray, parfit praktisour [true and perfect practitioner]" in part because he "knew the cause of everich [every] maladye."[1] According to the popular encyclopedia *De proprietatibus rerum*, compiled by Bartholomaeus Anglicus (d. 1272) and translated into Middle English by John Trevisa (d. 1402), a physician "nedith to knowe causis and occasiouns of eveles [diseases]" because "medicynes may never be sikerliche [securely] itake yif [if] the cause of the evel [disease] is unknowe."[2] These vernacular formulations reiterate a notion expressed by earlier medical writers. In the influential medical encyclopedia known as the *Canon*, an Arabic work written by the Persian philosopher and scientist Avicenna (Ibn Sina, d. 1037) and translated into Latin by the circle of Gerard of Cremona (d. 1187), knowledge of causes is made medicine's first task: "Since medicine considers the human body [*corpus humanum*] from the standpoint of how it is made healthy and how it sickens, and since we can have knowledge of neither unless it is known through its causes [*causas*], we must in medicine know the causes of health and of sickness."[3] The statement sounds commonsensical: it is useful to know *why* someone falls ill when reasoning out a cure. But it is also a testament to Avicenna's Aristotelianism. The *Canon* self-consciously sought to synthesize Galenic medicine and Aristotelian philosophy. It is no surprise then that the work found eager acceptance among European readers increasingly shaped by Aristotle's logic and theory of knowledge. Aristotle identifies true knowledge with a knowledge of causes: "We suppose ourselves to know something without qualification (as opposed to sophistically, accidentally) when we judge that we understand the cause upon which the thing depends"; and, more simply, "we know when we understand the cause [*tunc scimus cum causam cognoscimus*]."[4]

When Avicenna declared causation the sine qua non of medical knowledge, his statement appeared at the start of a vast and systematic tome. However, the meaning of the claim shifted as the *Canon* came to be digested by later medical writers. This happened, for instance, when the Italian surgeon Lanfranc of Milan (d. 1306) adapted Avicenna's dictum in his *Chirurgia magna*: "Avicenna said that one cannot understand something that has been caused unless we know it by the causes themselves [*ut dicit Avicenna, notitia rei quae causam habet non potest haberi nisi per suas causas sciatur*]."[5] In the hierarchies that organized medieval medicine, surgery was traditionally defined against *physica* as a lower form of knowledge, more manual and empirical. But Lanfranc's citation signals his bid to raise surgery's intellectual profile and to shift it from a craft to an art. In this newly "rational" surgery, which began in northern Italy and spread to France, surgical writers imported scholastic models while at the same time dislodging them from the university curriculum.[6]

During the fourteenth century, Lanfranc's treatise together with other works of rational surgery found their way to eager readers in England, and Middle English translations of Lanfranc's surgical writings survive in at least ten manuscripts. In these Englishings, practical instruction often took priority over theoretical schemes. One Middle English surgery, written in London in 1392, adapted Lanfranc's treatise by excising its theoretical material and emphasizing the redactor's own empirical findings.[7] "Avicen seith knoulechinge of a thing that hath cause mai nought be knowen but bi his cause [Avicenna says that knowledge of a thing that has a cause may not be known except by its cause]," reads another translation, completed by 1380.[8] In the phrase's new vernacular milieu, the importance of causal understanding is reiterated at an even greater remove from academic contexts. Causation here has less to do syllogisms and more to do with observed relationships and palpable results.

Learned medicine poured huge quantities of intellectual energy into understanding causation. Three major schemes were available to medieval thinkers to explain sickness and health: the Aristotelian, the Galenic, and the Joannitian. All three were deployed within the basic framework of bodily complexion, which was determined by the balance of the four elements and four humors, with their respective qualities of heat, cold, moisture, and dryness. The scheme with the broadest intellectual reach was no doubt Aristotle's model of the four causes: material, formal, final, and efficient (*materialis, formalis, finalis, efficiens*). While not strictly medical, it would have been familiar to anyone with a passing training in the liberal arts, and it was integral to the development of scholastic natural philosophy. Yet much in Aristotelian thought mitigated against its usefulness for medicine. Aristotle's emphasis on causal linearity and teleology, his wish to move swiftly beyond the evidence of the senses, and his expressed desire for certainty based on first principles set his thought at odds with the scenes of practice in which medicine was constantly entangled. Aristotle's causes, thanks to their emphasis on fixed and stable properties, tended to be best for defining identities rather than accounting for change.

Galen (d. c. 210), the most influential of classical medical writers, modified the Aristotelian framework and fitted it to the doctor's practical concern for bodily alteration. Galen subdivided Aristotle's most dynamic category, efficient cause, into three medical causes: a body's predisposition (in medieval Latin, the *causa antecedens*); the external factor leading to a harmful change in the body (*causa primitiva* or *procatarctica*); and the condition actually preventing the body's proper function (*causa coniuncta* or *contentiva*).[9] Later medical writers did not always employ this exact vocabulary, but their nosology tended to address all three topics in their discussions of causes. Yet the most popular and widely elaborated framework of specifically medical causation was the triad of categories known as the *res naturales*, the *res non naturales*, and the *res contra natura*, or, in a Middle English translation of Guy de Chauliac's *Inventarium*—"kyndely thinges and noght kyndely and thinges agenst kynde."[10] These were popularized in the *Isagoge* of Joannitius (Hunayn ibn Ishaq, d. 873), which was translated by Constantine the African (d. c. 1098). The *res naturales* encompassed what was intrinsic to the body; the contra-naturals consisted of diseases and their symptoms, which opposed the body's health; and the non-naturals stood in between. Neither good nor bad in themselves, the non-naturals were those elements of everyday life—air, diet, exertion, rest, excretion, and mood—that influenced somatic states. As Galen remarked of the six factors, "The body cannot but be altered and changed in relation to all these causes."[11] The highest expression of the medieval physician's art was thought to be the management of these non-naturals. English readers' interest in their proper handling is evident in the popularity of texts mixing medical and moral advice, like John Lydgate's most copied poem, the "Dietary" (discussed below), and recensions of the advice-for-princes manual the *Secretum Secretorum*, which included instructions on hygiene and regimen.

Even with these three flexible etiological schemata, medical writers in the late thirteenth century seized on a further causal rubric, that of "specific" or "occult" causation. It accounted for effects that could not be predicted in advance on the basis of primary qualities. For instance, no calculation of degrees of heat and cold, dryness and moisture could foretell the behavior of a magnet. Its properties of attraction could only be discovered empirically—although once discovered they were considered natural, not magical or supernatural. "Occult causation" made room for what could be learned from experience, beyond existent medical theory.[12]

These several schemes of etiological thinking—Aristotelian, Galenic, Joannitian, and (as an auxiliary) "specific" or "occult"—were products of learned medicine's etiological imagination. They show the science's restive puzzling over how to understand the nature of living bodies and the changes they undergo. Yet despite these many tools—or, in some cases, because of them—etiological explanation in *phisik* remained difficult. Causation cannot simply be observed. It is a relation that requires abstract thought to formulate. Medical experts needed to posit connections among causes, symptoms, and treatments. The intricacy of the task became an increasingly common topic of discussion in medical writing. For instance, the French surgeon Henri de Mondeville (d. 1316) drew attention to it in his *Chirurgia* of the early four-teenth century, which subsequently circulated in England.[13] According to Mondeville, it is only in the case of such thumpingly obvious causes as "a stick, or stone, a knife, or something of that kind" that ordinary people can perceive relationships of causation. When the harm results rather from "an intrinsic, interior, or antecedent cause [*a causa intrinseca interiore vel antecedente*]," the *vulgus* is at a loss.[14] Mondeville, like Lanfranc of Milan, was part of a tradi-tion that aimed to intellectualize surgery, and causal explanation was central to that project. His written expertise is laid out on the page like academic commentary: "I have presented the appropriate surgical procedure pure and simple, but next to it I have presented its causes and reasons and explanations in smaller letters than the text itself, as if in a commentary or gloss."[15] The manuscript layout insists on the connection between surgical practice and causal explanation. As he goes on, Mondeville declares that a practitioner who fails to realize that every illness derives from a general and rational system of causes will, as a result of this ignorance, attribute each sickness to an isolated cause and will therefore be no better than an empiric.[16]

Mondeville was an especially innovative medical thinker, and one of the points where he can be seen responding to the intellectual problems of the early fourteenth century is in his unusual enumeration of fifty-two *contingentia*, or contingent factors, in his surgical *practica*.[17] The list begins with the familiar Joannitian framework of naturals, non-naturals, and contra-naturals and then broadens to include miscellaneous factors not captured under any formal sys-temization of medical causes. Mondeville explains that the surgeon usually needs to know everything, omitting nothing, about all the details of a patient's past that may bear on his choice of treatment.[18] Each of these factors—"every individual condition as revealed in a patient, or in a wounded member, or in an illness, or wherever, whether it be favorable or harmful [*omnis particu-laris conditio existens aut reperta in patiente, membro laeso et morbo curando et aliis aliquibus inferius hic notandis, quae condicio nocet aut confert*]"—"creates a problem for the surgeon during treatment [*ponit difficultatem in curatione morbi curandi per cyrurgicos*]."[19] Mondeville's list of *contingentia* insists that in applying general scientific principles to particular cases, the surgeon has to be constantly alert to individuating factors.[20]

The difficulty of etiology found its paradigmatic expression in what was the most well-known piece of medical writing in the Middle Ages, the first aphorism of Hippocrates: "Life is short, art is truly long; the time is acute, experience treacherous, and judgment difficult" (*Vita brevis, ars vero longa; tempus autem acutum, experimentum fallax, iudicium autem difficile*).[21] Or, in the paraphrase most familiar to students of Middle English literature: "The lyf so short, the craft so long to lerne, / Th'assay so hard, so sharp the conquerynge."[22] While the narrator of Chaucer's *Parliament of Fowls* deploys the aphorism to comment on the labors of love, and indirectly, the labors of poetry, the phrase's first context of meaning was medicine. The latter half of the aphorism continues: "The physician must not only be prepared to do what is right himself, but also to ensure that the patient, the attendants, and the externals cooperate."[23] From its earliest versions, the *articella* (the collection of texts that served as the basis of academic medical education from the twelfth century to the end of the Middle Ages) included the *Aphorisms* alongside Galen's commentary on the same text. Galen directly links the meaning of the first aphorism to the ambiguities of causation: "If someone is treated with different medicines, and improves or worsens as a result, it is not easy to decide which of these helped or harmed him."[24] The first medieval expositors of the aphorism emphasized the difficulty resulting from both the numerousness of physical influences and the vastness of medical learning. Bartholomew of Salerno explains, "Art is long because of the multitude and difficulty of things comprehended in the art" (*ars vero longa propter multitudinem et rerum difficultatem huic arti subiacentium*), and Maurus of Salerno identified medicine's "length" with its dispersion into a multiplicity of rules and precepts (*Ars est longa, idest variis regulis et preceptis diffusa*).[25]

In 1301 Arnau of Vilanova (d. 1311), then perhaps the most famous physician in Europe, delivered a set of lectures to medical students at Montpellier concerning this single Hippocratic aphorism.[26] In the first *lectio* Arnau describes the factors that make the acquisition of medical art a project that exceeds the human lifetime. In the second lecture, he argues that this asymmetry of art and life can be addressed by studying the archive of medical thought. Accordingly, "it is necessary to communicate medical discoveries [*inventa de medicina*] to posterity in writing [*per scripturam*] . . . , and it is necessary for those wishing to be perfected in medicine to study those writings diligently."[27] Considered together, Arnau's first two *lectiones* express both wariness and optimism: what is proper to the art of medicine is overwhelmingly vast, but we can make progress by contributing to and relying upon medicine's textual tradition.

The third *lectio*, focused on medical practice, considers the difficulties of comprehending causation. Again and again in the course of the lecture, Arnau draws attention to the surfeit of causal factors that a physician faces. When a practitioner sets about diagnosis, he needs to know as much as possible about the patient—about symptoms (*accidentia*), lifestyle, and personal history. The properly knowledgeable physician should then be able to link all the symptoms to their causes: knowing the disease and its cause allows him to proceed to proper treatment. And yet, contingencies arise—on account of a patient's unique complexion, or the changing environment, or the preparation of medicines, or even the origins of a piece of fruit: "Will this patient be better helped by figs from Persia or India or Damascus, or by Alexandrine or insular dates? There is a great diversity found in things of the same kind, for example, plants that grow in the fields versus the same ones that grow in the mountains."[28]

As the *lectio* continues, Arnau praises Hippocrates for enjoining physicians to pay attention to external contingencies, and he warns his students to be on guard against whatever factors might impinge on patients' health, since "by anticipating future contingencies through their causes, physicians can usefully give commands that will allow [their patients] to avoid harmful effects."[29] To illustrate this ability, Arnau launches into a tour de force of etiological imagination, in which the litany of contingencies threatens to outpace any power of anticipation. The passage moves with metonymic agitation through the scene environing a patient, discovering in each detail the body's alarming vulnerability to its surround. "For example," Arnau says,

> the physician finds that his patient's home is situated at the foot
> of a bell tower; he can anticipate that the bells might cause a noise
> that would be unpleasant and harmful for someone suffering from
> headache. Likewise he anticipates that where there are many dogs
> there can be importunate and annoying barking. Likewise if he
> finds a north or south window in line with his patient's head, he
> knows that when those winds blow the patient's head will suffer
> unless his bed is moved or the window is tightly shut. Likewise if he
> sees that the bottle of syrup or decoction stands uncovered in some
> corner or window and he finds spider webs over it, he can anticipate
> that spiders may get into these vessels. If he finds his patient's
> house is roofless and open, subject to the gusts of the winds, he
> can foresee that a patient with dysentery who lives in such a place
> may incur gripes or other lesions of the stomach when any light air
> blows. Likewise if he is treating cancers or fistulas or swellings in the
> private parts and groin, and if these parts are exposed for any period

of time, remaining so as long as the physician is at work cleansing
or anointing or plastering, he can foresee that the patient may suffer
problems with a chill in his hips or pains in the thigh or belly or
other passions if he is not protected with hot air or warm cloths. If
a patient suffers from hemorrhoids, or has recently had a rupture of
the lungs, so that it would do him harm to get upset and he must
speak in a low tone, the physician can anticipate that the patient
will have reason to shout or perhaps to become angry if he has an
attendant who is deaf or careless or sleepy.[30]

A good physician on Arnau's account is one who recognizes that his patient's
environment is alive with causal forces and charged with contingencies that
might be anticipated and kept back from the patient's susceptible physiology. Urban soundscapes, the room's architectural axis, filaments of spider web
drifting in the corner: these quotidian details and many others are pulled into
potential contact with corporeality. The effect of the list is not to reassure
the audience of its exhaustiveness. "If I were to tell you all I have myself seen
and heard, the day would not be long enough to describe the cases to you,"
Arnau remarks.[31] Here he echoes the kernel of the Hippocratic aphorism in
connection to his own lecture: the day is short, but the art is long. Instead
of actual comprehensiveness, his catalogue evokes the endless differentiation
of circumstances, each one stirring with narrative potential, moving along
its anticipated trajectory and conjuring a near future that is simultaneously
treacherous and alterable. This is a causally volatile but also labile world.

　　This welter of potential influences cannot, finally, be exhausted. Arnau
understands *contingentia* to "make a fully rational course of treatment impossible," as McVaugh observes.[32] Indeed, the analogy that Arnau offers for the
physician's labors is intriguingly distinct from any bookish model of medical
expertise:

> Now the physician's role regarding a course of treatment is like
> a sailor's, because both govern what is committed to them not
> by following necessary and permanent rules but by weighing
> contingent and variable factors. For the sailor has to alter the
> sails and other things as the winds change; the physician has to
> modify his tools and practices in accordance with the changes and
> variations in the illness as well as in the dispositions of the air and
> the other circumstances by which the body is affected.[33]

The simile shows the medical practitioner buffeted by a maelstrom of circumstances. Just as the sailor has no stable ground to stand upon as he steers the ship and no place outside the wind wherein to set the sails, so the physician operates within ongoing "changes and variations." It is not adherence to certain rules that makes a good physician but rather the habitus of real-time adjustment and judgment, which can be only partially captured by rational discourse. Arnau's three lectures on the first Hippocratic aphorism argue for both the importance of medicine's growing archive of written expertise and this archive's insufficiency in the face of specific cases. The physician responds by altering the course of treatment, "modify[ing] his tools and practices," as the winds change. Illness can have no single fixed course of treatment for every patient.

The later Middle Ages was an age of etiological imagination. Within the broad context of causational fascination, academic medicine developed an especially elaborate vocabulary of forces, which was adapted and deployed to account for the interplay of environment, behavior, pharmacopeia, and bodily disposition as these factors met in patients' embodied present and shaped their future. From the fourteenth century, medical writers devoted more and more intellectual resources to rendering contingency, or the unpredictable confluence of heterogeneous causes, itself an object of thought. Mediating between natural philosophy's general principles and the particularities of an individual patient looked increasingly daunting: *Vita brevis, ars vero longa.* Scholastic schemes of explanation, lit up by the urgencies of pain, vitality, and life and death, circulated in new contexts and arguably made medicine the premier discourse of everyday etiology.

Authority

In late medieval England, the authority to cure was a decentralized and varied power. Medical practitioners came from many backgrounds and claimed the power to explain and heal on various grounds. The infirm might seek health care from physicians, apothecaries, astrologers, members of barber-surgeon guilds, itinerant "leeches" with or without formal education, midwives, tooth-drawers, oculists, parish priests, monastic communities, saints' shrines, or members of their own or other local households. These care-givers were varied in the actions they performed, in the basis for their efficacy or expertise, and in their accessibility and cost to patients. Medical *texts* in circulation likewise asserted their authority according to heterogeneous criteria. Some attached their contents to well-known authors, like Galen or Avicenna, and one popular remedy book claimed its discovery in Hippocrates' tomb.[34] Other works named prominent medieval surgeons like Lanfranc of Milan or Guy de Chauliac. Some incorporated bits of academic apparatus into practical instruction, signaling their legitimacy through scholastic mise-en-page. Still others claimed practical efficacy in the form of local testimonies, or *probatur* statements attributed to nearby individuals—as in the many verifications attributed to the Rector of Oswaldkirk in the remedy book of Robert Thornton.[35] If, as Emily Steiner has argued, "authority is never properly one thing" but instead is "something that one is always in relation to, that one is never absolutely identical to, and that one can only provisionally be said to possess," the discourse and practice of *phisik* were the occasions for authority's especially motley manifestations.[36]

Jostlings among the sundry models of authority formed the texture of late medieval medical discourse. With the exception of short-lived efforts by elite physicians in the early fifteenth century (discussed below), medical authority was neither newly consolidated nor newly centralized in late medieval England. Centralization came later, for instance, with the founding of the Royal College of Physicians in 1518. While guilds were common for barbers and for apothecaries (often as "grocers"), these trades were only partly medical in concern, and English towns lacked anything like the broadly medical guild that existed, for instance, in late medieval Florence.[37] In distinction from the rest of western Europe, English towns also had no tradition of providing physicians with salaries to help care for the poor and sick, nor did the crown fund charitable practitioners.[38] Apart from elite clients, then, there was little incentive in England for medical credentials. As a result, providing guidance to the sick remained a much less professionalized endeavor than it did on the continent, where medicine's secularization was well underway by the later thirteenth century. The numbers of physicians educated in England remained small—fewer than a hundred in total at Oxford before 1500, and about half that number in Cambridge.[39] Faye Getz's study of Oxford medical men in the fourteenth century discovers only four (out of forty) without record of ecclesiastical income, meaning that a minimum of 90 percent held benefices.[40] In the fifteenth century, Oxford medical graduates "did not change their essentially clerical and academic nature."[41] In addition to these few clerical graduates, it was often parish priests who were responsible for providing basic medical advice as well as access to written remedies, as manuscript evidence suggests.[42]

Medicine's entanglement with many different social roles meant that medical practice, and the authority that grounded it, was often available to local reinvention and negotiation. Though medicine assumed prominence in new contexts and the sheer number of medical manuscripts was soaring, caring for the sick and interpreting exceptional bodies were projects whose proper authorities were not known in advance. This fluidity gave rise to distinctive patterns of health care, including a certain *itinerancy* in one's course of treatment, as patients expected to visit multiple practitioners in the pursuit of care.

One writer and practitioner who exemplifies the protean character of English medical expertise is the surgeon John Arderne (b. 1307/8–d. 1377 or after), recently deemed "the most important English person in his field before the seventeenth century."[43] Arderne opens his best-known piece of writing, a treatise on the treatment of anal fistula, with biographical flourish. A Middle English translation of the original Latin reads, "I, John Arderne, fro the first pestilence that was in the yere of oure lord 1349 duellid [resided] in Newerk in Notyngham-shire unto the yere of oure lord 1370, and ther I helid many men of fistula in ano."[44] From there, Arderne lists the satisfied noblemen and clerics whom he cured, starting with "Sire Adam Everyngham of Laxton-in-the-Clay byside Tukkesford" and going on through nineteen further individuals, each named and specified in terms of geography and social rank. "All thise forseid cured I afore the makyng of this boke," he declares, thereby linking his composition to an impressive and locally detailed career of surgical success.[45] Arderne's *Practica* is unabashed in claiming the originality and value of his surgical technique, but it also stakes a claim to erudition. Arderne quotes extensively from the corpus of recent Latin *practicae*, including those by Lanfranc of Milan and Bernard of Gordon. His references indicate the availability of up-to-date continental medical texts for lay readers. Arderne is also the author of *De curo oculorum* (On the cure of eyes) and a less unified set of materials sometimes titled in manuscripts *Liber medicinalium*.

Being trained in surgery, a craft, it is unlikely that Arderne attended university. Yet he wrote in Latin, of a sort. Peter Murray Jones describes the surgeon's language as a "polyglot rather than a consistent Latin," with passages in Middle English and French, and its grammar "like that of a man thinking in English but writing in Latin."[46] The halting modulations of Arderne's prose testify to this English practitioner's belabored but also bravura entry into the learned tradition of European surgery. The *Practica*'s amalgam of manual expertise and learned synthesis was appealing in late medieval England—at least according to Arderne's account of the high fees he commanded and according to the large number of extant copies of his writings. A total of forty manuscripts survive. Of these, thirty-two preserve Arderne's Latin texts in whole or in part; the remaining eight are in Middle English and give evidence of four separate translation efforts.[47] Arderne's name appears more frequently in Middle English scientific and medical texts than does that of any other English practitioner.[48] His considerable authority, then, took shape between manual dexterity and erudition, vernacularity and Latinity, medical practice and medical writing.

Several manuscripts of Arderne's *Liber medicinalium* preserve a collection of *experimenta*, or case histories.[49] Some of these histories record the details of Arderne's own patients; others describe illnesses and treatments from a third-person perspective. One of the latter type illustrates the itineraries of care that are characteristic of late medieval *phisik*. The narrative is not so much the story of a cure as it is a tour of expertise. In it, a chaplain from "Colston faste by Byngham" is suffering from a painful, egg-shaped nodule on his chest. He receives medical advice from three sources in turn. First (in the words of a Middle English translation), "he was tawght of a lady [*a quadam domina edoctus*] to leye an emplastre ther to," and on her advice he takes to drinking a honey-based wound medicine, "the drynke of Antioche," for a "longe tyme."[50] But at a certain point the ineffectiveness of the lady's remedies becomes evident to the chaplain: "whan he perceyved that the forseyde medicines prevayled hym nowght he wente un to the Town of Notyngham to be leten blood." With this decision, his pursuit of a cure assumes a new direction: from local environs to nearby town, from nonprofessional woman to craft-trained man, and from noninvasive herbal concoctions to bloodletting.

The chaplain visits a barber (*barbitonsor*). In the hierarchy of medieval English medical expertise barbers played an emphatically manual role, being distinguished from surgeons in the relative simplicity of the procedures allowed to them. If figures like Lanfranc of Milan, Henri de Mondeville, and John Arderne were forging an intellectual identity for surgery, barbers by contrast tended to be relegated to the position of unreconstructed empirics. But in this story, the barber shows his medical ambition: when he sees the nodule on the chaplain's chest, he tells his customer that he recommends a more drastic course of procedure, "kuttynge or corrosyve [incision or corrosives]." The chaplain hesitates and decides to speak to an experienced surgeon (*sirurgicus expertus*) in the same town. This authority figure, who is also called *medicus* (*leche* in the Middle English translation), warns against any such *violentas medicinas* and explains that if the chaplain were to undergo them, "it wolde brynge hym to the deeth with owten ony rekevere [recovery] [*usque ad mortem ipsius langorem irrecuperabilem*]."[51] This is where the *experimentum* ends: the reader never finds out if the chaplain is cured. Instead the story rests with having sketched a provisional hierarchy of medical advice, a hierarchy emerging dynamically from the chaplain's itinerary—from a local lady to an overreaching barber-surgeon and finally to (in the Middle English) "awyse Sirurgyan."

The figure of the *domina* in Arderne's story is an interesting one. The title *domina*—or, in the Middle English translation, "lady"—indicates that this was a woman of means, probably propertied and respected, distinct from the figure of the *vetula*, or old woman, sometimes ridiculed by male medical writers. Upper-class women seem to have dispensed medicines quite regularly as part of their responsibilities in the household. The fifteenth-century commonplace book produced by the medical practitioner Thomas Fayreford, for instance, records the source of one recipe as Lady Poynings—who is elsewhere listed as one of Fayreford's patients. Fayreford also cites a successful treatment by "quidam domina," which succeeded even when "omnes scientes in Londyn" failed.[52] A brief letter from Sir John Paston II to his wife attests to her role as both a medical authority and, in this case, a medical writer. Sometime between 1487 and 1495, Paston wrote to "Mastress Margery":

> I prey yow in all hast possybyll to send me by the next swer
> messenger that ye can gete a large playster of your flose
> ungwentorum for the Kynges Attorney Jamys Hobart; for all hys
> dysease is but an ache in hys knee. . . . But when ye send me the
> playster ye must send me wryghtyng hough it shold be leyd to
> and takyn from hys knee, and hough longe it shold abyd on hys
> kne unremevyd, and hough longe the playster wyll laste good, and
> whethyr he must lape eny more clothys a-bowte the playster to kepe
> it warme or nought.[53]

> [I ask you to send me, in all possible haste, by the next reliable
> messenger that you can get, a large preparation of your poultice
> "flose ungwentorum," for the king's attorney James Hobart. For all
> his discomfort is but an ache in his knees. . . . But when you send
> me the plaster you must send me some writing about how it should
> be laid on and taken from his knee, and how long it should stay on
> his knee unremoved, and how long the plaster will remain good,
> and whether he should wind any more cloth about the plaster to
> keep it warm or not.]

Paston asks not only that Margery send him the medical preparation but also that she include written instructions, which marks her participation in the wide ranks of English medical literacy.[54] It is striking that Paston writes from his location among more elite court circles to seek out the medical expertise of his Norfolk home. In this, he perhaps echoes the perspective of his mother, who wrote to John Paston I in 1464, "fore Goddys sake be ware what medesynys ye take of any fysissyanys [physicians] of London. I schal never trust to hem."[55] One medical book that may have been made for the Paston family—the "litel boke of fisik" written by the professional scribe William Ebesham—contains Middle English texts about uroscopy, the plague, and astrology juxtaposed with roughly equivalent Latin versions.[56] This book, with its doubling of Latin and Middle English expertise, raises questions about how it might have been read and used in the Paston household.

Many further examples could be adduced to show how medieval patients moved among care-givers, testing whether this one or that one could help. Records of cures at saints' shrines tell a similar story: those healed often reported prior visits to medical experts, whose failures drove them to seek miraculous aid.[57] While such details of past treatment function to bolster saintly reputations and cannot be taken at face value, they do attest to the prevalence of conceiving healing as a winding, multistop route. Just as it was difficult to determine the exact chain of causes behind a symptom, it was hard to know just whose efficacy, or what kinds of expertise and influence, would lead to a cure. Whether the Nottingham surgeon trumps the local *domina*, or Margery Paston's cure outpaces those of court physicians, these and other examples suggest that medical discourse in late medieval England was composed of variegated and overlapping therapeutic competencies and that hierarchies of expertise often emerged locally through particular itineraries of care.

There were, however, two notable and closely related attempts at systematic change. In the first quarter of the fifteenth century, university-trained physicians twice tried to centralize the regulation of who could practice medicine. The first of these attempts was national in scope. In 1421 a group of physicians from Oxford and Cambridge petitioned Parliament and Henry V to establish them as a licensing body. Medical practice, they claimed, should be restricted to those who "have long tyme y used the Scoles of Fisyk withynne som Universitee, and be graduated in the same."[58] They demanded "that no Woman use the practyse of Fisyk." To enforce the new rule that all medical authority be academically ratified, the physicians asked that warrants be sent to "all the Sherrefs of Engelond" summoning anyone lacking academic credentials to "trewe and streyte examinacion" in "one of the Universitees of this lond." In other words, they called on the state's system of judicial power, its traveling courts endowed with an authority leading back to the crown, to make medicine a university-controlled pursuit.

One of the most insistent aspects of the petition's rhetoric is its effort to yoke *science* and *practyse*. The word *practyse* is used with hectic frequency, ten times in the petition's brief span. The physicians are eager to make the concrete business of healing depend on academic training. *Phisik*, they claim, is like theology and law; it "should be used and practised" only by those trained in it—but "in this Roialme is every man, be he never so lewed [ignorant], takyng upon hym practyse," leading to the "grete harme and slaughtre of many men." However, the petition continues, "if no man practised theryn" except "connynge [knowledgeable] men and approved sufficeantly y learned in art [the liberal arts], filosofye, and fisyk," then "shulde many men that dyeth, for defaute of help, lyve, and no man perysh by unconnyng [should many men who die for lack of help instead live, and no man perish on account of ignorance]." A university education here is cast as a matter of life and death, in a bid for the intellectualization of healing authority. The physicians' labor to link academic learning to the efficacy of care suggests that the connection was far from universally recognized. As we have seen, in the *Metaphysics* Aristotle admits that the empiric's know-how may top theoretical knowledge in the business of curing: "If, then, someone has the explanation without the experience, . . . he will often fail to cure." The ongoing significance of the Aristotelian comment is evident in Antonius of Florence (d. 1459), whose chapter on physicians in his *Summa Theologica* (a handbook for preachers) refers to what "the Philosopher says in book I of the *Metaphysics*" in order to remind readers that "we should choose experienced doctors to treat us, rather than those who have knowledge without experience." Antonius continues, "I consider it safer and better to commit oneself for treatment to practical physicians rather than theoretical ones."[59] The petitioning physicians were trying to counter just this idea and the social practices that went with it.

By all evidence, the physicians' petition came to nothing. For the tiny medical faculties at Oxford and Cambridge, the responsibilities described in the document were unfeasible, and there is no evidence that the act ever came before Parliament after the draft was prepared. Yet two years later, in 1423, university-trained physicians again attempted to secure the rights to medical practice, this time not in all the shires of England but in its most powerful city, London. In alliance with London surgeons, they asked the mayor and aldermen to establish "all Phisicians and Cirurgeans, withinne the libertees of London" as "oon Comminalte [one fellowship]."[60] In rhetoric similar to the draft act of Parliament, the petition cast practitioners' ignorance as a menace to public health: many people are "spillide be [ruined by] wreeched and pre-sumptuous practisours in phisyk, nought knowyng the treuthe or ground of that Faculte of Phisyk, and be [by] unkonnyng wirkers in Cirurgy, nought knowyng the trewe crafte of Cirurgy."[61] *Phisik* is called a "glorious konnyng [knowledge]" and surgery a "crafte," but both kinds of expertise require proper training; otherwise, the professions are "disclaundered [slandered]" and peo-ple hurt. Insistence on the dangers of medical ignorance in both the 1421 draft act and the London petition implies that the popularization of healing exper-tise was the occasion for anxiety and that elite physicians thought they could play on such anxiety to launch their ambitious reforms.

The ordinances of the London *comminalte* extend the vision of two com-plementary branches of expertise, medicine and surgery, to the physical archi-tecture of the group's meeting space. The document asks that "oon place" be established in the City of London "contenyng atte lest thre howses [chambers] severall."[62] One of these chambers would be for physicians exclusively ("oonly pertenynge to the Faculte of Physick") and one for surgeons exclusively ("oonly pertenynge to the Crafte of Cirurgye"). The third, however, would be a nonexclusive space of learning, "ichaired and desked for redyng and disputa-cions in Philosophye and in medicyns." "Medicine" seems to be the petition's preferred term for the unified field that physicians and surgeons shared. The common chamber for "redyng and disputacions" corresponds institution-ally to the highest office of the *comminalte*, the "Rectour of the Faculte of Medicyn," beneath whom are two "Surveiours of the Faculte of Phisyk" and two "Maistres of the Crafte of Cirurgye."[63] While the draft act of Parliament ignores surgery's independent footing, the *comminalte* carefully acknowledges it, even incorporating it into the built environment and structures of gover-nance—though the group reserved its highest post, that of rector, for someone with a university degree in medicine.

The only documented action of the *comminalte* after its establishment in 1423 is the ruling in a case brought by one William Forest, complainant, against three surgeons accused of an "alleged error of treatment of the wound in the muscles of the thumb of the right hand."[64] Eight physicians and surgeons made up the advisory jury, among whom were some of the most prominent medical men of late medieval England. The ruling recounts that "on 31 January last past, the moon being consumed in a bloody sign, to wit, Aquarius, under a very malevolent constellation," William Forest was seriously wounded in the muscles of his hand. On February 9, "the moon being in the sign of Gemini, a great effusion of blood took place." John Harwe, a "free surgeon," and two barber-surgeons, John Dalton and Simon Rolf, were involved in stopping the flow of blood, "which broke out six several time in a dangerous fashion, and on the seventh occasion, . . . the wounded man preferring a mutilated hand rather than death, the said John Harwe, with the consent of the patient, and for lack of other remedy, finally staunched the blood by cautery, as was proper, and thus saved his life." The advisory jury, "having diligently considered and fully understood the matter, on the evidence of the parties and the sworn testimony," determined that the surgeon and barber-surgeons "had acted in a surgically correct manner and had made no error, and that therefore they were absolved of all charges made against them by the said William." In addition, "They further imposed upon the complainant perpetual silence in the matter and, so far as possible, they restored to the defendants who were guiltless and had been maliciously and undeservedly defamed, the full measure of their good reputation, as their merits in the case required. Further they declared that any defect, mutilation or disfigurement of the hand was due either to the constellation aforesaid or some defect of the patient or the original nature of the wound." The ruling illustrates how the power to narrate mattered in late medieval medicine. William Forest is enjoined to silence, and his own version of events is left out of the ruling. As someone bearing the mark of both injury and treatment, he is forbidden from offering his own account. The jury's gag order as well as the wish to restore the defendants' reputations imply the fragility of the surgeons' standings. A patient's words mattered in London's medical marketplace. Although the ruling seems one-sided, with professional self-interest and allegiance stacked against the claimant, it is likely that William Forest soon had the chance to tell his story after all. The *comminalte* lasted just eighteen months before dissolving under pressure from the powerful guild of barber-surgeons.

The ruling also exemplifies how in late medieval England specialized knowledge of medical causation could trump other explanations. The jury's linking of astrological details with the "great effusion of blood" depends on the members' command of a learned system of correspondences between the positions of the stars and bodily flux. This esoteric system underwrites the judgment that the "malevolent constellation" is responsible for Forest's dangerous bleeding and so for the mutilating treatment, rather than any incompetence on the surgeon's part. When the expert jury deems that Harwe acted in a "surgically correct manner," they and he are announced to share this specialist proficiency, which exceeds the patient's understanding of the situation and so undercuts his account of causation and blame. As in the *Isagoge*, so in this case: "to the patient [*infirmo*] these are accidents, while to the doctor [*medico*], they are signs."[65] Faye Getz remarks of the case, "The fact that physic could offer an astrological explanation of this sort in the legal sphere is remarkable. Before this the layman was considered a sufficient arbiter in medical matters that came before the law, and the common law sufficient precedent."[66] If lay judgment usually sufficed, elite practitioners in London briefly created an alternative scenario, where they effectively wielded medical astrology in the elite regulation of London's medical practice. Yet the institution of the *comminalte* did not last, and Forest likely regained the right to tell his version of events, perhaps even armed with some of the expertise then circulating so plentifully in medical manuscripts. Medicine's explanatory systems were gaining ground, even if who was able to call on those systems, with what authority, remained a matter for contestation.

Sign

The perceptible qualities of bodies vary among individuals and among groups, and they also shift across an individual's lifetime. In the Middle Ages, some bodily characteristics were perceived to be fixed, like those codified through species, race, gender, or innate complexion.[67] Other traits were understood to shift with the body's ever-fluctuating internal state. Humors tinted the complexion; fever warmed the flesh; indigestion roiled the stomach; lethargy weighed the limbs. Changes like these were clinical signs. Diagnosis was the branch of pathology concerned with bodily signs, and Latin medical manuals included it alongside the other learned operations of medicine: nosological definition, etiology, prognosis, and therapeutics.[68] Handbooks generally advised that diagnosis should proceed by examining the patient's appearance, querying her personal history and experience of the illness, scrutinizing her excreta (especially urine), and feeling her pulse.[69] One symptom could point to many pathologies, and it was only via constellations of symptoms that disease could be reliably identified.

Symptoms are *signa naturalia*. While natural signs depend on direct or indirect causal relations, causation alone does not make a sign. Signification also requires a "mind apprehending [*animam apprehendentem*]," as Roger Bacon observes.[70] Learned traditions of bodily interpretation thus needed to train apprehending minds to recognize what features were meaningful as well as what they meant. This section focuses on two very different frameworks for late medieval corporeal hermeneutics: the diagnosis of leprosy and the practice of physiognomy. Examinations for leprosy regarded the body in terms of pathological change, while physiognomy interpreted it for fixed characterological disposition. Yet both practices faced similar uncertainties as they set about trying to parse living bodies into signifiers and to fix those signifiers with stable meaning. Uncertainties included how to recognize signs as signs, how to weigh conflicting signs against one another, who had the authority to interpret particular bodies, and what models of causation and selfhood undergirded these interpretive systems. Both leprous symptoms and physiognomic indices catalyzed the production of intricate textual aids to address such questions.

Leprosy was one of the most overdetermined bodily states of the later Middle Ages. It was regarded alternately as a medical, legal, moral, exegetical, thaumaturgical, and institutional matter, and according to surviving evidence, those diagnosed with leprosy played a variety of roles in medieval communities.[71] As Luke Demaitre has convincingly shown, medical writers in the later Middle Ages adopted a strongly naturalistic approach toward the disease.[72] Physicians and surgeons left out scriptural and moralistic glosses almost entirely and instead focused on material causes, diagnosis, and therapeutics. Nonetheless, leprosy's fraught status still mattered profoundly. Because serious social and legal consequences could follow from diagnosis, learned medicine developed an especially elaborate apparatus for identifying the disease. Scenes of examination could become flashpoints for conflict, and diagnosing leprosy emerged as a particularly high-stakes exercise in medical semiotics.

The official examination of someone suspected of having leprosy was called a *iudicium*, or "judgment," and those who were responsible for carrying it out were aware of the quasi-judicial character of their determinations. From the second half of the thirteenth century in France and Germany and on the Iberian Peninsula, university-trained physicians hired by city governments tended to be in charge of *iudicia*. However, because England had many fewer physicians and no tradition of retaining them for purposes of public health, priests and common-law juries remained the leading examiners of those suspected of the disease. This meant that a broader and more heterogeneous fraction of the population was responsible for diagnosis, and their authority was far from unimpeachable. For instance, William Mustardere, rector of Sparham in the late 1460s, diagnosed his parishioner John Folkard with leprosy, urging the man to "withdrawe hym from the compayne of other men."[73] Following this, Folkard "'manassed [menaced]'" the priest, warning him "that he shuld repent that ever he made any such noyse," and Mustardere soon found himself thrown in jail.[74] Carole Rawcliffe observes that "the false or malicious imputation of leprosy might also result in a suit for defamation. . . . Mistakes could thus inflict lasting damage on the person *making* as well as receiving the diagnosis."[75]

It is likely that such nonprofessional examiners were among the readership for the diagnostic guides that circulated both as parts of longer medical compendia and as independent texts in the later Middle Ages. Just prior to giving step-by-step instructions for a diagnostic exam, the surgeon Guy de Chauliac (d. 1368) warns his readers about the serious consequences of such an evaluation. The Middle English translation of Guy's *Chirurgia magna* reads:

> it is mykel to be taken hede aboute the examynynge and the dome of leprouse men, that is the moste iniurie (i. wrong) to sequestre or withdrawe tho men that schulde not be sequestred or withdrawen and leve leprouse men with the peple, for-whye it is a contagiouse sekenesse and infectynge. And therfore a leche that shal deme ham, he schall ofte byholde ham and turne and unturne the tokenes.[76]

> [It is much to be heeded in the examination and judgment of leprous men, that it is the greatest injury, or wrong, to sequester or withdraw those men that should not be sequestered or withdrawn, and to leave leprous men among the people since it is a contagious and infecting sickness. And therefore a medical practitioner who shall judge them, he shall often behold them and consider and reconsider the signs.]

A failure to diagnose would endanger those who do not have leprosy, while a "false positive" would unjustly force the patient to withdraw from social life. In response to these risks, Guy urges greater observational and interpretive effort, "turning and unturning" the symptoms. Indeed, the medieval medical accounts of leprosy consistently emphasize the painstaking labor of diagnosis.

One diagnostic treatise, often attributed in manuscripts to the fourteenth-century Montpellier physician Jordan of Turre, suggests that the examiner organize his observations according to a carefully rational scheme: "Proceed as follows: take a tablet and write the good signs on one side and the bad signs on the other, and you will not become confused."[77] Many treatises divided symptoms into "equivocal" and "unequivocal" categories, so that an examiner would not be misled by a *signum fallax*.[78] But even those distinctions were uncertain. In his *Lilium medicinae*, the Montpellier physician Bernard of Gordon (d. c. 1318) includes an extensive discussion of *dubia*, or doubtful matters, in his chapter on leprosy. At one point he recalls a patient who had fingers and toes "so deformed, disfigured, and falling apart that they had only one joint left." Yet over the course of twenty years, no facial symptoms appeared. While Bernard treated the man for leprosy, the physician changed his diagnosis in retrospect, since facial disfigurement is such an "unequivocal" sign: "Therefore, I guess, with conjecture in approximation of the truth, that it was not leprosy and that it could not have lasted for so long without disfigurement of the face. Even though I had once believed differently, now, after having labored diligently in this work, I am of another opinion and now I would not declare someone [like him] leprous. However, God knows the truth, I do not know."[79] Bernard's account is striking for its fretful uncertainty. Despite the spectacular disfigurements for which leprosy was known in hagiography and other literary representations, within learned medicine its discernment was treated as a difficult and anxious task.[80]

The volatility of leprosy's diagnosis is evident in a Chancery warrant from 1468. Written by three physicians of Edward IV, "William Hatteclyff, Roger Marshall and Dominic de Serego, doctors of Arts and Medicine," the warrant responds to an earlier petition demanding the removal of "Joanna Nightingale of Brentwood in the county of Essex from general intercourse with mankind, because it was presumed by some of her neighbors [*ex vicinis suis*] that she was infected by foul contact with leprosy [*foeda leprae contagione infectam*] and was in fact herself a leper."[81] Joanna apparently refused to accept this initial diagnosis and call for sequestration, and so a writ was prepared on account of the "grievous injury [*grave dampnum*]" and "manifest perils [*periculum manifestum*]" of her ongoing presence. The writ instructed the sheriff of Essex to assemble a common-law jury to make Joanna's diagnosis legally binding:

> having taken with you certain discreet and loyal men [*discretis et legalibus hominibus*] of the county of the aforesaid Joanna, in order to obtain a better knowledge of her disease, you go to the aforesaid Joanna and cause her to be diligently viewed and examined [*facias diligenter videri et examinari*] in the presence of the foresaid men. And if you find her to be leprous, as was recorded of her, then that you cause her to be removed in as decent a manner as possible,

from all intercourse with other persons, and have her betake herself immediately to a secluded place [*locum solitarium*] as is the custom, lest by common intercourse of this kind injury or danger should in any wise happen to the aforesaid inhabitants.[82]

As the writ indicates, the diagnosis that was initially "presumed" (*praesumeretur*) by her neighbors could be formalized and made binding by a local jury. Joanna was to be "diligently viewed and examined" in the jury's presence, though no mention is made of who should lead the examination. This initial writ is unconcerned with medical learning, and laymen and common law are treated as sufficient arbiters. Instead of medical expertise, the writ focuses on the perceived dangers to the community and to the customary status of sequestration.

However, Joanna was apparently supplied with friends in high places as well as suspicious neighbors. After the issue of the first writ, the Bishop of Bath and Wells and Lord Chancellor Robert Stillington (d. 1491) requested that the king's own physicians examine Joanna. They agreed and described their diagnostic exam in a second Chancery writ, which stressed the exam's methodical and learned character. As the writ recounts, "We examined her person, and, as the older and most learned medical authors have directed in these cases, we touched and handled her and made mature, diligent, and proper investigation whether the symptoms indicative of this disease were in her or not [*de persona sua consideravimus, et juxta quod antiquiores et sapientissimi medicinae auctores in hujusmodi casibus faciendum docuerant, ipsam tractavimus et palpavimus, per signa, hujusmodi morbi declarativa, discursum fecimus, si in ea reperirentur mature diligenter et prout oportuit inquisivimus*]."[83] The physicians provide their reader, nominally Edward IV, some background information to appreciate their method: "We are taught by medical science that the disease of leprosy is known by many signs [*Docemur equidem ex scientia medicinali morbum leprae in communi per plurima signa*]." And so, they continue

in the case of the woman brought before us, upon going through upwards of twenty-five of the more marked signs of general leprosy we do not find that she can be proved to be leprous, by them or a sufficient number of them. And this would suffice, generally, to free her from the suspicion of leprosy, since it is not possible for any to labor under the disease in whom the greater part of these signs are not found [*in hoc casu, mulieris nobis oblatae per viginti quinque &*

ultra signa leprae in communi famosiora discurrentes, non invenimus
ipsam ex illis aut eorumdem sufficienti numero posse convinci leprosam,
tt hoc quidem generaliter pro liberando ipsam a dicta praesumptione
sufficeret, cum non sit possibile leprae morbo quempiam laborare in quo
non multa pars hujusmodi signorum reperiatur].[84]

We can discern in this passage the influence of treatises like Jordanus of Turre's, with its instructions to notate symptoms on a chart of "good signs" and "bad," as well as Bernard of Gordon's careful parsing of equivocal and unequivocal signs. The physicians even recount an otiose further step in their exam, when they search for the symptoms of leprosy's four subvarieties: "going through upwards of forty distinctive signs of the different varieties of leprosy, we do not find that this woman is to be marked as suffering under any of the four kinds, but is utterly free and untainted [*liberam prorsus et immunem*]." They conclude their diagnosis, "We are prepared to declare the same more fully to your highness by scientific process [*per processum scientificum*], if and wherever it shall be necessary."[85] With this last statement they promise an even greater display of learned rigor, should the occasion demand it.

In this document, then, the practice of bodily interpretation appears in its deeply social aspect. Joanna's neighbors are the first to diagnose her, drawing on the traditions of sequestration in canon law (and ultimately Mosaic Law) as well as novel rhetorics of contagion.[86] It is impossible now to determine the reasons behind this initial diagnosis. Were there visible symptoms that called for it, or was it motivated by the desire to lay hold of a woman's property, or to bridle her willful behavior? Joanna's neighbors, finding their diagnosis ignored, petitioned the court of Chancery to lend it legal force. But against the normal course of common law, in which a jury's judgment was adequate to determine leprosy, the king's own physicians were solicited. Thanks to the exceptional intervention of Joanna's apparent ally Robert Stillington, scientific discourse gained a foothold in the situation, and the physicians answered the earlier writ with their own exam, rendering "the truth [*veritas*] on this subject most plain and clear [*clarissima*]."[87] None of the documents includes Joanna's own account, but her refusal to accede to her neighbors' diagnosis is a statement in itself. Though the patient's speech is given no particular authority in the document, it is her diagnostic dissent that gathers a conflicting set of interpretive practices around her. The situation illustrates how the parsing of bodily signs was the occasion not only for interpretation but also for the extrasemiotic negotiation among different authorities and systems of bodily discernment.

Physiognomy, like leprosy's diagnosis, occasioned the fraught recoding of medieval bodies into legible signs. The physiognomic art sought to discover a person's character on the basis of bodily features, and in late medieval England it circulated in the discursive borderlands between medicine, natural philosophy, magic, and literary pleasure. Like *phisik*, physiognomy derives from the Greek term *physis*. As one Middle English treatise remarks, "This word *phisonomea* ys said of *phisis*, that is nature, and *gnomos*, that is dyvynynge [divining, discerning]."[88] In his influential commentary Roger Bacon (d. 1294) gave the word a slightly different gloss: "'Physiognomy' is the rule of nature in the complexion of the human body and in its composition—because in Greek 'nomos' is 'law,' and 'phisis' is 'nature' [*Phisonomia est lex nature in complexione humani corporis et eius composicione, quia Grece 'nomos' est 'lex,' 'phisis' est 'natura'*]."[89] Whether grounded in *gnosis* or *nomos*, medieval physiognomy presumed the ordered lawfulness of nature, which undergirded the correspondence of physical features and character. This mutual entailment of body and behavior was usually explained with a nod to astrology. James Yonge, in his translation and redaction of the *Secretum Secretorum* in 1422, states that "al bodely thyngis [all bodily things] be governyd and ordaynyd by the Planetes and the Sterris [stars]," and accordingly everyone is "disposid dyversly [diversely] to vertues and to vices."[90] Astral determinism does not sit comfortably with Christian theology, and Étienne Tempier's well-known condemnations of 1277 insisted anew that stars merely incline and do not determine human behavior. But physiognomy leaned heavily on this inclination and elaborated the fantasy that bodies, by virtue of being natural things, made persons legible.

Medieval English readers appear to have been eager for physiognomic writings. The catalogue *Scientific and Medical Writings in Old and Middle English* lists 113 manuscript witnesses for Middle English texts of physiognomy from the fourteenth and fifteenth centuries (although this number is somewhat inflated by separate entries for prologues and texts). Anglo-Latin physiognomies survive even more plentifully. Physiognomy's manuscript contexts indicate its flexible generic identity, moving between the medicoscientific and the fantastic. Those in straightforwardly medical contexts include, for instance, three Latin tracts in a medical compilation owned by St. Mary's Priory, Coventry, which bears annotations and signs of use, like the addition of recipes by the *infirmarius*.[91] One of the remarkable "Sloane Group" of medical manuscripts—identified by Linda Voigts as the productions of a bookmaker specializing in medical compilations—includes a physiognomy, as do three closely related manuscripts.[92] Roland l'Ecrivain, a member of the

Parisian medical faculty, presented an original physiognomy to the Duke of Bedford in 1430. However, physiognomic instructions also appeared alongside more esoteric and exotic materials, like texts on alchemy and divination.[93] In two manuscripts, a physiognomy is incorporated into a romance, the *Buik of King Alexander the Conquerour*, in a combination implying that the pleasures of fantastic narrative and physiognomy were thought congruent, or even mutually amplifying.[94] Exoticism is also emphasized in John Metham's mid-fifteenth-century book, written for Sir Miles Stapleton: a love plot set in Persia is sandwiched between a palmistry and a physiognomy. One late thirteenth-century Latin physiognomy, owned and annotated in the library of Bury St. Edmunds, is preceded by a letter from the legendary figure of Prester John.[95]

Physiognomy's fungible generic identity reflects medieval readers' uncertain sense of what to do with physiognomy's implications for embodied subjectivity. If the heavenly bodies or other natural forces imprinted personality and left its indices all over the face to be read, where did this leave moral deliberation and free will? However, to critique physiognomy too stridently, or to insist too vehemently on the untrammeled freedom of human behavior, destroyed physiognomy's alluring promise that learned expertise could turn the treacherous world into a domain of natural signs. Friction between the desire for knowledge and anxiety about physical determinism is variously legible in physiognomic texts, but I focus here on one Middle English example— the unexceptional seventh chapter of a treatise on natural philosophy. The treatise was written around 1400 in a compilation of medical and scientific texts, now London, British Library, Sloane MS 213. The chapter claims that its physiognomic lore is drawn from Aristotle's teachings to his pupil Alexander, marking its source as the *Secretum Secretorum*, the pseudo-Aristotelian treatise translated (in full) from Arabic to Latin around 1230. More than six hundred manuscript witnesses of the *Secretum* survive, in Latin and various European vernaculars; it was a remarkably popular text.[96] The physiognomic portion often circulated separately from the rest of the book, as it does in Sloane MS 213.

"Here sues certeyne rewles of phisnomy" (Here follow certain rules of physiognomy) reads the rubric at the start of the chapter, and its contents mostly take the form of rules, or straightforward principles for translating between body and character:

Nose when it es sotyl and small, he that owes it es wrathfull and angry. Who that has a longe nose straght to the mouthe he es

gentill, worthy and hardy. Whose nose es like an ape, he es hasty.
Schorte nose toknes a schrewe, and if the noseholes be wyde also,
that es a synger and liccherous.[97]

[When a nose is subtle and small, he that owns it is wrathful and
angry. He who has a long nose, straight to the mouth, is noble,
worthy and strong. He whose nose is like an ape's, he is hasty. A
short nose signifies a rogue, and if the nose-holes are also wide, then
he is a singer and lecherous.]

A long list of such physiognomic signs was the quintessential form of the
genre. The repetitive sentences that make up the bulk of physiognomic treatises tend to follow one of two formulas: either *whoever has x is y*—as in, "Who
that has right litel eares he es foltisch, thevysch and liccherous [foolish, thieving, and lecherous]"—or, alternatively, *x signifies y*—as in, "Many heres upon
aither [either] schuldre signyfies foly [foolishness, madness]."[98] Both constructions imply a model of embodiment that is static, deterministic, and inter-
pretable. Physiognomy, as the treatise claims, gives the power "to knowe by
only [only] thoght when men lokes on any man, of what condicions he es."[99]
Quotidian perceptions of bodily form are transformed into esoteric insight
into someone's true identity, thanks to the insights of the physiognomic text.

In actuality, numerous factors mitigated against the straightforward usefulness of physiognomy. Many observations were difficult to make, like the
close scrutiny of the eye's iris or a view of body parts ordinarily hidden from
sight. Even if a slew of physiognomic observations were gathered, how did one
harmonize them into a comprehensive sense of the person? What if someone
had a long nose, making him noble and worthy, and small ears, meaning he
was thieving and lecherous? The treatise instructs its readers, "set noght thi sentence [understanding] ne dome [nor judgment] in one of these signes allone,
bot gader the wittenes [gather the evidence] to-gider of ilk [each] one."[100] But
exactly *how* to synthesize the evidence was far from clear. Still, the idea that
physiognomy really *was* practicable, that its list of rules could make the social
field legible, was essential to its appeal. Physiognomic texts were suffused with
what might be called an otiose practicality.

If physiognomy then gives literate expression to an ethos of determined
character and legible embodiment—and if this ethos must have been part of
its attraction—most physiognomic texts also bear within them an antidote to
this idea, an antidote in the form of a story. This is the remarkably widespread

exemplum of Hippocrates and Philomon (or Polemon), the ancient masters of medicine and of physiognomy, respectively. The tale begins with a group of curious medical students, the "disciples" of Hippocrates, who decide to seek out the philosopher rumored to be the "chefe mayster and hyest doctur" of physiognomy.[101] From the start, two disciplines of bodily interpretation, medicine and physiognomy, are set in tense and inquiring relation.

Secretly the students have a portrait made of their teacher, depicting the "fourme and schappe of Ypocras [Hippocrates] in parchemyne [parchment]," and they bring this image to Philomon. They demand, "'Byholde this figur, and deme [judge] and schewe to us the qualités of the complexion of it.'"[102] Philomon studies the portrait and then declares that the man depicted in it is lecherous, deceitful, and greedy. The students are shocked. Their adventure in cross-disciplinary knowledge testing has gotten away from then, and they nearly kill Philomon on the spot. To appease them, he explains that he was answering them merely according to "'my sciens'" but that after all, he does recognize that the picture "'es [is] the figure of the wyse Ypocrase.'" The confused students rush back to their master, seeking his explanation and reassurance. Hippocrates listens to their account and then remarks:

> "Trewly Philomon saide sothe, and he lafte noght of the leste letter
> of the treuthe. Nevertheles, sithen I biheld and knewe me schapli
> to these thynges filthy and reprovable, I ordeyned my soule kyng
> above my body, and so I withdrewe my body fro thise thynges and I
> overcome it in withholdyng of my foule luste."[103]

> ["Truly Philomon spoke the truth, and left out not the least letter.
> Nevertheless, since I beheld and knew myself inclined to these filthy
> and blame-worthy things, I ordained my soul king over my body,
> and so I withdrew my body from these things and I overcame it by
> withstanding my foul desire."]

The exemplum then draws to a close with a striking redefinition of Hippocratic medicine: "This es the praysyng and wisdome of the werkes of Ypocras, for phisik es noght elles bot abstynens [abstinence], and conquest of foule covetus lustes [desires]."[104]

The exemplum emphasizes the abstract and formal character of physiognomic knowledge and how such abstraction limits what physiognomy can know. Philomon examines "it," a picture, rather than "him," Hippocrates. The depicted face is a matter of "fourme," "schappe," "figur," and "qualités," and it is this image that grounds Philemon's two contradictory judgments—first, that the man in the portrait is wicked, and second, that the image represents "wyse" Hippocrates. The antithesis between Philomon's pronouncements testifies to an incoherence in physiognomy's way of understanding other people, the object of its gaze: it ignores their social identity to insist on their somatic legibility. The Hippocratic triumph over physiognomy consists in setting Philemon's two aporetic pronouncements into dynamic and transformative relation. If physiognomy never resolves the tension between knowable bodies and volatile agencies, Hippocrates masters that tension within the self. He says of his disposition to vice, "I biheld and knewe me schapli to these thynges." The word "schapli"—meaning conformed or inclining—echoes the "fourme and schappe" of Hippocrates' portrait, yet the physician shows not only that "schap" can be comprehended but that its consequences, and therefore its meanings, can be controlled. Hippocrates' "I" and "me" ("I . . . knewe me") are further troped into soul and body: "'I ordeyned my soule kyng above my body.'" Into the static equations of physiognomic rules, Hippocrates injects temporality, reflexivity, and agency.

Though Philomon's pronouncement departs from the truth "nought the least letter," one may suspect that this letter kills (*littera enim occidit*, 2 Cor. 3:6). The Pauline echo is given support by the fact that the treatise's physiognomic chapter concludes with a quotation from "seynt Poule": "'No man sale [shall] be crouned [crowned], bot als [unless] he has lawfully and stalworthly stryvene [heartily struggled]'" (2 Tim. 2:5).[105] Just prior to this biblical quotation, the treatise switches to a second-person address:

> And thus ther thou knowes thi self or any other schaply and
> bowable to any vice by way of thi compleccion, do thi self and
> councele other to do as Ypocras did, and make thi soule to reule thi
> body by gode resoun and discrecion, withstandyng by vertue tho
> vyces to whilke thou art conable borne of compleccion.[106]

> [And where you know yourself or any other shaped and inclined to
> any vice because of your complexion, do for yourself—and counsel
> others to do—as Hippocrates did, and make your soul rule your
> body according to good reason and discretion, withstanding by
> means of virtue those vices to which you are disposed on the basis
> of complexion.]

Here the treatise veers toward penitential self-discipline and leaves behind the semiotics of small noses, little ears, and hairy shoulders that occupy the bulk of the physiognomic text.

The significance of Hippocrates and Philomon can only be evaluated if the exemplum's position in the physiognomic text is taken into account. This narrative, arguing for the determinative power of self-governance, constantly circulated alongside physiognomic rules. It is recounted in the works of such medieval thinkers as Albertus Magnus (d. 1280), Roger Bacon (d. 1294), Pietro d'Abano (d. 1316), and Michele Savonarola (d. 1468), all of whom treated physiognomy with intellectual seriousness and respect.[107] Physiognomic rules imply, in their very syntactic form, the mutual determination of physical body and moral disposition. They promote the fantasy that readers can be inducted into an esoteric knowledge that transforms the apprehension of bodies into characterological insight. What this means for readers' own corporeality the rules leave unexamined. The exemplum, by contrast, shows self-cultivation triumphing over natural disposition to the point that physiognomy's pronouncements become futile. It refocuses attention away from knowing others to knowing oneself. The point is not that the story makes the science conformable to dogma. The adage *astra inclinant, sed non obligant* was sufficient to squeeze physiognomy into orthodoxy. Instead, the popularity of this disjunctive conjoining shows that medieval readers found the compound of exemplum and rules good to think with. Story and treatise articulate starkly different versions of embodied subjectivity, and so whatever understandings of the physical self emerge from reading the text as a whole are informed by their dissenting interplay. This is a both/and model of writing about the body, which calls for readers' active parrying of colliding models of causation, signification, and subjectivity.

Book

What did medieval men and women understand *phisik* to encompass? Medieval English book-making functions as an important source for recovering contemporary understandings of the discourse. Compared to theology, for instance, medicine generated relatively little commentary about its audience, purpose, and discursive status in late medieval England. While people fiercely debated what counted as religious doctrine and who had a claim to read and write it, medicine catalyzed few polemical articulations. The 1421 and 1423 efforts at elite reform are among the only ones. Instead, epistemological evaluation and metapragmatic reflection were often recorded in the material artifacts of books. Manuscripts embody in their contents and layout medieval ideas about medical genres, intellectual traditions, and the relation between literacy and healing. Take, for instance, the redefinition of *phisik* that concludes the story of Philomon and Hippocrates: "Phisik es noght elles bot abstynens, and conquest of foule covetus lustes [Medicine is nothing other than abstinence and the conquest of foul, covetous desires]."[108] With this line, the exemplum seems to subordinate the scientific and technical aspects of the Hippocratic art to the project of moral self-governance. Set in contrast to physiognomy's somatic determinism, *phisik* is made the standard-bearer for the subject's freedom from nature.

Yet, just as the story's constant attachment to the physiognomic rules tempered its critique of them, so *phisik*'s redefinition here was qualified by the textual and material frameworks in which it was articulated. A quick tour through the contents of the codex in which the words appear, now Sloane MS 213, gives a sense of the discursive environment in which it assumed meaning. The chapter on physiognomy is part of a larger vernacular treatise on natural philosophy, which also treats astrology, meteorological and calendrical prognostics, the four humors, and uroscopy. The treatise helps constitute the Middle English portion of the manuscript, a section of more than thirty folios that also includes texts on medicinal oils and waters, bloodletting, and geometry. Most of the Latin texts in the manuscript appear to be in the same hand, datable roughly to 1400.[109] The Latin works probably by the same scribe include the popular herbal *De virtutibus herbarum*, a lapidary, a translation of the Sevillian physician Ibn Zuhr's (d. 1164) regimen of health, Arnau of Vilanova's translation of a treatise on medicinal simples by the Andalusian polymath Abu al-Salt (d. 1134), a survey of medicinal simples by Jean de Saint Amand (fl. late thirteenth century), and part of the cosmological treatise *Imago mundi* by Honorius Augustodunensis (d. 1154). A portion of the *Isagoge* of Joannitius is written in another hand and inserted, and a plague treatise by a later scribe is appended at the end.[110] The manuscript is quite finely produced, large in size with initial capitals decorated in blue, green, and red. Around the turn of the fifteenth century someone in England invested considerable expense in this book that unites a wide array of authorities in Latin and vernacular to account for how material substances and physical processes interact with one another and affect the human body.

The contents of the manuscript, then, stand at odds with the moralistic redefinition of medicine offered at the end of the story of Hippocrates and Philomon. The tacit argument from the collection of texts is that *phisik* is a specialized and technical art, one that entails familiarity with cosmology, herbal and lapidary lore, diagnosis from urine, phlebotomy, and sophisticated accounts of pharmacopeia. When the physiognomic treatise turns from bodily signs to the management of vices, it does so within the horizons of a very learned medical manuscript. In an important essay on scientific and medical books, Linda Voigts picks out Sloane MS 213 as especially representative of this new class of books.[111] The essay analyzes 178 English scientific and medical manuscripts produced between 1375 and 1500 to show that they share not only a common archive of texts but "physical features that set them off from belletristic, theological, philosophical, chronicle, legal, pedagogical and household manuscripts."[112] These manuscripts testify to an apparently broadly shared sense of what constituted scientific and medical books in late medieval England. Voigts has elsewhere uncovered evidence that this common sensibility supported a medical "publisher," who in the 1450s and early 1460s produced "a specific *kind* of manuscript, uniform in appearance and scientific and medical in subject matter."[113] All of these codices made implicit claims about how medical writing should be used and understood.

Sifting through even a fraction of the medical manuscripts that survive from late medieval England soon reveals that they fail to sort according to ready-made categories. There is no strong or consistent divide between Latinate academic learning and vernacular practicality. The cases where ownership can be traced demonstrate that in plenty of cases elite physicians owned simplistic practical texts and manual practitioners possessed elaborately theoretical ones. For instance, a remarkably learned treatise of nearly two hundred pages in Cambridge, Gonville and Caius MS 176/97—which cites from Joannitius's *Isagoge*, Constantine's *Pantegni*, Galen's *Tegni*, the *Canon* of Avicenna, Isaac Israeli, Giles of Corbeil, Rhazes, Hippocrates, Galen's commentary on the *Aphorisms*, and Walter Agilon and which expounds on a technical difference between Galen and Avicenna on the nature of synochal fever—is, according to its preface, addressed "nought to clerkys, but to myn dere gossip [friend] Thomas Plawdon, citiseyn and barbour of London," so that he might "betir entre into the worchynge of fisyk in tyme of lakkyng [scarcity] of wise fysicians."[114] Traditionally, barbers held an unexalted position in the hierarchy of medical practitioners, performing at most bloodletting and minor surgeries, but the preface assumes that with the treatise's help, Plawdon could perform "the worchynge of fisyk."

Conversely, a medical manuscript known to belong to the elite physician John Argentine (d. 1508) contains "unsophisticated calendrical, uroscopy, bloodletting, and remedy material in the vernacular."[115] Argentine was among the most eminent physicians of fifteenth-century England, having studied medicine in Italy (probably at the medical school in Ferrara), practiced at the English court from 1478 onward, and become provost of King's College, Cambridge in 1501.[116] In his own medical commonplace book, Argentine cites the craft-trained English surgeon John Arderne more than any other medical authority and seems to give equal credence to *experimenta*, or the empirical cures he comes across in the course of his practice, and the prescriptions of written authorities.[117] In England, as these examples suggest, there was no automatic correlation between a reader's social status and the degree of intellectual sophistication in the medical texts he or she owned. This variability points to the remarkably dynamic and heterogeneous nature of medical literacy in England.

Medical writings affected not only those who read them but also those who experienced the care that was influenced by them. The medical compendium that is now London, British Library, Harley MS 2390 includes a particularly fascinating document mediating between the practioner-reader and his potential patients. Apparently compiled for an itinerant care-giver, the book originally opened with the words of a public proclamation, or banns, advertising services:

> Hoyit, hoyit, yiff there be any man or wymman that is dyshesyd in
> any dyversse seknesses, that is for to sayne, al maner wonddes, hurttes,
> wit hegge tooll, swerd or daghard, here is a man that is a conyng man
> in leche-craftis bothyn in ffysykke & surgere that wylle curyn alle
> manere off seknesses be the grace off god the qwiche ben curabele.[118]

> [Hear ye, hear ye! If there is any man or woman diseased with any
> of these diverse sicknesses, that is to say, all kinds of wounds and
> hurts—with hedge tool, sword, or dagger, here is a man that is a
> knowledgeable man in leechcrafts, both in *phisik* and in surgery,
> who will cure all manner of sicknesses which are curable, by the
> grace of God.][119]

The banns originally occupied the first pages of a compilation of primarily Latin medical texts, including an herbal, two guides to diagnosis from urine, and a collection of medical recipes. After the opening call to attention—*hoyit, hoyit*—the crier's script launches into a list of more than thirty ailments that the doctor could cure—from mormals to migraines, from toothache to flux, deafness to gout, scalding to saucefleme, morphew to mouth-worms, epilepsy to hemorrhoids—in other words, "all maner wounddis and dyshesys [diseases] in any partes of mankende qwyche is possybele for to ben curyd [which are curable] be [by] the grace off god and mannys connynge [expertise]."[120] In the manner of effective advertising, the list both conjures anxieties and offers the possibility of their relief. The disturbing evocation of bodily vulnerability is balanced against the promise of expertise. All these disease names signal simultaneously the teeming plethora of illness and the specialized knowledge of the "connyng man." In case listeners missed the point, the banns run through a second, similar list: constriction of breath, pains at the heart, aposteme, bladder, stomach, phlegm, costiveness, gas, spleen, swelling, stopping of the kidneys. The paratextual apparatus of the book has a peculiarly immediate relationship with the banns' vernacular orality. As Voigts has demonstrated, the banns' catalogue of ailments corresponds almost exactly to the list of rubrics heading the manuscript's Latin *receptarium*. The table of contents, it seems, is the source for the startling litany of ailments. Here, a Latinate finding aid is thus turned outward, reaching past the boundaries of the manuscript to address a broader audience, "any man or wymman that is dyshesyd." Broadcast into the town's public soundscape, the list of disease names seeks to draw members of the community into contact with the healing knowledge of the book and its user.

What the leech actually offers, according to the banns, are not surgical procedures or prepared medicines. Rather, for a penny a patient can have his or her "water," or urine, evaluated—"and he xall demyn thoo watteres & tellyn hem of thoo evellys in any man or womanis body & qwatte maledy soo evere it be [and he shall judge those waters and tell them about those harms in any man's or woman's body and whatever disease it is]." For another penny, the doctor will "wryttyn hem here medycynes in a bylle [write them their medicines in a document]."[121] The medical practitioner traffics in words—the spoken words of diagnostic consultation and the written words of remedies. The banns show how the language of medical learning might have entered the lives of individuals in the fifteenth century, even those who did not own or read books. If they paid their two pennies, they would have come away with new information about what was going on inside their bodies, information framed in the terms of "leechcraftis." They would also possess a "bylle" inscribed with a remedy aimed at improving their health by "the grace off god and mannys connynge." Or, if passersby chose not to consult the visiting doctor, then one imagines they continued onward with a litany of infirmities ringing in their ears.

This section has thus far focused on coherently medical manuscripts from late medieval England. Less commonly, however, medical works might appear in the same manuscripts as works of devotion or entertainment. One well-known example is Lincoln, Lincoln Cathedral MS 91, written by the Yorkshire landowner Robert Thornton, which includes three large thematic sections, dedicated respectively to romances, to moral and devotional materials, and to medical and pharmaceutical knowledge.[122] Another similar manuscript, which echoes Thornton's in its deliberate planning and in its codicological divisions by genre, has been reconstructed by Kathleen L. Scott; I refer to it here as the "Rawlinson-Sloane" manuscript.[123] It was originally divided into five sections: a didactic and moralistic part; a historical part; a sequence of narrative and literary works; a sequence of "functional and informative" texts, first on hunting and hawking and then on medicine; and finally a religious text, the confessional guide *Manuale curatorum*.[124] It was probably assembled for a family of the provincial gentry.[125]

The medical portion of the Rawlinson-Sloane manuscript is exceptional in its searching attitude toward the status of medical knowledge itself. George Keiser has drawn attention to the uniquely moralistic bent of the plague treatise attributed to "Master Thomas Multon," which alone among Middle English plague texts begins by designating "plague as divine retribution for sin."[126] That text's unusual mingling of religious and medical explanations has a parallel in the manuscript's dialogue on surgery. The dialogue, unfolding between two "brothers," is an engaging device added by the translator to frame the contents Roger of Parma's *Practica Chirurgica*. However, the dialogue's opening departs from the surgical source-text to pose unusual questions about the place of medicine in a divinely controlled world. One "brother" queries the other:

> Brother, seth thou sayst that God sendeth men syknes and helth
> hem aftirward when Hym liketh, wherto shuld eny man studien in
> lechecraft syth God, yf Hym liketh, may hele a man wythout leches,
> and yf He wil that a man be nat heled, travayle of leches nys but in
> vayne?[127]

[Brother, since you say that God sends men sickness and heals
them afterward when it please him, why should any man study
medicine?—since God, if he likes, may heal a man without doctors,
and if He wishes that a man *not* be healed, the work of doctors is
but in vain?]

The speaker wants to know—in light of God's omnipotence, how one to
understand the utility of *phisik*? More broadly, how does one resolve the different versions of causation offered by medicine and religion? The other brother
answers quite conventionally by explaining that God imbues his "vertu in
word, in ston, and in grasse and bestis, for profite of mankynd" and "men
shuld studien in lechecrafft" to help their "bretheren."[128] Nonetheless, the
question asked explicitly by the first brother continues to be posed tacitly by
the very shape of the Rawlinson-Sloane manuscript. Its wide-ranging contents would have required readers to decide when and how to use its differing
generic sections. Do romance, religion, and medicine have anything to say to
one another? Their material unity in the manuscript suggests that they do, and
the nature of that relationship would have been negotiated in the book's use.

A final example illustrates the textual dynamism of *phisik* in late medieval
England. John Lydgate's poem the "Dietary" is a close translation of an anonymous Latin *Dietarium*.[129] Evidently, the "Dietary" was remarkably appealing
to late medieval and early modern readers. It survives in fifty-nine manuscripts
and is Lydgate's most widely attested composition—"topping everything in
popularity," as A. S. G. Edwards comments.[130] As I have argued elsewhere, the
"Dietary" was copied and read as part of at least three distinctive categories of
Middle English writing.[131] Two are familiarly Lydgatian: it was treated as a work
of literary art, frequently found in poetic anthologies centered on Lydgate's
and Chaucer's verse, and it also circulated as a piece of moralistic didacticism, for instance accompanying Benedict Burgh's rendering of the Distichs
of Cato. The third tradition of the poem's circulation is within medical compilations. At least eleven witnesses of the "Dietary" appear within medical and
scientific manuscripts, in the company, variously, of Latin, Anglo-Norman,
and English medical works, in verse and in prose. Neighboring texts include
recipes, charms, phlebotomies, uroscopies, prognostication aids, astrological
charts, alchemical instructions, herbals, a treatise on the virtues of rosemary, a
lapidary, plague tracts, mnemonics for the four humors, and a Middle English
poem on embryology.

In its own contents, Lydgate's poem itself cannily capitalizes on medicine's wavering between a specialized, technical discourse and a more general model of moral didacticism and poetic wisdom. The first stanza provides a kind of physiological "hook," seeming to establish the poem on straightforwardly medical grounds:

> For helth of body cover fro cold thi hede.
> Ete non raw mete—take gode hede therto—
> Drynke holsom drynke, fede thee on lyght brede,
> And with apytyte ryse fro thi mete also.[132]

> [For bodily health, cover your head from cold. Eat no raw meat—
> take heed of that; drink wholesome drink, feed yourself on light
> bread, and with appetite remaining rise from your food.]

The "Dietary" invites its audience into the poem for the sake of "helth of body," and the reader embarks amid the typical precepts of medical regimens. Of course, the personalized regimens that physicians would provide to noble clients were tailored to each patient's particular humoral disposition and way of life. Lydgate's poem, by contrast, transmits advice so general as to be applicable to everyone. The "Dietary" even eliminates the broad distinctions found in closely related works like the *Regimen sanitatis Salernitanum*, which differentiates advice for sanguine, choleric, phlegmatic, and melancholic types. This abandonment of physiological nuance facilitates the poem's blithe weaving between medical and moral advice:

> If so be that lechys do thee fayll,
> Make this thi governans if that it may be:
> Temperat dyet and temperate traveyle,
> Not malas for non adversyté,
> Meke in trubull, glad in poverté,
> Riche with lytell, content with suffyciens,
> Mery withouten grugyng to thy degré.
> If fysyke lake, make this thy governans.[133]

> [If doctors fail you, make this your rule if you can: temperate diet
> and work, no resentment for adversity, meek in trouble, glad in

poverty, rich with little, content with the necessities, merry in your rank without complaining. If *phisik* is lacking, make this your rule.]

The remaining eight stanzas continue the pattern, weaving between physiological advice and ethical and spiritual precepts. This generic flexibility, which apparently helped make Lydgate's "Dietary" so popular, is internal to the poem's meaning: its theme is the inextricability of *phisik* and ethics, body and soul, and medicine and broader practices of self-governance.

The books that spoke of English *phisik* in the later fourteenth and fifteenth centuries were diverse, but as an aggregate they materialized a new sense of what medical codices could encompass and how they could be designed and used. Books of practical science, including *phisik*, became a prevalent genre that appealed to a broad spectrum of readers and affected an even wider number of medieval men and women. The banns in Harley 2390 show the technical vocabulary of medicine put to use as aural advertising in late medieval towns. The surgical dialogue in the Rawlinson-Sloane manuscript dramatizes medicine's subordination to theological rubrics. From the redefinition of Hippocratic medicine as "noght elles bot [but] abstynens, and conquest of foule covetus lustes" to the contents of Lydgate's most popular poem, writers showed themselves interested in integrating the newly prominent discourse of medicine into other models of self-governance. We should also be alert to the corporeal benefits of literary pleasure, or what Glending Olson has called the "hygienic justification" of narrative and poetic delight.[134] John Arderne, after all, recommends that a "leche" should "talke of gode tales and of honest that may make the pacientes to laugh."[135] Attending to the aesthetics of information in medical texts, or what Lisa H. Cooper has memorably called the "poetics of practicality," highlights the enjoyment of feeling knowledgeable and of imagining oneself ready to act in the face of the body's intractable materiality.[136]

PART II

Playing with *Phisik*

Chapter 3

Satire and Medical Materialism

"Guk guk, gud day, schir!" begins the rollicking medical satire "Sum Practysis of Medecyne" by the late fifteenth-century Scottish poet Robert Henryson.[1] With these words, the poem's narrator launches the boasting preface to a small collection of medical recipes he claims to have authored, a "sedull" addressed to his rival medical practitioner. "Guk guk" is a Middle Scots onomatopoeia imitating the cry of the cuckoo and, by extension, signifying nonsense.[2] In invoking the cuckoo's voice, Henryson casts the deviant medical language of his composition—its lexicon of *materia medica* and disease, of filth and excretions—under the sign of birdsong. The poem's trill, however, is not that of the lyric nightingale or courtly tercelet but rather that of the bird known for its repetitive, nonsensical call—known, one might say, for its *jargon*.

The etymological roots of jargon lead back to Old French *jargon*, meaning the sound of birds, from the onomatopoeic base *jarg-*, *garg-*, related to *la gargouille*, the throat, and its "gargling." The *jargoilliant* of birds points to "langage en général," or the babble of speech stripped of any particular meaning.[3] Jargon is the material of language, devoid of sense or reference. When words strike a listener or reader as mere jargon, it marks the threshold of a community of knowledge, where insiders are distinguished from outsiders, experts from novices. Words that have precise significance for some are for others so many empty phonemes rattling past. The "guk guk" that commences "Sum Practysis of Medecyne," this chapter contends, refers to the peculiar musicality of medical language turned aside from its healing purpose and flaunting its own poetical energies—a perverse sonorousness that other literary works explore as well. Satire was one of two literary paths that the discourse of medicine traveled on its way into fictional narrative and poetry; the other, exemplary narrative, is discussed in the following chapter. Both satire and exempla provided to medieval thinkers opportunities to play with *phisik* and to turn its concepts, terms, and intellectual operations to literary ends.

What was the learned poet Robert Henryson up to in his nonsensical parody of medical textuality? What would its import have been for the poem's fifteenth-century readers? So copious is the medical learning on display in another of Henryson's works, *The Testament of Cresseid* (the topic of Chapter 6), that scholars have speculated that the poet might also have been a physician.[4] While this remains mere conjecture (at odds with the sixteenth-century tradition that he was a schoolmaster in Dumerfermline[5]), "Sum Practysis of Medecyne" is evidence of his thorough familiarity with the conventions of medical discourse, a familiarity that he would have shared with many contemporary readers. By the second half of the fifteenth century, Scotland as well as England saw the growing textualization of medical learning in Latin, Gaelic, and Scots, and Henryson no doubt would have had passing familiarity with medicine's role in English manuscript culture.[6] The present chapter sets Henryson's "Sum Practysis of Medecyne" within both the corpus of medical satire and the circumstances of late medieval *phisik*'s expanded accessibility. I do the same for Chaucer's "Nun's Priest's Tale," in which the hen Pertelote speaks a particularly unauthoritative version of *phisik*, and for the East Anglian miracle play the *Croxton Play of the Sacrament*, where the role of an itinerant quack doctor has long puzzled interpreters. These works were written in a period when medical discourse functioned as a novel textual laboratory for configuring words, bodies, and substances into new relations.[7] The materiality of the physical body and the materiality of medical language were increasingly bound up together, and medical satire exaggerated and commented on that nexus.

Medieval satire was a literary mode concerned with the exposure and condemnation of vice. It usually assumed a stance of censure in the service of reform, though variations like estates satire were occupied more with generalizing characterization. At one extreme satire verged toward complaint and lament; at the other, toward grotesquerie and comedy.[8] Initially a decidedly clerical undertaking, satire in the later Middle Ages shifted away from its academic and ecclesiastic footing as vernacular poets adopted its disparaging comportment and ironic narration to many situations and purposes.[9] Accordingly, satire operated less as a genre than a literary mode, a stance that texts of many types might assume when it suited their purposes. *Medical* satire takes as its target medicine's failure to live up to its central promise, that the technical manipulation of the body qua physical thing relieves suffering and restores health. The textual tradition of medical invective is a long one, and unpacking its late medieval significance requires tracking the accumulated legacy of its literary associations as well as its points of contact with the contemporary medical milieu.

This chapter argues that running throughout the corpus of medical satire is an obsession with materiality, from bodily substances to language's noise, from the countless stuffs of *materia medica* to physicians' greed. In many cases, satire's materialism works by exaggerating tendencies in actual medical practice and exacerbating those things that made care seem dangerous or difficult. In what follows, I map the sources and contours of medieval ambivalence about *phisik* and then follow the expression of that ambivalence into satire, including the "Nun's Priest's Tale," "Sum Practysis of Medecyne," and the *Croxton Play of the Sacrament*. Medical satire evinces both fascination and furious skepticism toward *phisik*'s vocabulary of materiality. When the physician's techniques falter and remedies fall short, medicine's cannily physicalizing regard—what might be called its *strategic materialism*—becomes the object of critique. In its moments of failure, *phisik* suddenly looks grotesque or dehumanizing, as though allied with the physical limitations it was meant to temper and relieve. At its limit, medical materialism assumes the status of violence, and scientific jargon is that violence's speech. Satire was the occasion to decry but also, and backhandedly, to *relish* medicine's materialist stratagems.

Incomprehensible language has the potential to function, in the words of Daniel Tiffany, "not simply as a failure of meaning, but as a productive phenomenon in its own right." Tiffany's wide-ranging study of "lyric obscurity" makes the case that perplexity is essential to poetry. By "displaying its obscurity" and "making a spectacle of incomprehension," verse precipitates an encounter with the very substance of language.[10] Medical satire can be understood to execute a special version of this lyric task. When medieval men and women turned to medical discourse to learn what to do about the body, they also confronted the obscurities and shortcomings of *phisik*—its jargon, expense, disgust, pain, and proximity to death. Medical satire, in parading *phisik*'s opacity and making a spectacle of its jargon, offers an encounter with medical discourse's "phenomenology of unknowing," to borrow Tiffany's phrase.[11] Medical satire takes as its starting point the convergence of language's inscrutability with experiences of sickness, injury, corruption, and death. It plays these two dimensions of human limitation off of one another in an exercise of poetic invention. If the literate creativity of practical medical writing strove to elucidate the obscure materialities of embodiment and expression, satire set about simultaneously censuring and enjoying them.

Materia Medica and *Materia Poetica*

As medical texts became ever more numerous over the course of the fifteenth century, largely for audiences outside of universities, experiences of medicine's incomprehensibility were also, inevitably, on the rise. The "vernacularization, or laicization, or popularization" of medicine was not a matter of mechanically transferring information to new audiences.[12] It also redistributed the labors of medical reading, shifting them away from university students who followed a set curriculum to the makeshift and variable undertakings of lay medical education. George Keiser, in his detailed study of the remedy book copied by the Yorkshire landowner Robert Thornton (d. c. 1465), remarks that the text is "replete with evidence that Thornton frequently did not understand the medical material he was copying," which was "perhaps because of his unfa-miliarity with the technical language—a common problem in the copying of vernacular medical books in 15th-century England."[13] Like Thornton, most readers and writers fell along a continuum of medical literacy and medical ignorance. John Arderne thinking in English while writing in Latin, Margery Paston penning medical instructions to send along with her poultice, and a customer clutching a penny's worth of scribbled advice from an itinerant doc-tor: these are all encounters with the literate mediation of healing expertise.[14] The increase in the proportion of people who relied on *phisik* to interpret their bodies, imagine causation, and effect cures also entailed an uptick in the effortful work of attempting to turn medical discourse into efficacious action.

Several circumstances worked to make medicine at once especially dif-ficult and especially urgent to comprehend. One factor was medicine's poly-glot vocabulary, stemming from its long history of transmission. Much of the classical medical learning that made its way to the medieval West had been preserved, redacted, and elaborated by physicians and natural philoso-phers writing in Arabic. When Latin translations by Constantine the African, Gerard of Cremona, and others began circulating in western Europe in the twelfth century, they bore the linguistic traces of (at a minimum) Greek and Arabic. Writing in the mid-thirteenth century, the Franciscan intellectual and Englishman Roger Bacon (d. 1294) linked the failures of contemporary physi-cians to their linguistic incompetence: "because they are ignorant of the Greek and Arabic and Hebrew languages from which an infinite number of words in the Latin books are taken, they are not able to understand drugs nor how to make them."[15] Translation into the vernacular added yet another layer of lin-guistic mediation. Relative to other vernacular traditions and to other genres of English writing, the degree of multilingualism in medical writings was exceptional.[16] Even when Middle English alone was used, it was often a clumsy medium for scientific exposition, and translations could occasion plentiful Latin borrowings, awkward grammatical constructions, and other compromises in conveying technical information from one language to another. For the late medieval reader, medical knowledge threatened to coagulate in the very density of its signifying medium.

Even the apparently simplest of medical genres, the therapeutic recipe, demanded dizzyingly broad terminology. A rangy lexicon was required to enumerate recipes' variegated ingredients—their nuanced repertoires of flowers and seeds and minerals and oils and animal parts, which collectively embodied the plenitude of the natural world. "God yeveth [gives] His vertu in word, in ston, and in grasse and bestis, for profite of mankynd," as one medieval surgical text explains, invoking a medieval commonplace.[17] However, patterns of textual circulation meant that words could end up geographically very far from their referents. Remedies originating in the Mediterranean world, for instance, sometimes called for flora and fauna alien to England. For evidence of how seriously readers took the problem of pharmaceutical jargon, one might look to the production of synonymies in Britain, or glossaries that attempted to stabilize the meaning of, most commonly, plant names. Tony Hunt describes sixty-four surviving herbal synonymies produced in England between 1280 and 1500, which were intended to coordinate the various botanical terms in circulation in Latin, French, and Middle English.[18]

The proliferation of terminology into ever-finer capillaries of naming is part of a pursuit of precision, but it simultaneously tends to obscurity. To use a basic concept from information theory, the potential both for "information" and for "noise" grows with the expansion of the lexicon. This is the ironic reversal inherent in the nature of jargon: at some point, technical exactitude bends back around into senselessness, to the cuckoo's *guk guk*. The fact did not escape the notice of those critical of medicine. Pliny the Elder, whose *Naturalis historiae* is perhaps the most influential work of medical invective up through the early modern period, writes, "The Mithridatic antidote is composed of fifty-four ingredients, no two of the same amount. . . . It is plainly a showy parade of the art, and a colossal boast of the science [*ostentatio artis et portentosa scientiae venditatio*]. And not even the physicians know their facts; I have discovered that instead of Indian cinnabar there is commonly added to medicines, through a confusion of names [*inscitia nominis*], red lead."[19] Red lead, Pliny goes on to reveal, is a poison (*venenum*).

A couple of examples from the small corpus of Middle English satirical remedies, or what Denton Fox has deemed "medical burlesques," likewise foreground what Pliny calls *inscitia nominis*, ignorance or confusion of
names. "A good medesyn yff a mayd have lost her madenhed [virginity]" calls
for "the kreke [cluck] of a henne" and "the neygynge [neighing] of a mere
[mare]."[20] Such fancifully sonic ingredients stage the disjunction between
naming a thing and actually possessing it, between sound and substance. In
a miscellany produced around 1470 in the West Midlands, the manuscript's
compiler (who also copied the majority of its remedies) composed an original
piece of medical satire, in which a leech bids his patient "to gaydere an erbe he
wyst never where and make a plaster he wyste note whereof and he schuld be
hoole he woste never when upponn warranttys [to gather an herb, he did not
know where, and make a plaster, he did not know of what, and (the patient)
should be well, he did not know when—guaranteed!]."[21] The faux prescription
implies the ultimate interchangeability of all the *materia medica* that remedies
ordinarily take pains to distinguish: herbs from wherever, mixed with whatever, administered however. Part of the barb and pique of medical satire, then,
derives from the violence of its language against reference. It turns emphatically away from the outside world and instead toward the literary occasion of
the words' own enunciation. What referentiality could be more urgent than
that of the suffering body? Yet in these mock recipes, literary momentum is
found in riding roughshod over logic and discarding meaningful relationships
between words, bodies, and things.

Over the course of the Middle Ages, then, writers took up *materia medica*
not only as a problem of practical reference but also as a poetic resource. The
French genre of *herberies*, or parodies of healers' self-promotion, is one aspect
of this satirical tradition.[22] The *Dit de l'Herberie* by Rutebeuf (d. c. 1285) is the
most well-known example. In it, an itinerant doctor (*mires* in Old French)
offers herbs, precious stones, and remarkable elixirs from around the world:
"I'm bringing you carbuncles and 'garcelar' stones, which are entirely blue-
violet, along with herbs from the Indian deserts and the isle of Ceylon [*Car-
bonculus et garcelars / Qui sunt tuit ynde, / Herbes aport des dezers d'Ynde / Et de
la terre Lincorinde*]."[23] He boasts, "In Apulia, in Calabria, and over at Palermo,
I've collected herbs that are rich in great virtue. No matter what illness you
use them for, the illness runs away and takes cover [*En Puille, en Calabre, en
Palerne, / Ai herbes prises / Qui de granz vertuz sunt emprises: / Sus quelque mal
qu'el soient mises, / Li maux c'en fuit*]" (21–25). The speaker's inventory includes

both conventional treasures and what one translator calls "a little esoteric dust in the eyes," in the form of otherwise unattested words.[24] The wandering doctor's speech is an opportunity for wild poetic invention, for rhyming obscure materials and distant place-names in lines that strain comprehensibility. The promise of these multiplicitous materials is health, portrayed alternately in fantastical terms—"stones that bring the dead back to life [*pierres . . . Qui font resusciteir le mort*]" (32–33)—and in earthy ones: "If your rump vein gets throbbing, I'll cure that item too [*Ce la vainne dou cul vos bat, / Ie vos en garrai sanz debat*]" (71–72). The *herberie* promises that the far-flung wonders of the globe will overcome the body's indignities. Its brazen irony is that the opposite is likely the case, at least for this speaker's wares—and all the curlicues of the doctor's pharmaceutical rhetorical are probably no match for kidney stones or a toothache.

Closely related to *herberies* are the scenes in French and German religious plays of an apothecary advertising his wares. As early as the eleventh century, the liturgical dramatization of the three Marys on their way to Jesus' sepulcher gave rise to the character of the *mercator* or *ungeuntarius*, a merchant of spices and medicaments; he is the first nonbiblical character to appear in such dramatic works.[25] By the fourteenth century, vernacular versions of this scene had taken on a special vitality. The *espicier* in the *Passion du Palatinus*, for instance, delivers a boastful forty-three-line monologue hawking his goods.[26] The *apothicarius* in the passion play of Sainte-Geneviève runs through an even longer catalogue of merchandise, organized around the anaphora *J'ay* (I have):

> J'ay poivre, gingenbre et canelle,
> Poudre de saffran bien nouvelle,
> Nois muguettes, pomes garnates,
> Giroffle, citonal et dates,
> Garingal, folion, pénites,
> Cubèbes, rasis, nois confytes;
> J'ay gingenbrant et pignolat,
> J'ay trop bon sucre violat,
> J'ay grosse et grêle dragie
> De girouffle et d'anis glagie,
> Poivre lonc, commin, reguelice,
> Amendes, ris et verdegrice.[27]

[I have pepper, ginger and cinnamon, fresh saffron powder, nutmeg
seeds, pomegranates, clove, white turmeric and dates, galangal,
Indian leaf, barley sugar, pepper berries, white lead, candied nuts.
I have candied ginger paste and pine nuts; I have exquisite violet-
tinctured sugar; I have heavy and light sweets made from clove buds
and anise powder, long pepper, cumin, licorice, almonds, rice, and
verdigris.]

There seems to be no reason why his listing should ever stop. When it finally
does, his words have suggested both the endless variety of material things and
the endless profusion of their names. The enumeration of spices evokes the
vast sensual world even as the words come unstuck from that world, propelled
by their own prosodic materiality. *Mercator* speeches are also defined by their
basic structural irrelevance in the context of the biblical narrative. Being bound
by the Gospel record, the Marys will purchase only myrrh and aloe, and even
these, of course, will not anoint the corpse for which they are intended. The
apothecaries' monologues, then, are a kind of festive, worldly dross. They revel
in the sensory pleasures of words and in the pungent, expensive substances to
which those words refer—but their delights are gently ironized by the larger
salvation plot in which they feature.

Patient Readers

Another circumstance that helped tinge medicine with dubiousness in the later
Middle Ages was its context of bodily distress. Then as today, medical care was
most urgent in situations of somatic breakdown. Medieval medical science, as
a rule, addressed sickness and injury by regarding the patient (at least temporarily) as a material thing, susceptible to the influence of physical processes and
substances. *Phisik* bracketed other frameworks for understanding the human
in order to explain and implement techniques like purgation, pharmaceutical preparation and application, surgical procedures, and the manipulation of
regimen. While medicine's provisional reification of the person grounded its
claims for practical efficacy, it was also at the root of its unsavory associations.
It was one reason that medical satire was so rude about doctors, associating
them with the brute materiality it was their task to overcome.

Jill Mann's tour through physicians' satirical depictions turns up several
common themes. The satirical archetype is a bad healer, even dangerous; he

colludes with apothecaries, and his greed means that he is glad to hear of sickness; his authority depends largely on empty rhetoric; and he leans toward atheism.[28] To this list based on Mann's observations can be added physicians' perennial association with bodily excretions—paradigmatically urine but also waste in general, drawn off in purgative procedures or otherwise secreted by the sick—and with worthless medicaments, prescribed for profit and for bluster. Together these satirical themes add up to a materialist economy of bad *phisik*, which appears when physicians trade on vulnerable bodies for gold, as payment "wan in pestilence"[29]; when they parrot the lingo of medical science, degrading it to empty chatter; when they reduce their patients to excretory metonymies, jordans of urine held up to the light; and when they prescribe expensive amalgams of who-knows-what. Gold, excrement, jargon, and material stuffs circulate in deleterious exchange.

This materialist economy could look downright murderous. Pliny remarks, "Only a physician can commit homicide with complete impunity [*medicoque tantum hominem occidisse inpunitas summa est*]."[30] Petrarch (d. 1374) writes vitriolically to the physicians attending Pope Clement VI that "in your work, you often use dangerous hocus-pocus to prescribe the death of your wretched patients [*periculosis ambagibus dictare soles miserorum mortes*]."[31] The association of physicians with violence takes on spectacular form in Chrétien de Troyes's *Cligès*, dated to 1176. The main plot of the romance concerns the love between Cligès and his uncle's wife, Fenice. Fenice hatches a plan to fake her own death and escape her marriage with the help an ointment that makes her appear dead. As Fenice is lying in her coffin and the whole kingdom mourns her, "three wizened doctors arrived from Salerno [*Sont venu .iii. fisicien / De Salerne molt ancien*]."[32] By the late twelfth century, Salerno had become shorthand for expertise in diagnosis, prognosis, and cure. Physicians from Salerno began popping up in romances, *lais*, *dits*, and satires.[33] Hearing that Fenice refused medical care prior to her death, the Salernitans grow suspicious. Their leader, "the most learned doctor [*qui plus saveit*]," covertly palpates her as she lies in her coffin and apprehends that she is alive.[34] The visiting physicians then promise they can restore the queen to life and so are left alone with her to exercise their art. At this point, suspecting that Fenice is pretending death, they attempt to revive her with treatments that devolve quickly into torture. They "pulled her out of the coffin and began to beat her [*Lors la getent fors de la biere, / Si la fierent et si la batent*]."[35] When this fails, they beat her with whips and finally pour molten lead in the palms of her unmoving hands and threaten to "set her entire body on a grill until she was well roasted [*Ja endroit la metront en rost / Tant qu'ele iert tote greïllie*]."[36] The story parrots the torments of the martyrs, with Salernitan physicians in the place of the pagan emperor and Fenice, a servant of love, playing the virgin saint.

One thing that might be observed of these satirical portrayals is that they concentrate medical authority in a professional figure, usually that of the physician but occasionally a surgeon or apothecary. They expose the contingency and fallibility of the physician's authority, but they do so by focusing on his expertise as a distinctive vocation. Readers are called to be in sympathy with patients, even as they are allowed to stand shrewdly beyond the practitioner's predations. But this sharp demarcation of roles does not address the plural and diffuse forms of medical expertise that characterized much of the later Middle Ages. In fact, the wildly varying expertise of medical readers was another factor contributing to medicine's equivocal status. Most British practitioners were not university trained, and many practiced only on occasion, amid other vocations and roles. Yet this heterogeneous aggregate of readers became the engine of *phisik*'s large-scale textualization. The simultaneously pedagogical and practical role that medical writings played—transforming readers' understanding while also directing their action—placed enormous stress on these texts' intelligibility.

Medical works often remark on their own role in making care possible. The Dominican Friar "Master Thomas Multon" explains that he was moved to "gader [gather]" his "trety" on the plague "and sette it in Englissh" in the hopes that "every man, bothe lerned and lewde [uneducated]," might "the better understand hit, and do [act] thereafter, and to be his owne phisicien in tyme of nede ayenst the venym and the malice of the pestilence."[37] Here Multon extends even to the unlearned the chance to act as rational healers. Similarly, the authorial persona in an Englished gynecological treatise explains the treatise's usefulness in terms of helping women avoid untrustworthy male practitioners: "And therfore, in helping of women I wyl wright of women prevy sekenes the helping, and that oon woman may helpe another in her sykenesse & nought diskuren her previtees to suche uncurteys men [And therefore, to help women, I will write about the care of women's private illnesses, so that one woman may help another in her illness and not reveal her secrets (or, secret parts) to such discourteous men]."[38] The preface conjectures that women, with the aid of the translated text, will be able to help one another and eschew suspect masculine authorities. While the preface's statement needs to be contextualized within the history of masculine, clerical titillation at women's secrets, it also illustrates the idea that vernacular medical texts could transform their readers into care-givers.[39]

John Lydgate's most popular poem, the "Dietary," announces its utility in similar terms. "If so be that lechys do thee fayll, / Make this thi governans," it announces, and, again, "If fysyke lake [fails or is absent], make this thy governans."[40] Emphasizing its skeptical distance from esoteric jargon, the poem concludes, "Thys resate is of no potykary, / Of mayster Antony ne of master Hew; / To all deserent it is Dyatary [This recipe is from no apothecary, not from Master Anthony nor Master Hugh. To all who desire it, it serves as regimen]."[41] Named "masters" and apothecaries are dismissed, and the text takes its authority instead from its readers, who are *deserent* (desirous) of instruction. As Jake Walsh Morrissey observes, the closest analogues of Lydgate's "Dietary" are works of proverbial wisdom, like the *Distichs* of Cato or Lydgate's own "Mesure Is Tresour," rather than the sophisticated regimens of contemporary physicians.[42] The "Dietary" draws on what Faye Getz has called the "encyclopedic medical tradition," which harkens back to Pliny the Elder's *Historia naturalis* and other Roman writings that treat medicine as part of a general knowledge of estates management and self-care.[43] This tradition expresses unrelenting skepticism about what it portrays as the intellectualist excesses of Galenic medicine, even as it circulates alongside works from the Greek tradition—much like Lydgate's verses, despite their proud eschewing of university masters, travel in compendia of learned medicine.[44] Pliny's simple remedies and Lydgate's advice act as medical learning that skewers learned pretensions. They suggest there is no clear line between medical satire and medical textuality.

One feature notably shared by the "Dietary," Multon's preface, and that of the gynecological treatise is that they reinscribe the power differential between doctor and patient into the *self*-relation of the literate audience. The imbalances that typically define the roles of physician and patient are made to lose their stability; perhaps, with the help of the text, the sick can provide their own care. The medical reader being addressed has an identity suspended *between* patient and practitioner, sufferer and authority. The audience's position is dynamic: they have the potential to become care-givers themselves. But such attempted leaps of competence bring with them the chance of their failure. Another brief medical satire, found in the Vernon Manuscript (Bodleian Eng. poet. e. 1), consists in a false recipe titled in a manner indistinguishable from "straight" remedies—"A good medycyn for sor eyen."[45] This prescription "for a man that is almost blynd" lays out a dubious course of treatment, like

At evyn wrap hym in a cloke,
and put hym in a hows full of smoke
And loke that every hol be well shett.
And whan hys eyen begyne to rope,
Fyll hem full of brymston and sope.[46]

[At evening, wrap him in a cloak and put him in a house full of
smoke and check that every hole is well shut, and when his eyes
begin to weep, fill them with brimstone and soap.]

Who is the joke on, exactly? Certainly on the blind person, who is hypothet-
ically to be subjected to such treatments. However, the reader also wobbles
in and out of the satire's crosshairs. Satire's community of readers "in" on the
joke is formed against the naïve users of recipes, precisely those who might
earnestly copy "a good medycyn for sor eyen" onto a manuscript flyleaf. The
imperative mood characteristic of recipes casts the reader in the role of healer.
However, in this burlesque, the reader is conscripted to be either an unwitting
dupe or a menacing joker who is allied with the parodic instruction.

In Chaucer's "Nun's Priest's Tale," the hen Pertelote shows herself to be
an aspiring but unsteady medical authority. When the rooster Chauntecleer
awakens frightened from a dream, Pertelote seizes on the terminology of digestion and humors to dismiss the dream's prophetic significance. She claims it
has a purely physiological explanation:

Swevenes engendren of replecciouns,
And ofte of fume and of complecciouns,
Whan humours been to habundant in a wight.
Certes this dreem, which ye han met to-nyght,
Cometh of the greete superfluytee
Of youre rede colera, pardee,
Which causeth folk to dreden in hir dremes
Of arwes, and of fyr with rede lemes,
Of rede beestes, that they wol hem byte.[47]

[Dreams are engendered by excess and often by vapors and by
people's complexions, when humors are too abundant in a creature.
Truly this dream that you have dreamed comes from an excess
of your red choler, which causes people in their dreams to fear

arrows and fire with red flames and red beasts that would bite
them.]

Pertelote's is thuddingly materialist dream interpretation, in which the color
of the dream image indicates the humoral etiology. Chauntecleer's nightmare
is made a symptom, a bodily disturbance inciting interpretation. As the avian
couple debate its causes and significance, they bring a plethora of arguments
and authorities to bear on it, in a charmingly absurd episode of etiological
imagination.

In her spouting of medical terminology, Pertelote is a trebly undercut
mouthpiece. She is a chicken spouting human learning, a woman teaching
a man, and an English-speaker trying to master Latinate medical vocabulary.
The second and third points are knit together by Chauntecleer's joke at her
expense: "*Mulier est hominis confusio*— / Madame, the sentence of this Latyn
is, / 'Womman is mannes joye and al his blis'" (3164–66). Together with the fact
that Chauntecleer's dream *does* turn out to be prophetic, these factors ironize
the medical expertise Pertelote offers, associating it with a clumsy materialism
that is expressed as much in her feminine person as in her etiological ideas.
The satire seems to turn upon questions of reading. Curiosity about the kind
and degree of Pertelote's literacy is raised by her use of learned vocabulary and
citation of authorities, by Chauntecleer's Latinate trick at her expense, and
by the rooster's references to his own reading practice (3064, 3110) and wish
that she "hadde rad [this] legende, as have I" (3121). The world of the story is
apparently one where chickens peruse books, albeit roosters more than hens.
The "Nun's Priest's Tale" is marvelously alive to the pleasures of mismanaged
idiolect, and Pertelote's combination of dodgy literacy and materialist medical
advice echoes (in a satirical key) many of the issues raised by the vernacular
medical texts discussed above.

Like Lydgate's "Dietary," Pertelote dismisses the need for professionals: "I
conseille yow the beste," she says, "Though in this toun is noon apothecarie,
/ I shal myself to herbes techen yow" (2945, 2948–49). Her subsequent advice
combines some of the jargony pleasures of a *mercator* speech with homespun
provincialism. It is "in oure yeerd" (2951) that she promises the proper herbs
can be found, for a "laxatyf" that will purge Chauntecleer "bothe of colere and
of malencolye" (2943, 2946). She advises:

Ye been ful coleryk of compleccioun;
Ware the sonne in his ascencioun

Ne fynde yow nat repleet of humours hoote.
And if it do, I dar wel leye a grote,
That ye shul have a fevere terciane,
Or an agu that may be youre bane.
A day or two ye shul have digestyves
Of wormes, er ye take youre laxatyves
Of lawriol, centaure, and fumetere,
Or elles of ellebor, that groweth there,
Of katapuce, or of gaitrys beryis,
Of herbe yve, growyng in oure yeerd, ther mery is;
Pekke hem up right as they growe and ete hem yn. (2955–67)

[You are very choleric in your complexion. Beware that the sun
high in the sky does not find you full of hot humors, for if it does,
I would bet, you will have a tertian fever, or an acute fever that
may be your killer. For a day or two you shall have a digestive aid
of worms before you take your laxatives of spurge laurel, centaury,
and fumitory, or else hellebore, which grows there, of caper spurge
or dogwood berries, of ground ivy growing in our yard, which is
pleasant. Peck them up just as they grow and eat them down.][48]

The barnyard comedy of the lines does not allow us to forget that these are
chickens: Chauntecleer should eat a few worms before "pecking up" his *materia medica*. Despite her animal nature, Pertelote moves freely through the
operations of diagnosis, prognosis, and remedy, taking into account factors
that range from her lover's complexion to the sun's position in the heavens.
Some scholars have argued that Pertelote's prescription would have been toxic
had Chauntecleer followed it, but what is perhaps more to the point is that
her interpretation of the symptomatic dream is dangerously wrong and leads
straight to the fox's jaws.[49] While readers are meant to laugh at hen and cock
both, it is clear that she is more wrong than he. The "Nun's Priest's Tale" is
medical burlesque, but not in the vein of estates satire. Instead, Pertelote's
markedly technical lexicon of etiology and *materia medica* marks her as speaking a discourse she does not command. Feminine pretensions to vernacular
medical authority yield a materialism that is both dangerous and comic. Here
as elsewhere, satire is the opportunity to play with, and enjoy, *phisik*'s failures
of explanatory and curative power. Language is shown giving over to obscurity, and medical discourse flaunts its opaque materials.

"Sum Practysis" of Medical Satire

Readers coming upon the only surviving manuscript witness of Robert Henryson's "Sum Practysis of Medecyne" confront a set of crisscrossing generic cues.[50] The carefully constructed Bannatyne Manuscript—compiled in 1568, probably for printing and circulation among the "mercantile and legal classes of Edinburgh who shared a conservative taste for a variety of medieval literary forms"[51]—situates "Sum Practysis of Medecyne" squarely in an assortment of "ballettis mirry [merry ballads]," including satires, poems of insult, and other comic pieces. Yet the mise-en-page of Henryson's poem asserts a different discursive identity (Figure 3). The four remedies that make up the bulk of the poem conform to a manuscript layout typical of medical recipes, with a separate heading for each cure. Each rubric begins with the Greek root *dia-* ("Dia culcakit," "Dia longum," "Dia glaconicon," and "Dia custrum"), meaning "made of" or "consisting in," often used for medical compounds in medieval Latin.[52]

The diction of the remedies is also recipe-standard. Action is cast in the simple imperative verbs well-worn from *receptaria*: "*cape* [take]," "put," "*recipe* [take]," and "myng [mix]." Linguistic ingenuity is concentrated instead in the stock of nouns, naming a repertoire of *materia medica* like wine dregs, sorrel, sage, laurel, linseed, pitch, and mustard. The recipes even conclude in standard fashion, with efficacy phrases, or certifications of their usefulness: "Is nocht bettir I wis, / For the collik [There is nothing better I know for colic]" and "Is nocht bettir be God, / To latt yow to sleip [There is nothing better, by God, to allow you to sleep]."[53] At a glance, then, the poem's claim to convey practical information possesses a certain plausibility. Remedy collections were among the most popular genres of *any* kind of writing in the fifteenth century, and small sets of recipes found their way into odd spots in manuscripts of all kinds. The Bannatyne Manuscript elsewhere includes some perfectly serious "preceptis of medecyne" as well as Lydgate's "Dietary" (fols. 72–74).

The first words of the composition are the "guk guk" of the cuckoo. Yet no sooner has the narrator trilled this note of nonsense than he begins to justify his act of medical writing as a countermeasure against claptrap: "Your saying I haif sene and on syd set it, / As geir of all gaddering, glaikit nocht gude [I have seen your advice and set it aside, as a compilation of nonsense, foolish, not good]" (5–6). The authorial persona, boasting of his own curative powers, claims to send the remedies that follow "Becaus I ken your cunnyng in to cure / Is clowtit and clampit and nocht weill cleird [because I know your

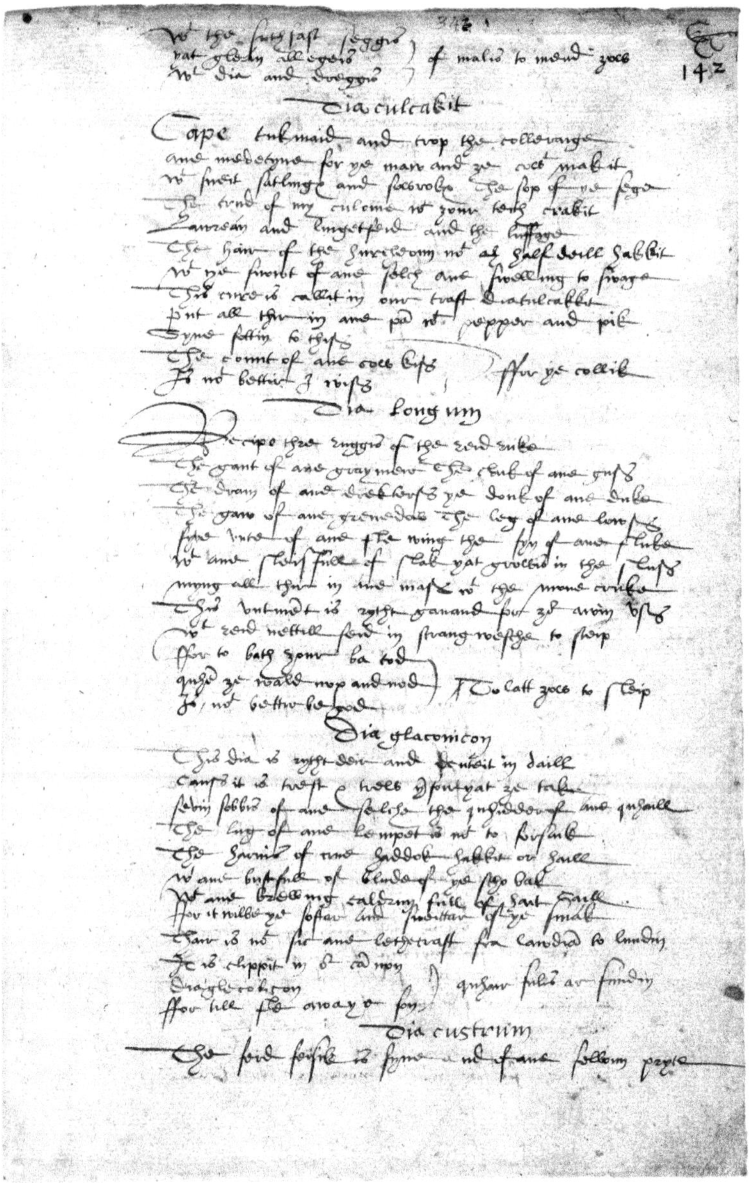

Figure 3. Robert Henryson's "Sum Practysis of Medecyne." Advocates'
MS 1.1.6 (Bannatyne Manuscript), fol. 142. Scottish, 1568. Reproduced
by permission of the National Library of Scotland.

skill in curing is patched and botched and not well enlightened]" (14–15). The writer's opening gambit, then, seems aimed at drawing a distinction *within* medical writing, between his own efficacious prescriptions and the "lawitnes [ignorance]" of the *you* whom he addresses (17). The condemnation of others' foolish or deceptive language was a commonplace of medieval medical texts, especially of those meant to make medical expertise more accessible. For instance, in the preface to his Middle English translation of the *Liber uricrisiarum*, Henry Daniel contrasts his own charitable uses of medicine with the "pompouse lif or bostful, ful of wordes, ful of fables and ful of lesinnges [lies], as leches [doctors] that bene now ar wonte [accustomed] to done."[54] Toward the end of the fourteenth century, the London priest John Mirfield justifies his compilation of a Latin medical encyclopedia for the "poor followers of Christ" by impugning "the fraudulent practices of modern physicians" (*varias fraudes modernorum medicorum*).[55] Invective was internal to the project of transmitting medical knowledge. Initially, then, "Sum Practysis of Medecyne" acknowledges medicine's propensity for jargon and confusion only the better to guard against them.

Soon enough, however, these familiar features of medical textuality are shown to be parodic simulacra. It is not just his rival in *phisik* but the author himself who lacks control over his *glaikit* (idiotic) language. The recipe for "Dia custrum [Cough medicine]," for example, calls for "thre sponfull of the blak spyce, / With ane grit gowpene of the gowk fart, / The lug of ane lyoun, the gufe of ane gryce [three spoonfuls of black spice, / With a great double-handful of cuckoo fart, / The ear of a lion, the grunt of a piglet]"—all to be administered along with "nurice doung for it is rycht nyce, / Myngit with mysdirt and with mustart [nurse dung, for it is quite exquisite, / Mixed with mouse droppings and with mustard]" (68–73). In the line's jangling musicality, consonance and rhyme are foregrounded as the selection criteria for the recipe's ingredients. These sonic qualities in turn are echoed in the imagery of meaningless noise, a pig's grunting and a cuckoo's fart. These empty sounds mix with mouse droppings and a woman's excrement, a combination in which bodily waste comes to constitute an analogue for the matter of language, stripped of meaning. When medical language loses its sense, the implicit analogy runs, it becomes empty sound, farts and grunting and nonsense—just as when *materia medica* loses the specificity that makes it salubrious, it becomes base *materia*.

The poem's first recipe is for "Dia culcakit," which Denton Fox glosses as "befouled-buttock drug." Its first line instructs, "*Cape* cuk maid, and crop the colleraige [Take excreted crap, and harvest water-pepper]" (27). *Colleraige*, or water-pepper, is a plant with irritant medical properties, and its French etymology (*cul* + *rage*) corresponds to its alternative English name, "arse-smart."[56] Henryson taps into the painful potential embedded in the very constitution of the word, etymology proving an irritant as much as the referent. "Cuk maid," or (as Fox translates it) "defecating done," is the only ingredient to precede water-pepper, making excrement the poem's first and, as it turns out, most essential substance. The motif of bodily waste functions to thematize one of the underlying principles of medical burlesque. In the grip of satire, the language of medical expertise dissolves simultaneously into the materiality of *verba* and the materiality of *res*, its substance becoming indistinguishable from song and from excrement.

"Sum Practysis of Medecyne" thus deploys the forms of practical instruction to undo them. It sets up an antagonism between its two organizing forms, the recipe on the one hand and the thirteen-line alliterative stanza with wheel on the other, a stanzaic form associated with flyting, or the poetic exchange of insults.[57] It is flyting's ludic, aggressive inventiveness that governs "Sum Practysis"—a manic poesis that takes as its occasion the wrenching of recipe conventions to new purposes. Of course it is not inevitable that the practical and the poetic should be set at odds with one another. Medical works were sometimes versified for mnemonic reasons or to give organization and interest.[58] As the prologue of the poetical "Manuale de Physica et Chirurgica" explains, the text was written "in metir . . . rather than in prose / That it be lustiere to lere & lightere to kunne [so that it would be more pleasant to learn and easier to understand]."[59] "Sum Practysis of Medecyne," however, sets *lust* and *lore*, verse and information, in conflict. Throughout the poem, the phonetic composition of words takes precedence over the logic of denotation. Poetry emerges from medical rationality's destruction. "Dia longum" (Long prescription) begins:

> *Recipe* thre reggis of the reid ruke,
> The gant of ane gray meir, the claik of ane gus,
> The dram of ane drekters, the douk of ane duke,
> The gaw of ane grene dow, the leg of ane lows,
> Fyve unce of ane fle wing, the fyn of ane fluke,
> With ane sleiffull of slak that growis in the slus;
> Myng all thir in ane mas with the mone cruke. (40–46)

[Take three pulls of the red rook, the yawn of a gray mare, the cluck of a goose, the penis of a drake, and the dive of a duck, the bile of a green dove, the leg of a louse, five ounces of a fly's wing, the fin of a flounder, with a sleeve-full of algae that grows in the sluice. Mix all these in a mass with the crescent moon.]

The first line is enticing to pronounce, its alliterative compression bursting out from the germinal "r" of *recipe*. The list of impossible and wretched objects that follow—from a duck's genitals to the scum on the weir—seems conjured by the demands of alliteration and rhyme. Gestures (pull, yawn, dive) escape objecthood and suggest the futility of trying to gather these named things: no one could actually carry out the verbal imperatives, *take* and *mix*, that govern them. The concoction they are set to constitute, stirred with the crook of the moon, is simply "ane mas [a mass]," an unmeasured and unspecific amalgam of stuff.

Perhaps the most shocking ingredient in the poem is "the crud of my culome [arse, fundament], with your teith crakit" (30). In the context of medieval diagnostics, a patient's "crud," urine, or blood often functioned as his or her self-representation within the medical encounter—a metonymy that, for the skilled interpreter, could convey the patient's entire embodied state. Such excretory figurations are disturbingly stripped of any resemblance to the body as a form for ethical or humanist recognition. Medical writers and satirists alike were sensitive to the potential disjunctions between the self and its waste. Professional advice at the outset of the treatise *De cautelis medicorum* cautions physicians against wily patients, eager to test a healer's skill by bringing a faulty diagnostic sample: a physician should first of all determine "whether the urine be of man or of another animal or another fluid."[60] Satires regularly mocked medicine's tendency to rely on the specimen more than the proof of the person. However, in Henryson's poem, the ubiquitous exchange of bodily materials is reversed, and the patient receives the doctor's waste along with his words. The inclusion of the first- and second-person pronouns ("the crud of *my* culome, with *your* teith crakit") renders the image pertinent not just to the patterns of scatological imagery throughout the poem but also to the confrontation between two physical bodies that underlies both the medical encounter between doctor and patient and the rhetorical interchange between writer and reader. Words, waste, bodies, and remedies form one obscene circuit. The narrator, the would-be medical expert spinning out the exuberant nonsense of

"Sum Practysis," shows his advice to be similar to his own excrement, which he offers as *materia medica*. He does not transcend the indignities of embodiment or even mediate them through discursive knowledge. Rather, his language of information is swallowed up in materiality.

The reversal of the usual exchange of bodily waste further erodes any situational superiority of the "leech." As discussed above, the late medieval medical reader occupied an unstable role. Vernacular works of *phisik* oscillated between addressing a "lewde" patient and a "lerned" medical practitioner; a reader could be the one who suffers *or* the one who heals. Henryson reinscribes that rhetorical instability in "Sum Practysis of Medecyne" by muddling the identity of the ostensible addressee of the verses. Initially the narrator seems to direct his words to another practitioner, whom he chastises for his foolishness ("Als your medicyne by mesour I haif meit met it, / The quhilk I stand ford ye nocht understude [And your medicine by measure I have precisely judged—which I guarantee you've not understood]" [7–8]). However, this rival is soon conflated with a suffering patient, as the writer shifts from criticizing "your cunnying in to cure [skill in healing]" to rhyming the lines "this sedull *I send you*" in order "Of malis *to mend you* [to cure you of ailments]" (14, 22, 26). "You" encompasses both the medical practitioner and, it turns out, a sick person in need of remedies. The stress on the second-person pronoun and the addressee's body continues in these lines from "Dia longum":

> This untment is rycht ganand for your awin us,
> With reid nettill seid in strang wesche to steip,
> For to bath your ba cod,
> Quhen ye wald nop and nod;
> Is nocht bettir be God,
> To latt yow to sleip. (47–52)

[This ointment is highly suitable for your own use, to steep in stale urine, with red-nettle seed, for bathing your scrotum, when you would nap or nod; there is nothing better by God to prevent you from sleeping.]

Even after this thorough conscription of the reader into the role of the medical patient (exposed down to his very genitals), the narrator returns at the poem's conclusion to the posture of educating a fellow healer: "Bot luk on this lettir and leird gif ye can, / The prectik and poyntis of this pottingary [But look

on this letter and learn if you can, / The practice and details of this apothe-
cary]" (81–82). Just as so many vernacular readers "looked on the letters" of
medical writing in an effort to fashion themselves into informed healers, here
the reader of the poem is cast in a likewise changeable role. Henryson plays
with the slippage between literary reader, medical practitioner, and patient in
a manner that echoes and exaggerates the instability immanent to the whole
field of late medieval medical textuality.

Henryson's writer wraps up his "sedull" of prescriptions with an aphorism: "It is ane mirk mirrour, / Ane uthir manis ers [It is a dark mirror, another
man's arse]" (90–91). This is a parody of the Scottish proverb, "It is a dark mirror, another man's thought (or mind, or meaning)."[61] Characteristically for the
poem, mind and meaning are exchanged for the corporeal and scatological.
By rendering the medical encounter one in which a man's thought is replaced
by his "ers," the narrator seals his composition with a pithy completion of the
patient's and medicine's reduction to base materiality.

Henryson's parodic aphorism finds a striking parallel in a unique author-
portrait at the outset of one fifteenth-century medical text (Figure 4). The
text is a Middle English rendering of John Arderne's surgical treatise on anal
fistula, one of the most frequently translated medical writings in late medieval Britain, with four distinct Middle English renderings of Arderne's Latin.[62]
The picture cannot help but recall the long tradition of medieval sodomitical
satire, even as it functions to bolster the authority of the medical text that follows. Arderne is shown seated on a *cathedra*, or professorial chair, despite the
fact that he was not a university physician but a craft-trained surgeon.[63] Richly
clothed, he holds in one hand a tool of his trade, and his other hand points
with the didactic gesture of the *maniculae* frequently found in the margins
of late medieval manuscripts. The meeting of doctor and patient takes place
through the "mirk mirrour" of the completely, even obscenely, materialized
body. The index of Arderne's authoritative gesture intersects exactly with the
anus of his patient, the "nether eye" of the physicalized body that faces surgeon and reader in a position of radical vulnerability. The illustrator did not
draw the upper half of the patient's body, which is not in itself remarkable: the
elaborate program of illuminations that appeared in manuscripts of Arderne's
treatise frequently depicted only the patient's lower region, relevant to the
cures Arderne set forth. However, in this case, the illustrator did choose to finish off the partial figure with a face emerging just at the waist, suggesting the
patient's actual identity, his ontological status, as grotesque. The image renders
absolute the intersubjective asymmetry of the medical encounter.

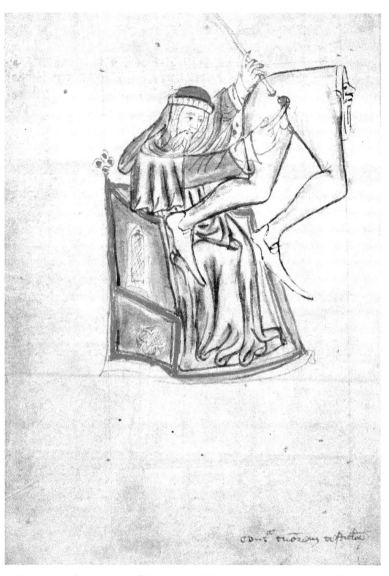

Figure 4. Author-portrait of the surgeon John Arderne. English, early fifteenth
century. © The British Library Board, Sloane MS 2002, fol. 24.

Arderne confidently addresses his reader with the didactically pointing finger, including him or her in the community of medical expertise. However, as I have suggested, the late medieval medical reader might well also have identified with the partial, emphatically somatic, arse-first body—in other words, with the reflection in the dark mirror that Henryson invokes to conclude his poem. While the author-portrait of Arderne radicalizes the division between expert and patient, readers found themselves in an uneasy wavering between the two roles. The very difficulty of medical language, of the multiplicity of *materia medica* and the numerousness of the body's parts and diseases' forms, tended to make the acquisition of medical knowledge difficult and to transform the language of healing into jargon. While Arderne's authoritative confidence might have provided a motivating fantasy that fueled the production of medical writings, one can imagine readers feeling uneasy with the stark distinctions that structure the portrait. Henryson's "Sum Practysis of Medecyne," by contrast, ultimately implies that no stable medical authority is available. The satirical remedies, rather than elevating readers to an elite community of expertise, bind them all the more tightly in the conditions of embodiment and materiality that medicine has pretensions to overcome. In this burlesque universe, knowledge is shown to be jargon through and through. The only way that normative medical discourse could recuperate "Sum Practysis of Medecyne" is to deliver a dose of cathartic laughter.

Medical Materialism in the *Croxton Play of the Sacrament*

At the center of the East Anglian miracle play the *Croxton Play of the Sacrament* is a scene of dismemberment. The play's archvillain, the Jewish merchant Jonathas, has his hand first nailed to a post and then pulled right off his body. He and his compatriots flee, but the hand remains onstage, a reminder of the grotesquely material nature of fallen flesh. It is into this scene, electric with the body's partible corruption, that medical satire enters the play. In the ensuing episode, *phisik* joins mercantilism and rationalistic skepticism as the play's challengers to sacramentality and faith. The *Croxton Play*, like the broader tradition of medical satire, sets up a series of reductive equivalences among corporeality, money, tangible stuffs, and language to evoke the bad materialism that the play's central miracle, the animated eucharistic host, triumphantly overturns.

The play dramatizes what happens when a Christian merchant, Aristorius, steals a consecrated eucharistic wafer and sells it to the Jewish merchant Jonathas. Jonathas and his companions subject the host to a battery of tests as they try to prove the ordinariness of the bread and justify their skepticism toward Christian doctrine. Instead of destroying the host as they intend, however, the Jews unleash its uncanny liveliness. At the play's midpoint, Jonathas and his panicked friends accidentally sever his hand while trying to remove the wafer stuck to it. At the point when these misfiring eucharistic experiments reach their climax, the host miraculously transforms into a bleeding, speaking "image" of Christ's person, who restores Jonathas to bodily integrity and sparks the Jews' conversion.[64] Although the main action of the plot can be summarized without any mention of medicine, *phisik* actually plays a surprisingly prominent role. The plot takes an abrupt turn when Jonathas loses his hand: a quack doctor, Master Brundyche, is suddenly being heralded by his servant Colle. Master Brundyche and Colle transform the play's concerns with commodification, naturalistic explanation, and materialism by yoking these more closely to the condition of corruptible embodiment, a condition that the play's audience members are shown to share with the dismembered figure of Jonathas.

The action of the play opens with a pair of dramatic monologues, one by Aristorius, who in the list of dramatis personae is called *Christianus mercator* (Christian merchant), and the other by the Jewish merchant Jonathas. Between the two of them, they take on many of the functions of the figure of the *apothecarius* or *mercator* in the liturgical plays discussed above. They boast of foreign travel, commercial prowess, and expensive, exotic wares. Aristorius's speech comes first, with twenty-seven alliterating lines chock-full of place-names. Much of it is ordered alphabetically, as though to imply a commercial reach as encompassing as an encyclopedia:

> In Antyoche and in Almayn moch ys my myght.
> In Braban and in Brytayn I am full bold.
> In Calabre and in Coleyn ther rynge I full ryght.
> In Dordrede and in Denmark, be the clyffys cold,
> In Alysander I have abundawnse in the wyde world.
> In France and in Farre fresshe be my flowerys.
> In Gyldre and in Galys have I bowght and sold.
> In Hamborowhe and in Holond moch merchantdyse ys owrys.
>   (97–104)

[In Antioch and Alemannia, much is my might. In Brabant and
Britain I am very bold. In Calabria and Cologne, there I move
about freely. In Dordrecht and in Denmark, by the cold cliffs, and
in Alexandria—I have abundance in the wide world. In France
and in the Faeroe Islands, fresh are my flowers. In Gelderland and
Galicia I have bought and sold. In Hamburg and in Holland, much
merchandise is ours.]

In all these places and more Aristorius's fame "spryngyth" and his merchandise "renneth [circulates]" (91, 94). David Lawton suggests that the speech's
"length is its point: it serves to overshadow the play it initiates."[65] And indeed,
like the bombast of the *mercator* before he sells his myrrh and aloe, the scale of
the boasting comes to be ironized by the action that follows.

Jonathas's speech follows Aristorius's by enumerating the exquisite goods
he trades. Two stanzas about precious stones and two stanzas about spices do
what *herberies* do well: they conjure teeming material variety, but they also
swamp comprehension with a dizzying pile-up of vocabulary. The things he
names begin to sound more and more similar—stuff and sound, all of it finally
exchangeable:

> Gyngere, lycoresse, and cannyngalle,
> And fygys fatte to plesere yow to paye;
> Peper and saffyron and spycys smale,
> And datys wole dulcett, forto dresse;
> Almundys and rys, full every male,
> And reysones, both more and lesse;
>
> Clowys, greynis, and gynger grene,
> Mace, mastyk, that myght ys,
> Synymone, suger, as yow may sene,
> Long peper and Indas lycorys;
> Orengys and apples of grete apryce,
> Pungarnetys and many other spycys. (175–86)

[Ginger, licorice, and galingale, and fat figs to please you to buy;
pepper and saffron and tiny spices, and very sweet dates for serving.
Almonds and rice fill every bag, and raisins large and small. Cloves,
grains of paradise, and green ginger, mace, mastic that is strong,

cinnamon, sugar, as you can see, long pepper and Indian licorice, oranges and apples of great price, pomegranates and many other spices.]

In the unfolding of Jonathas's speech, the lexicon of material particularity accumulates and begins to blur together. The reduction of specificity to an abstract sameness—which is the logic of jargon as well as the merchant's warehouse—implicates the cash economy that the play seeks to bring into crisis. When Jonathas approaches Aristorius to buy the consecrated host, his first allusion to it is simply as a "thyng," one thing among others: "'I have clothe of gold, precyous stons, and spycys plenté: / Wyth yoll a bargen wold I make. / I wold bartre wyth yow in pryvyté / On lytell thyng [I have gold cloth, precious stones, and abundant spices; I want to make a bargain with you. I would barter with you privately for a little thing]'" (274–77). That the pair can agree on a fair price of one hundred pounds for the "lytell thyng" demonstrates their co-implication in this economy. Even the most singular of objects can be reduced to cash value and to the stockpile of things. Though one merchant is Christian and the other Jewish, their transaction places them in moral equipoise; to each of them, the body of Christ is worth just this much.

Following their agreement, each of the men participates in a perverse, materialist iteration of the Last Supper. Jonathas and his Jewish compatriots lay the wafer on the table and then mockingly recount the main tenets of Christian doctrine (389–441). Their ironic recapitulation is of course ironized again by the larger Christian framework within which they are contained. For his part, Aristorius dines with his local priest on wine and bread. Aristorius's clerk tells them proudly, "'Syr, here ys a drawte of Romney red— / Ther ys no better in Aragon— / And a lofe of lyght bred: / Yt ys holesom, as sayeth the fesycyon [Sir, here is a drink of red Rumney wine—there is none better in Aragon—and a loaf of light bread: it is wholesome, as the physician says]" (340–43). Aristorius agrees, reiterating the wine's medical virtues to his dining companion: "Thys Romney ys good to goo with to reste: / Ther ys no precyouser fer nor nere, / For all wykkyd [unhealthy] metys yt wyll degest [digest]" (345–47). Thus, servant and master offer an entirely materialist account of the meal's salubriousness. Wine and bread are so much fodder for good digestion. The scene's reductive physicalism is rendered additionally ominous by its dramatic suspense: the unwitting priest imbibes what "ys good to goo with to reste" and will fail to notice the thief at the pyx. Mention of "the fesycyon" foreshadows two ensuing events in the play: the appearance of another materialistic servant-master pair, Colle and Master Brundyche; and the literalization of the commonplace metaphor of Christ as physician (from Mark 2:17) when the host comes to be miraculously anthropomorphized near the end of the play, to heal Jonathas.

Jonathas finds himself in need of such a cure thanks to a peculiar bit of eucharistic slapstick. The Jews have decided to boil the wafer in "fowr galouns of oyle clere," but when Jonathas tries to throw it in the pot, the thing sticks to his hand. In what is clearly meant to be an antic set piece, he "renneth wood [mad]," as the stage directions specify, shouting, "Out, out! Yt werketh me wrake [does me injury]! / I may not awoyd [remove] yt owt of my hond!" (499–500). Trying to help Jonathas in his panic, his friends catch him and restrain him. Yet they apparently share his sense of the wafer's phobic intolerability. In an unwitting imitation of Christ's Passion, they drive nails through the wafer—and Jonathas's hand along with it—to bind it to a post, so that "with mayne [strength] and myght," they can "pluke hys armes awey" (512–13). The outcome of their heaving and tugging, as the stage directions reveal, is that "Here shall thay pluke the arme and the hond shall hang styll with the Sacrament." Hand and wafer together remain, a spectacle for the characters and the audience alike. At this point Jonathas beats a temporary retreat, urging his companions, "Now hastely to owr chamber lete us gon, / Tyll I may get me sum recuer [cure]" (521–22). The dismemberment marks a point of inflection in the plot: the violence that the Jews have sought to exercise on the host turns back around on their leader. The Jews disappear from view, but the suspended hand maintains a set of uncertainties before the audience's eyes. Will this body be reconstituted? How do the two fleshly fragments stuck together there, hand and bleeding wafer, relate to one another? What will transpire in the grotesque space stretched open between the hand and the wounded body that now lacks it? It is into this tension of dismemberment, at a high point of burlesque, that Colle, the doctor's servant, enters the play.

"Aha, here ys a fayer felawshyppe," Colle begins (525). Colle most likely comes forward out of the audience, shifting attention to what has before seemed like nondiegetic space, the gathering of spectators. The phrase "fayer felaw-shyppe" probably refers to the audience, since Jonathas and his companions have retired. With his comment, then, Colle abruptly implicates the assembled onlookers in the action of the play, "eras[ing] the temporal and geographical distance between the imagined world of the stage and the real world of the audience," as Stephen Wright observes.[66] Though the play is set in Aragon, Colle is a distinctly English name, and while "Master Brundyche" is Flemish, he is announced as residing near the neighborhood landmark "Babwell Myll"

(621). This local color insists on the immediacy of the episode's context, which is ultimately grounded on each audience member's embodied presence.

"I have a master I wolld he had the pyppe ["the pip," a disease], / I tell yow in counsel [in secret]," Colle remarks confidentially (527–28). Indeed, Colle makes a habit of jumping back and forth between pronouncing publicly and "in counsel," intermittently boasting about his master and then undercutting those claims with sly disparagement:

> Mayster Brendyche of Braban—
> I tell yow he ys that same man—
> Called the most famous phesycyan
> That ever sawe uryne!
> He seeth as wele at noone as at nyght,
> And sumtyme by a candelleyt
> Can gyf a judgyment aryght
> As he that hathe noon eyn. (533–40)

> [Master Brundyche of Brabant, I tell you he is the same man called the most famous physician that ever saw urine! He sees as well at noon as at night, and sometimes by candlelight can give a judgment just as well as he who has no eyes.]

The physician's skills in uroscopy are compared to those of a blind man. More ominously Colle remarks, "He had a lady late in cure, / I wot be this she ys full sure: / There shall never Cristen creature / Here hyr tell no tale!" (549–52). *Sure* can mean both "safe" and "discreet," but the second clause disambiguates the first: the punning implication is that the lady is dead. The point is made again after Master Brundyche enters. Colle asks, "how dothe yowr pacyent / That ye had last under yowr medycament?"—and the physician replies, "I waraunt she never fele anyoment [discomfort]" (581–83). Cheekily, Colle returns, "Why, ys she in hyr grave?" (584). The servant characterizes his master not just as a buffoon but as the agent of death, rushing the natural body to its terminus.

Even with his master beside him, Colle continues his double entendres. His irony constantly sets up and overturns the organizing boundaries of who is in on the joke. Like jargon, irony foments distinctions on the basis of exactly how much different auditors understand. Here, onlookers are treated like confidants and like dupes in quick alternation, as Colle conspires with them against his master, and against them in his master's service. Colle's speech renders the

spectators aware of themselves as a "fayer felawshyppe," apprehensible to those
in the play and perhaps vulnerable to its events. More subtly, his quick shifts
of disclosure hail them as interpreters whose position is unsteady, vibrating
between naiveté and knowingness. Master Brundyche similarly addresses the
audience so as to bring them to uncomfortable self-consciousness. Echoing
Colle's first line, he turns his gaze on them, as though to size up his prospects:
"Here ys a grete congregacyon, / And all be not hole [healthy, whole]" (601–2).
Ironized though it may be, the physician's gaze catches up the assembly in a
negative diagnosis—they are "not whole," or not healthy—a condition literalized onstage in Jonathas's hand. The hand remains nailed there, a tense
emblem of the mortal body awaiting its restoration. The historical time and
place of the story's represented events have broken down in this episode, but
the setting has not yet given way to the liturgical, sacramental temporality
of the play's processual conclusion.[67] Now, as the leering physician speaks, is
rather the lived time of the spectators' bodies, when "alle be not hole."

Master Brundyche hurries Colle into delivering his official proclamation
to this promisingly unwholesome-looking bunch. The catalogue of diseases
that ensues is an exuberant play of medical jargon, though it includes plenty
of conditions that would have been recognizable, if not familiar, to the assembled audience. Colle's speech is a means of catching up the entire assembly
into the bumbling, menacing purview of Master Brundyche's expertise. His
words address their corruptible embodiment, which they share with the play's
central villain, the dismembered Jonathas. Colle announces:

> All manar of men that have any syknes,
> To Master Brentberecly loke that yow redresse.
> What dysease or syknesse that ever ye have,
> He wyll never leve yow tyll ye be in yowr grave!
> Who hat the canker, the collyke, or the laxe,
> The tercyan, the quartan, or the brynnyng axs,
> For wormys, for gnawyng, gryndyng in the wombe or in
>   the boldyro,
> All maner red eyn, bleryd eyn, and the myegrym also,
> For hedache, bonache, and therto the tothache,
> The colt-evyll and the brostyn men he wyll undertak.
> All tho that have the poose, the sneke, or the tyseke,
> Thowh a man were ryght heyle, he cowd soone make hym sek.
>   (608–19)

[All manner of men that have any sickness, see that you address
yourself to Master Brundyche. Whatever disease or sickness that you
have, he will never leave you until you're in your grave. Whoever
has cancer, colic, or diarrhea, the tertian fever, quartan fever, or the
"burning ashes," for worms, for gnawing or grinding in the belly
or whatever body part, all manner of red eyes, inflamed eyes, and
migraines also, for headaches, for bone-aches, and in addition to
the toothache, the swelling of the penis and men suffering from
hernia he will undertake. All those that have the catarrh (cold), the
head-cold, or the phthisis (tuberculosis)—though a man were quite
healthy, he could soon make him sick.]

Colle's proclamation stages the emptiness of his self-aggrandizing lexical distinctions. Medical language becomes jargon. This is the third massive list
delivered in the play, and its form connects it back to the opening pair of mer-
chants' speeches. Colle's litany of pathologies forms a parallel with Aristorius's
far-flung trade routes and Jonathas's exotic wares. All are jargony testaments to
the reduction that their worldview effects, through their shared commitments
to commerce and materialist explanation. Here, the audience is invited to
recognize themselves in the catalogue of infirmities, even as they are repelled
by how empty, if not deadly, the physician's expertise is.

Just after this invitation for the audience to join the ranks of Master Brundyche's patients, the action shifts back to the main plot. Colle spots Jonathas
returning to the scene and offers him his master's services: "Men that be masters of scyens be profytable. / In a pott, yf yt please yow to pysse, / He can
tell yf yow be curable [Men that are masters of science are beneficial. If you'll
piss in a pot, he can tell you if you're curable]" (647–49). The juxtaposition
of science and pissing again emphasizes the materialism of Brundyche's operations. Even Jonathas, desperate though he may be, rejects the leech's services.
He dismisses the pair, shouting, "Avoyde, fealows, I love not yower bable!"
(650). The "bable" of *phisik* as well as the jargon of merchandise are, at the
end of the play, replaced by the euphony of prayer and hymn. *Christus medicus*
heals both body and soul, rather than narrowly and dangerously concentrating on physicality. It is striking, however, that Colle and Master Brundyche
do not return at the play's end to participate in the redemptive community
of *Corpus Christi*. They disappear as suddenly as they have appeared, after
exhausting their dramatic function. In contrast to the conversion of the Jews

and Aristorius's new penitential identity, the doctor remains an unredeemed irony of the community.

The role of this medical interlude has puzzled critics, although its literary precedents, I hope, are clear. The apothecary of the French *herberies*, the *mercator* of liturgical dramas, and (at a greater generic distance) the physician of estates satire all provide ready precedents.[68] Some scholars have argued that Colle and Master Brundyche are part of a later interpolation, introduced sometime between the drama's composition after 1461 and the sixteenth century. The scene has metrical variety not found in the rest of the play, though the variations could correspond to the scene's change in subject matter.[69] As David Lawton quips, "It is as if Shakespearean clowns never existed."[70] The narrative extraneousness and poetic exuberance of the *mercator* episodes in liturgical drama suggest that we ought to be cautious in presuming uniformity in dramatic action and style. Whether original or added in subsequent decades, however, the episode would have been significant to whatever audiences saw it. For a time, it interrupts the plot's forward motion, and it ultimately disrupts its closure since Brundyche and Colle do not return for the concluding procession.

The role of the satirical apothecary or physician has in effect been divided among four characters in the play, Aristorius, Jonathas, Colle, and Master Brundyche. Together they evoke a closed circuit of materialism, an economy trading in bodily, monetary, sacramental, material, and lexical substances as though everything could be reduced to mere stuff—as though the eucharist were nothing but bread. The play uses medical satire to dramatize the urgent dangers of such materialism. If audience members might have maintained a feeling of moral superiority vis-à-vis the doubting Jews or blasphemous Aristorius, they are less liable to escape the medically vulnerable corporeality into which Colle and Master Brundyche summon them. It is the intimate proximity of this violent materialism that the play uses medical satire to establish and *Christus medicus* to overcome. The miraculous human "image" that the eucharist assumes tells Jonathas, "Go to the cawdron—thi care shal be the lesse— / And towche thyn hand to thy salvacion" (776–77). The stage directions suggest a solution to Master Brundyche's diagnosis that "all be not hole": "Here shall Ser Jonathas put hys hand into the cawdron, and yt shal be hole agayn." The "bable" of *phisik* in the *Croxton Play of the Sacrament* reminds us of medicine's and our own limits and so turns us to a different disposition of bodies and words, meaning and matter.

Jargon's Dream

After the four scatological, nonsensical, and metrically frenetic recipes that make up most of "Sum Practysis of Medecyne," the authorial persona begins the poem's concluding stanza with another invocation of the cuckoo: "Gud nycht, guk guk, for sa I began" (79). From start to finish, Henryson's medical satire has been spoken in the avian tones of nonsense. The relationship between birdsong and poetry in medieval literature is of course a richly traditional one, birds' conventional role being that of the sweet spur to the entwined tasks of love and lyric—from the troubadour's lark to the singing birds of May at the outset of the *Romance of the Rose*. However, in "Sum Practysis of Medecyne," the cuckoo's voice shows the way to an alternative literary trajectory for birdsong. Jargon's catalyzing desires are not erotic but epistemic; jargon's drive is toward encyclopedism and a way of speaking about the world that would finally be adequate to its variety and the intricacy of its operations. Medicine's opaque materials are written and copied as part of an effort to bring bodies' shadowy workings into speech and the realm of practical action. The nonsensical birdsong that defines the limits of Henryson's jargon-filled poem—*guk guk*—conjures two antagonistic limits, or dreams, of language: one, perfect precision and specificity, a complete expression of complete knowledge; the other, pure sound, a language that leaves behind meaning and becomes music. Medical satire capitalizes on jargon's proximity to song, to the vibratory stuff of language, but it does so at the acknowledged cost of language's referential and practical functions, its curative connections between body and world.

At the outset of the Middle English translation of Lanfranc of Milan's *Chirurgia magna*, Galen is quoted as advising, "he that wyl knowe sothfastnes of a thing, bisie him nought to knowe the name of a thing, but the worchinge and the effete of the same thing."[71] Late medieval medical textuality and its satirical rearticulation demonstrate the simultaneous desirability and difficulty of following Galen's advice, of passing beyond names to functions and effects and mastering the circulation of medicine's multiple materialities. For its part, medical satire explores what it might mean both to suffer and to sing the limits of *phisik*.

Chapter 4

Embodying Causation in Exempla

Deep in a chapter on leprosy in his 1305 medical encyclopedia, the *Lilium medicinae*, Bernard of Gordon tells a story.[1] While discussing the causes of leprosy, Bernard lists numerous factors that might induce the disease, like pestilential air, conception during menstruation, eating "melancholic" meat like fox or hare, and consuming milk and fish together at the same meal. When the list reaches leprosy's sexual transmission, it shifts abruptly into narrative. Bernard writes:

> Caveat igitur quilibet coire cum muliere leprosa. Recitabo modo quid accidit quadam vice. Quedam comitissa venit leprosa ad montempesulanum et fuit finaliter in cura mea. Et quidam baccalarius in medicina ministravit ei & iacuit cum ea et impregnavit eam. Perfectissime factus est leprosus. Igitur felix quem faciunt aliena pericula cautum.[2]

> [Then let everyone beware having sex with a leprous woman. I will recount what happened once. A certain leprous countess came to Montpellier and wound up in my care, and a certain bachelor of medicine attended to her, lay with her, and impregnated her. He became completely leprous. Indeed, lucky is the person made cautious by the perils of others.]

Bernard recounts this anecdote to communicate a piece of medical knowledge and an admonition: sex with a leprous woman can cause leprosy, so avoid it. The story, then, is an exemplum, defined by Joseph A. Mosher as "a short narrative used to illustrate or confirm a general statement."[3] The diction of the tale is alive to the traffic between general axiom and narrative specificity: Bernard's nouns pass between the universal to the particular, from *quilibet*, "anyone," to a certain (*quedam*) countess and a certain (*quidam*) medical student, and the verbs shift from the jussive mood (*caveat*), opening on to future occasions, to the perfect indicative of the remembered incident, which "happened one time" (*accidit quadam vice*). What undergirds the story's linking of precept and narrated event is their mutual connection to a principle of causation. It is *because* the bachelor of medicine sleeps with his patient that he becomes leprous, and this causal relation pertains not only to the world of the story but to that of readers as well, making it possible for us to learn from such *aliena pericula*.

Exempla, this chapter contends, are technologies of etiological imagination. They are narrative instruments for relating general to particular through the mediation of causality. By definition, examples stand in relation to broader categories or principles, and exempla, because they are narratives, figure such generality through the depiction of causes: things happen as they do *because* some more general force is at work. In this way, exemplary stories perform some of the same intellectual work as medicine, which seeks to parse nature's overarching causes as these are at work in individual patients. Exempla and *phisik* both traffic between general principles and idiosyncratic cases, for practical ends. The medieval histories of medicine and exempla are also marked by crossings and borrowings. Narrative became an increasingly prevalent technique of medical writing in the later Middle Ages, and medical theory found its way into sermons, miracle stories, and didactic tales.

While not all exempla rely on characters' bodies to illustrate their *sententiae*, an enormous number do. Falling ill and being healed, disfiguration and restoration, are not just common elements in exemplary plots but are among the basic techniques by which such stories communicate meaning. The human body makes a good medium for depicting cause-and-effect relations because bodies are switchpoints between action and vulnerability, doing and undergoing. This is evident in Bernard's exemplum. The *baccalarius* initially is defined by action: he gives medical care to the countess, he sleeps with her, and he impregnates her. Then comes the plot twist, when he is made (*factus est*) leprous. From three active verbs to a passive—the reversal is typical of exemplary narratives, as the central agent comes to be acted upon. With neat irony, the student's paradigmatically form-giving act of insemination leads to loss of bodily form in leprosy, and medical authority sows sickness. In a pattern that many exempla follow, macrocosm recoils upon microcosm, and the governing forces of the narrative world become apprehensible in a character's flesh. The final sentence of Bernard's story, the aphoristic "lucky is the person made cautious by the perils of others," acts as a hinge between the events of the plot and its readers, completing the text's rhetorical circuit.

Exempla constituted perhaps the most widely disseminated narrative form of the later Middle Ages. They were recounted in sermons, compiled in collections, and appeared in almost every sphere of late medieval discourse. Exempla hovered between rhetorical device and literary mode. Like a device, an exemplum usually circulated as a component part of a larger work, and it was treated as a figure in rhetorical and poetic treatises. But exemplarity was also a stance, a disposition, that various narrative genres could assume. Romance, fable, *miraculum*, historical anecdote, medical case: all could be turned to exemplary ends. Despite these protean qualities, the exemplum had strong ties to established genres like sermons and "mirrors for princes," which gave consistency to the stories' style and subject matter. In the Middle Ages, exempla functioned as one pathway that the discourse of medicine traveled on its way into fictional narrative and poetry. Like satire (the topic of the previous chapter), exemplary stories offered medieval thinkers the chance to play with *phisik* and its accounts of sickness, injury, healing authority, and the causes of bodily change. Forms of didactic narrative meanwhile traveled into medical writing, as Bernard's anecdote in the *Lilium* suggests. Especially in the later Middle Ages, growing awareness of medical contingency, or the almost innumerable causal factors that could affect someone's embodied state, encouraged medical writers to rely on illustrative narratives, which made room for etiological uncertainty and speculation in a way that precepts alone did not.

The present chapter argues that exempla were important forms of etiological thought and shared much with the discourse of medicine. The first section offers an overview of medieval exempla from the vantage of etiological imagination. I then examine the crisscrossings of medicine and exemplary narrative in genres ranging from medical *practicae* to sermon collections. The *similitudo* of body and soul gave rise to particularly complex accounts of medical and spiritual care, and I argue that it was the fundamental instability of the soul's relation to the body in pastoral rhetoric that made the literary traffic between them so generative. The chapter concludes with readings of two tales from the *Gesta Romanorum*, a widely used collection of exempla compiled around 1300 and translated variously into Middle English. The models of bodily change that circulated in these stories changed little with the novel understandings of bodies, nature, and causation of the later Middle Ages. Instead, baldly

unrealistic episodes of sickness and healing continued to carry out sophisticated semantic work. What precisely exemplary characters' bodies were good
for becomes clearer when the dynamics of abrupt infection, sudden disfiguration, and deus-ex-machina cure are redescribed in terms of the exemplum's
distinctive narrative poetics.

Exempla as Etiological Technologies

Medieval practices of recounting and interpreting exempla emerged from
multiple traditions.[4] In Aristotle's *Rhetoric*, the example (*paradeigma*) is
described as an inductive argument leading not just to a universal principle
but to that principle's re-application in another case, namely, the occasion at
hand (*Rhet.* I.2, 1357b25ff.). The device of *narratio* in Cicero's *De Inventione*
and exemplum in the pseudo-Ciceronian *Rhetorica ad Herennium* adapt the
Aristotelian model, and these were important sources for medieval thinkers.[5]
In classical rhetoric, collections of exemplary loci established an archive of
familiar historical figures and episodes, intended for widely varied argumentative ends. But beyond this classical legacy, recourse to illustrative stories was a
nearly universal practice. The parables of Jesus, recorded in the Gospels, derive
in part from Jewish narrative traditions. The Church Fathers recognized the
didactic power of exempla, with Ambrose declaring them "more persuasive
than words alone," Augustine's sermons peppered with them, and Gregory
the Great's *Dialogues* eventually coming to serve as an exemplum collection
for preachers.[6]

Exempla were thus in circulation throughout the Middle Ages. However,
they were reconsolidated as a distinctive genre when, in the late twelfth century, they began to be gathered into collections for preaching, as part of what
James J. Murphy has called the "rhetorical system" of the *ars praedicandi*.[7] As
they circulated with the new mendicant preaching orders, exempla increasingly
answered to the desires of lay audiences. Production of exemplum collections
as reference works was at its height between 1250 and 1350.[8] Following this
clerical aggregation, the collections gradually spread to more secular and vernacular contexts, and works like Boccaccio's *Decameron* and Gower's *Confessio
Amantis* bear a teasing and troping relation to earlier collections of virtuous
tales. In addition, Larry Scanlon has drawn attention to "public exempla," or
the classicizing, political stories that served as building blocks for the "mirror
for princes" genre that thrived in the high and later Middle Ages.[9] By the end

of these developments, as Scanlon remarks, the "narrative form dominated later medieval culture, particularly in England."[10]

The semantic task that defines the exemplum is its transformation of a general principle or *sententia* into an efficient cause in the narrative world. Or (to describe it from the opposite direction) the text promises to make the force of its emplotment, or the principle of its ordering and interrelation of events, available as an idea applicable in other situations. At the moment that a norm acquires narrative efficacy—say, when *lying is wrong* becomes *the liar is struck blind*—the norm takes on narrative force, and emplotment is linked to practical reason. By becoming determinate in a particular situation, ideas becomes *causes* and therefore part of the current of mutual entailment that flows through the events of a story, holding them together as plot. The fundamental role of causation in constituting narrative is captured in E. M. Forster's well-known distinction between what he calls mere "events arranged in their time-sequence" (e.g., "The king died and then the queen died") and what is truly "a *narrative* of events, the emphasis falling on causality," as in "The king died, and then the queen died *of grief*."[11] In an exemplum, the story's final cause, its point, is made an efficient cause, or the logic of events. "The exemplum illustrates a moral because what it recounts is the enactment of a moral. The moral does not simply gloss the narrative," writes Scanlon.[12] J. Allan Mitchell likewise argues for the "reciprocal movement between narrativity and normativity": "Exemplary narratives generate morals 'from below' even at the moment morality engenders them 'from above.'"[13]

It is in this way that medicine and exempla negotiate the same conceptual terrain, the space stretched open between concepts and particulars, or between "a systematically interconnected set of generalizations" and "all the occurrences of the world . . . in their concrete particularity."[14] An exemplum's plot is something like an individual patient, in that it becomes an object of knowledge when joined to a generalizing claim—just as the patient is comprehended medically when her body is recognized within broader scientific categories. Yet the fit between particularity and generality (between body and science, or between tale and moral) is never perfect, and their slippage makes way for the contingencies that bedevil—but also constitute—medical and interpretive practice. It is medicine's indissociability from individual cases that leads J. Allan Mitchell to describe it as paradigmatic of the long history of what he calls "casuistic thought": "Law gives us one useful vantage from which to view casuistry at work, medical practice another. Given that the dilemmas judges or juries and physicians confront can be unprecedented, it makes sense that practitioners in both areas should prefer a kind of deliberation that works from the 'bottom up,' deriving practical precepts from case-analysis rather than reading off principles from some pre-established moral code."[15] For Mitchell, the importance of the "bottom-up" approach in medicine makes it an analogue for the late medieval rhetorical culture of exemplary tales.

What kinds of causation did medieval exemplary narratives deal in? One of the few medievalists to think comprehensively about this question was the Germanist Frederic Tubach, who in a 1962 essay argued for an important change in causality's narrative representation in the Middle Ages. Tubach claims that before the thirteenth century, the model of cause-and-effect emplotted in medieval exempla worked according to "a dynamic principle *beyond* the phenomenological sphere," which he calls "the metaphysical principle of ethics."[16] By contrast, in later exempla, from the thirteenth century forward, the "accidental substance of the narrated world" became primary in exemplary stories, "and narrative progression drew its causality from it."[17] The metaphysical principle withered, and "the divine order became merely an abstract, static principle relegated to an extraneous schematic moral, or else it was ignored all together."[18] Medieval exempla, on this account, turn from God to the world.

The secular-humanist bent of Tubach's history is obvious: the "rigid structure" of an "absolute ethical norm" gives way to the "proliferate growth" proper to the "unending variety of tangible phenomena."[19] The story backdates to the Middle Ages the origins of literary realism and the epistemic secularization usually ascribed to later periods. More surprising than this familiar historiographic arc, however, is the fact that Tubach seems to ignore what his own scholarship would have made him uniquely well positioned to notice. Tubach is also responsible for compiling one of the most comprehensive resources for the study of medieval exempla—the *Index Exemplorum*, a collection and summary of 5,400 "medieval religious tales."[20] Skimming through the entries in the *Index Exemplorum* reveals countless plots that recur in multiple medieval sources, early and late. Neither the form nor the content of the stories changed punctually with the rise of mendicant orders, although some came to be recounted in new contexts and styles. Tubach's essay implicitly acknowledges that consistency across time, even as he seeks to minimize its consequences. He cites a pair of contrasting exempla, one illustrating "the metaphysical order of divine ethics" that he associates with the earlier age of exempla, and the other, "the relative norms of social propriety and expedience," supposedly of interest to the later era. However, *both* come from Jacques de Vitry's preaching.[21] Part of what makes exempla challenging to theorize is their durability across contexts and their ability to mean differently in different frameworks. Perusing a collection of exempla like the *Gesta Romanorum* or the *Alphabetum narrationum*, each compiled around the year 1300, readers in fact encounter a grab bag of causational models, some unfolding according to the "accidental substance of the narrative world," some governed by supernatural forces, some transpiring according to an allegorical logic, and some occupying a zone of uncertainty among these.

But if Tubach's central claim about exempla and causation fails to convince—namely, that late medieval exempla in the aggregate turned away from divine power and toward natural and quotidian causes—he nonetheless raises important questions about the historically varying ways that didactic stories represent and shape understandings of reality. After all, change *was* afoot in medieval discourses of causation. Twelfth- and thirteenth-century modifications in the understanding of nature produced increasingly exacting accounts of the miraculous. Many theologians, influenced first by Plato's *Timaeus* and then Aristotle's natural philosophy, came to agree that the physical world had a rational structure and that once created it had the capacity to operate by its own laws.[22] Of course, God could intervene in this order of secondary causes—but it was knowledge of nature's regularities, established by natural philosophy, that made it possible to recognize these regularities' contravention. Even later anti-Aristotelian developments, which emphasized the freedom of the human will and God's absolute rather than ordained powers, did not dampen the zeal for parsing miracles from ordinary occurrences. Canonization proceedings grew ever more exacting in their distinction of natural from supernatural causes, and in the late Middle Ages the discernment of spirits focused new etiological scrutiny on visionary experience.[23]

Thus, rather than accepting Tubach's neat but inaccurate story of a sea change for exempla, when they supposedly turned away from divine power toward this-worldly causes, literary history might learn more from the lushly chaotic picture painted by the *Index Exemplorum*. Its evidence of recirculation, modification, and repurposing implies that exemplary stories should not be taken as straightforward evidence of "what medieval people thought," as they are sometimes construed in the "history of mentalities." Instead, the narrative modality of the exemplum was a way of thinking about, and playing with, the claims of normative order. Some exempla sought to persuade through historiographic models of evidence, citing eyewitnesses and proper names, but plenty of others were patently unconcerned with conventions of verifiability or plausibility. Semantic malleability was part of the exemplum's identity as a rhetorical device, and collections of exempla often contain stories in underdetermined forms, awaiting the usage that will flesh out their significance. In frame stories, like the *Canterbury Tales* or Gower's *Confessio Amantis*, it is possible to see writers experimenting with this contextual flexibility of narrative. Exempla, then, constituted a zone of semantic fine-tuning for medieval interpreters, where, in the instantiation of didactic propositions, and in the clamoring plurality of such instantiations, the claims of various etiological and ideological traditions mingled with another.

One illustration of the later Middle Ages' crisscrossing regimes of narrative authority can be found in the account of Henry IV's supposed leprosy, written by the fifteenth-century theologian and university administrator Thomas Gascoigne (d. 1458). The fiercely partisan story links Henry's infection to the execution of Richard le Scrope, Archbishop of York, in 1405.[24] The intended purpose of Gascoigne's text is uncertain, and it appears only in a personal manuscript, though it was apparently the source for Clement Maidstone's *Martyrium Ricardi Archiepiscopi*.[25] The text is a balancing act, aiming to convey both the clear moral polemic of an exemplum and the evidentiary authority of a historical document. Thus, Gascoigne emphasizes the circumstantiality of his narrative and the authoritative observation of eyewitnesses. He names the king's exact location when leprosy strikes and the town where he stops for the night. He lists several witnesses by name and stresses the reliability of his information, as with the firsthand account of *magister Georgius Pluntum*, who saw (*vidit*) the king's condition and then swore to Gascoigne concerning it (*michi dixit and juravit*).[26] However, Gascoigne is at the same time eager to reinforce the teleological shapeliness of his narration, to make clear that these facts are organized and emplotted by divine judgment. Thus Henry is struck with leprosy at exactly the same time that the execution takes place (*eodem tempore quo archiepiscopus fuit decollatus*). Gascoigne makes clear that Henry's disease is no gradual succumbing to infection, which might then have multiple causes. Rather, "it seemed to him that someone sensibly struck him" as he rode (*videbatur sibi quod unus sensibiliter eum percussit*).[27] Here, the unremarkable idiomatic expression "struck by disease" (*fuit percussus*, occurring twice earlier in the passage) is concretized with agential and violent force. The image brings to mind Chaucer's "Man of Law's Tale," when a knight falsely swears Constance's guilt: at once a supernatural hand "hym smoot upon the nekke-boon, / That doun he fil atones [struck him on the neck, so that he fell down at once]."[28] While in Chaucer's tale the event has an archaic air, bespeaking a vanished age of God's direct justice, in Gascoigne's account the gestural impact of the king's leprosy heightens its shock in the present era.

The king, figure of secular sovereignty, becomes in the course of Gascoigne's story saturated with another, divine order of law, which shows its dominion through disease, not unlike King Uzziah's leprosy (2 Chron. 26:16–21). Gascoigne was part of a self-consciously orthodox group of Oxford theologians who valorized preaching as a means to reform, and for much of his life Gascoigne was at work compiling a preacher's aid, his *Dictionarium theologicum*, gathering scriptural and theological passages together with his own moral and anecdotal commentary.[29] Gascoigne was someone who would have thought keenly about the rhetorical power of exempla. In the contest of church and state that this exemplary story recounts, first the archbishop's and then the king's body are made violently subject to juridical one-upmanship. The story stages a contest over who makes things happen, who holds the reins of the plot's causation. In the end, it is Scrope who is cast as a martyr, whose death is to the glory of God, and Henry is made an example of divine justice.

Narrative Medicine

As the causal forces understood to determine the material world became more multifarious in the later Middle Ages, medicine's task of interpreting individual bodies became more delicate.[30] It required picking out relevant threads of explanation and mapping particularized itineraries of implication and consequence. As Henri de Mondeville explains in introducing his catalogue of medical contingencies (*contingentia*), surgeons need to know every detail, "every individual condition as revealed in a patient, or in a wounded member, or in an illness, or wherever, whether it be favorable or harmful."[31] Arnau of Vilanova's comparison of the physician to a sailor—"because both govern what is committed to them not by following necessary and permanent rules but by weighing contingent and variable factors"[32]—vividly imagines how the unpredictability of the material world impinges on the physician's art.

By the fourteenth century, when *medicina* was firmly established as an academic discipline, some continental masters of medicine were coming to worry less about medicine's status vis-à-vis Aristotelian science and more about the lessons of their professional practice. In a commentary from 1339, the Parisian master Pierre Chauchat remarks, "In order to have success in the art of medicine, it is better and more useful to verify principles through operations than to question these principles using demonstration *propter quid*."[33] In downplaying the proofs of reason in favor of those of practice, Chauchat indexes an important trend. Debates in learned medicine began to show "a more acute awareness of the difficulty of applying authoritative general rules to individual cases," as Danielle Jacquart observes.[34] And the trend continued; Nancy Siraisi notes that "especially in the late fourteenth and the fifteenth centuries, discussion of specifics pertaining to disease and treatment seems to have absorbed an increasing amount of the time and attention of the most highly educated physicians."[35]

It is in this context, amid the intellectual ascent of practice and the growing awareness of causal contingency, that medicine's novel uptake of narrative should be understood. Stories incorporated into medical writing could convey the interaction of multitudinous factors more effectively than the enumeration of scientific precepts alone. This is because narrative, as a mode of scientific discourse, could recreate the process of moving between concrete particularities and the relevant medical causes. One newly prominent genre in late medieval medicine was the *practica*, an encyclopedic medical or surgical work integrating fundamental theoretical information with practical instructions for treatment. The authors of *practicae* generally included a number of *casus* or narratives of their own experience and that of their peers. Meanwhile, *consilia*, or didactic accounts of cases, became a newly prominent academic genre. *Consilia* developed in Bologna, probably under the influence of the prestigious jurists writing opinions on legal cases. They could be based on real or fictitious patients, and they tended to present the "personality of the patient (sometimes his or her name), social standing, age, complexion, symptoms of the disease, supposed causes of the disease, and diet and prescribed treatment."[36] Over the fourteenth and fifteenth centuries the genre spread from Bologna to the rest of Europe. The circulation of medical *casus, consilia*, and *experimenta*[37] gradually altered the tenor of medical authority, as "it became common practice in the fifteenth century to ridicule the sophisticated refinements that one gladly attributed to one's colleagues" and to foreground one's own practical know-how.[38] The upshot of these narrative forms, according to one historian of medicine, is that by the end of the Middle Ages, "the part of medicine designated as 'practical'" had become "strangely overgrown," and the new "attention focused on *particularia*, which were meant to 'verify' the principles [of learned medicine], did nothing but assist their progressive disintegration."[39]

Surgical manuals were especially likely to be stocked with illustrative narratives, which were often signaled with labels of *narratio* or *exemplum*.[40] Although Latin surgical writers drew on translations of Arabic sources, their use of anecdotes was their own.[41] Surgeons' common recourse to narrative corresponds to their special relationship with medical *practice*. Since the thirteenth century, learned surgery had had a vexed relation to academic faculties of medicine, one of alternating emulation, dialogue, and subordination.[42] While surgeons like Lanfranc of Milan, Henri de Mondeville, and Guy de Chauliac promoted the "rational" or theoretical basis of surgical expertise, they also vaunted surgery's special practical acuity, as a distinctively manual art that was taught through apprenticeship. Surgical exempla were a means to record the intellection immanent to curative action. The English surgeon John Arderne represents an apparent intensification of the already prevalent practice of surgical storytelling. As Peter Murray Jones notes, Arderne "developed the use of narrative in surgical writing far beyond that of other surgical authors in the scholastic tradition."[43] Arderne's form of storytelling, Jones continues, "somewhat resembles the exempla recommended as means of instruction and moral edification by the preaching order of friars."[44] This recourse to the tactics of lay pedagogy makes sense insofar as Arderne was writing at an even greater remove from elite university medicine than were his Italian and French predecessors. The audience for his text was decidedly mixed, and exemplary narratives would have been a technique of instruction familiar to the breadth of his readership. Narrative was also a medium well-suited to presenting his own experiences, which were central to his cultivation of authority. Less calcified forms of medical writing—indeed more improvised and vernacular ones—seem to have attracted narrative exemplification.

The case of Arderne illustrates England's idiosyncratic position vis-à-vis the narrativization of medicine in the later Middle Ages. Medical curriculum at Oxford and Cambridge remained decidedly old-fashioned, composed mostly of texts from the Salernitan *articella*, the oldest stratum in medieval Europe's revival of classical medicine.[45] The English faculties are unlikely to have been responsive to the fourteenth-century continental trends described above. But Oxford and Cambridge played only a minor role in English *phisik*. Elite practitioners often trained abroad, and many of those who remained in England nonetheless showed themselves to be in touch with continental developments. John Arderne's *Practica*, for instance, includes copious excerpts from Lanfranc of Milan and Bernard of Gordon. The *Breviarium Bartholomei*, a medical encyclopedia written for hospital use by the ecclesiastic

John Mirfield, cites Arnau of Vilanova and Bernard of Gordon among other recent authorities.[46] In any case, given the weakness of academic medicine in England, *phisik* tended to favor nonspecialist rhetorical devices like the exemplum. When English readers did manage to encounter the continental vogue for narrative medicine, it reinforced their own already-established tendencies.

A surgical exemplum that typifies the rhetorics of healing and medical instruction in circulation in late medieval England appears in a chapter on hemorrhages in the Middle English translation of Lanfranc's *Chirurgia magna*, which survives in at least ten manuscripts. In Oxford, Bodleian Library, Ashmole MS 1396, this story is labeled an "ensaumple," and it recounts what happens to a young man stabbed by a small knife. Lanfranc describes the dangerous state of the wound, which damaged both veins and nerves, and he recalls his own advice: "Thanne I demede nessessarie," he reports, the tying off of the vein and the application of oil of roses to the damaged nerve. But his advice is not heeded:

> the modir of that child sente for a lewde leche which that reprevede foule my doom, & he behighte to heele safly the child. He dwellide on the cure, & I wente my wey / The which leche took hede to him .x. daies, that neithir the akynge ceesside ne the blood was not staunchid, & so the siik man was nygh deed / & at the laste I was clepid, & I wolde not come to the pacient / Thanne a fiscian that was frend to the freendis of the pacient blamede the modir & hir freendis that thei hadden left counseil for thilke idiotis biheeste.[47]

> [The mother of that child sent for an ignorant practitioner who disparaged my judgment, and he promised to heal the child safely. He reflected on the cure, and I went my way. This practitioner took care of him for ten days, during which neither the aching ceased nor the blood was staunched, so the sick man was near death. And at last I was called, but I would not come to the patient. Then a physician that was a friend of the patient's friends blamed the mother and her friends on account of their having abandoned good advice for this idiot's promise.]

Lanfranc's *practica* warns against unlearned practitioners at other points as well, for instance when he admonishes, "He that knowith not thes canones [principles], wel yvele [very poorly] schal he heele woundis."[48] In the *ensaumple* just quoted, in a narrative pattern that is repeated elsewhere in Lanfranc's *Chirurgia*,[49] another practitioner is called in after Lanfranc's initial prescription has been made. The recourse to several doctors illustrates the multistop itineraries of care that seem to have characterized medieval treatment. It also gives the author an opportunity to demonstrate the practical efficacy of his own expertise. After the "lewde leche" disparages Lanfranc's judgment, the master surgeon proudly withdraws to watch the disaster play out. It is only when Lanfranc's prescribed cure is finally applied, albeit in his absence, that the youth improves: "and so bi this counseil he was restorid agen to heelthe." The efficacy of his "counseil" emerges as the moral of the story: his methods are the decisive factor, tipping the condition of the patient toward health. Notably, it is not Lanfranc's manual skills but his verbal advice, put into action by someone else, that saves the patient from danger—and thus legitimates his treatise's authority. As he declares elsewhere in the *Chirurgia*, there are many who "mighte ful long tyme have lyved" if their surgeons had "kept aftir my teching in this book."[50]

Lanfranc's anecdote and the surgical exempla it typifies have an important analogue in miracles of healing. Nancy Siraisi describes such medical and surgical narratives being "almost like secular parallels" to miraculous cures.[51] Both kinds of stories tend to emphasize the desperateness of the patient's condition, and they contrast the ultimately successful cure with others' failures: saints triumph where doctors fall short, and physicians and surgeons cure where rivals have faltered.[52] The two narrative types share the common blueprint of the exemplum and use its conventions to manage the etiology of bodily change. Physicians and divine healers have shared plotlines ever since the Gospel story of the hemorrhaging woman, healed by the touch of Jesus' cloak; she had previously spent all her money in vain on physicians (*medicos*) who were unable to stop her flux.[53] The miraculous cure was perhaps the most widespread paradigm of healing in the culture of medieval Christendom. Accounts of miraculous cures make up the bulk of most shrines' thaumaturgical records and conventionally are the first items mentioned among a saint's posthumous powers. Ronald Finucane has found that at English shrines between the twelfth and fifteenth centuries, more than 90 percent of the miracles documented are cures for human illness.[54] There is some evidence for medical practitioners' rivalrous skepticism toward saintly powers—for instance, Guy de Chauliac ridicules the ranks "of wommen and of many ydeotis or foles [idiots or fools], the whiche remitten seke men for all manere of sekenesse onliche [only] to seyntes."[55] Yet the general relation between medicine and the saints seems to have been one of complementarity, since infirmity was sometimes susceptible to natural amelioration, sometimes to divine succor, and sometimes to neither.

Medical writers, like the authors of devotional and hagiographic works, were well aware of the power of narrative simultaneously to convey truths and to shape reality rhetorically. *Consilia* could be true or fictional, but either way they illustrated how out of a welter of circumstances, the relevant factors of diagnosis and treatment could be discerned. Exempla in *practicae* like Lanfranc's concretize instructions about how to treat particular conditions while also reinforcing the authority of the surgeon. Rhetorically managing a patient's sense of the forces at play in her body is sometimes discussed explicitly by medical texts. In the deontological prefaces that often appeared at the start of *practicae*, care-givers are advised about how to talk to patients. Lanfranc instructs (in the Middle English translation), "curteisli speke to the siik man, and in almaner siiknes [in whatever kind of sickness] bihote him heele [promise him health], though thou be of him dispeirid [though you depair for him]; but never the lattere [nevertheless] seie to hise freendis the caas as it stant [tell his friends how the case really stands]."[56] This two-part strategy, telling the patient one thing and his friends another, reflects the conviction that optimism and pessimism can affect health, and so the patient must be kept in good spirits. John Arderne carries this advice further, advising the practioner to *double* the predicted time to the cure because the risks of a tardy remedy are so great: it "giffeth [gives] cause of dispairyng to the pacientes."[57] If the patient then inquires about the unexpected speediness of the cure, the surgeon should answer that it is because "the pacient was strong-herted, and suffrid wele sharp thingis, and that he was of gode complexion and hadde able flesshe to hele; & feyne [feign] he othir causes pleseable to the pacient."[58] Practitioners thus have a responsibility to guide their patients' understandings of causal processes, even if they must *feyne* some of what they convey—because such etiological understanding can give rise to physiological effects.

A delightfully extreme version of medical fiction-making is recounted in the *Reductorium morale*, a preachers' encyclopedia compiled by Pierre Bersuire (d. 1362). The story originated in Arnau of Vilanova's *De parte operativa* and then found its way, with some elaboration, into Bersuire's stock of exempla. Under the encyclopedia's entry on melancholics, the story tells how Arnau devised a treatment for one of his melancholic patients. The patient refused to eat because he believed himself to be already dead (*mortuum se credebat*) and, as he reasoned, the dead do not eat (*mortui comedere non debebant*).[59]

In response, Arnau dressed himself in black, announced himself to be dead also, and asked the patient to go with him to a cemetery, where, by design, others were waiting there dressed in black, pretending to be dead and feasting lavishly. Arnau invited the patient to join the meal, and so the man was cured of his self-starvation (*et ita eum sanavit*). In the tale, the physician draws on the power of fiction to influence bodily reality. To avoid his patient's death, Arnau puts on death as a costume. Allowing the patient's melancholic delusion to remain intact, Arnau rather enters into it with him and peoples it with a benevolent conspiracy of revelers. The story is memorable for its ingenious gentleness. It shows the authoritative physician joining the patient's fantasy so as to make it survivable, and it values sustenance above distinctions of truth and falsehood. Arnau wards off the threat of the graveyard by transforming it into a festive spectacle of care. Bersuire cites the story to illustrate the vain beliefs of melancholics, but it produces meaning in excess of that—exemplifying, for instance, that with the right companions, and a little art, illness can be transformed into a condition of thriving.

Body and Soul

In the middle of an English sermon from the first half of the fifteenth century, which was likely written in Oxford for a mixed clerical and lay audience, there appears a citation from the *Viaticum*, the medical treatise by the "skillful doctor Constantine [*artificiosus medicus Constantinus*]." The quotation provides the theme for the sermon's second half, and it describes the sequence of fevers supposedly caused by dietary intemperance: "through the misuse and excess of food and drink men fall into the cotidian fever [*in cotidianum febrem*], from the cotidian into the quartan or acute [*a cotidiana in quartanam vel acutam*], and then there is nothing else but death, [which] only a few avoid."[60] The sermon's modern editor points out that the *Viaticum*'s discussion of fevers actually includes no such reference to gustatory excess, so this plausible-sounding etiology is perhaps a moralistic flourish, the first in a series of transformations that the sermon works on its medical source text.

As soon as the sequence of fevers from Constantine's *Viaticum* is invoked, the sermon turns to interpreting them *moraliter*—morally, scripturally, and allegorically. In the course of the sermon, these fevers pass over multiple bodies. The progress of disease starts with Adam: after eating the forbidden fruit, he "fell into the cotidian [fever] of original sin that just like a fever [*sicut febris*]

made his tongue lose taste so that he could not savor God."[61] In the macaronic mixture of Latin and Middle English that makes this sermon collection distinctive, the writer explains that at one moment the fever "made him
shiver with the cold and sorrow of fear [*tremere frigore of soroo et timoris*]" and
at another made him burn with carnal desire. The corporeal symptoms of
fever are transformed into spiritual conditions. But it is also the case that in
medieval Christianity Adam was understood to have fallen physiologically at
the moment of sin. Before, as the sermon recounts, he had been "pure without corruption, healthy in every way without any bodily infirmity [*purus sine
corupcione, sanus in omni parte sine aliqua infirmitate corporali*]." With the bite
of forbidden fruit, his complexion became imbalanced and his body vulnerable to infirmities. The sermon plays on the mutuality of Adam's corporeal and
spiritual corruption, allowing them to stand as a pair of real, coincident events
as well as vehicle and tenor.

The sermon then passes to the body of "man [*homo*]," who enters the
phase of acute fever. This fever burns him corporeally as well as spiritually
(*tam corpus quam animam*), and all the physicians (*phisici*) predict death: "In
this burning fever man lay and burned for many thousand winters [*In ista cal-
ida febri homo iacuit and brent mony thousant wynter*]," the sermon reports.[62]
Other "physicians," patriarchs and prophets, gave the sick man "many great
medicines [*plurimas medicinas et magnas*]," including the "prescription [*recep-
tum*]" of the "Old Law," but these prove unsuccessful. Finally, the heat of
the man's acute fever was so strong that neither Hippocrates, Avicenna, nor
Galen (*nec Ypocras, Avicenna, nec Galienus*) dared to touch the patient. It was
then that the "experienced doctor Jesus [*peritus medicus Iesus*]" arrived and,
following the doctrine of contraries, "gathered cold herbs [*frigidas herbas*]
in the field of his humanity to reduce our burning fever." The shift into the
first-person plural (*nostrum*) signals that *we* are now those who burn with
fever. This medical case has run all the way up to the present of the sermon's
Christian auditors.

In discussing Jesus' "very beautiful cures [*pulcherrimas curas*]," the sermon
writer mentions the miracles of healing in the Gospels, like Jesus' curing of
the ten lepers and the blind man.[63] These are literal, physical cures, miraculous
in their transgression of nature's ordinary workings. But they are interwoven
with metaphors of natural healing, like the figurative "plaster [*emplastrum*]"
that Jesus made from the "cold herbs" of hunger, thirst, poverty, and sickness. After such remedies, Jesus then turned to the "main cure [*principalem
curam*] for which he had come" and so prepared a "syrup of his precious blood

[*surripum sui preciosi sanguinis*]"—"And with this precious medicine he fully healed his patient." In the final turn of this extended conceit, the sermon addresses the audience directly:

> Go to your spiritual doctor [*spiritualem medicum*], your curate, to whom Jesus gave the power of healing you [*potestatem sanandi te*]. Show him your sore [*Schew him thi sore*], tell him the burden of your conscience, and do penance for it. And even if the medicine of penance [*medicina penitencie*] be sharp, corrosive, even if it stings you, it is for your [good]. Suffer a little, it is for your benefit. If you use this medicine, you heal your sore [*sanas thi sore*], if you punish your body [*punias corpus tuum*], you save yourself [*sanas te*] from eternal death.[64]

Penitentially punishing one's physical body saves the body of metaphor, which is fevered and hurt. This is the soul's figurative body, which has been elaborated in the sermon's allegorical exposition at varying proximities to literal flesh.

In a very short span, then, this sermon plays across an extraordinarily dynamic apparatus of meaning-making, a series of interlocking analogies between disease and sin, physician and Christ, medical and pastoral care, and body and soul. These metaphors are made to encompass much of salvation history as well as an urgent call to penitential succor in the present. As the unfolding of the conceit demonstrates, these analogical pairs do not remain on discrete levels as signifier and signified, or vehicle and tenor. Instead, physiological and spiritual realities are constantly repositioned relative to one another. The sermon shows itself interested in the fact that bodies may *really* be sickened or healed—that Adam did suddenly become susceptible to illness, Jesus really healed the blind man, and eating too much can give you a fever—and also that bodies serve as a figural resource, one that physicalizes spiritual and theological conditions that on their own lack sensory immediacy.

Joseph Ziegler, in an analysis of the role of medicine in late thirteenth- and early fourteenth-century writings for preachers, has tracked what he calls the "medical model" of spiritual analogy, formed by "similes which portray the relationship between God and his ministers and the believer in terms of the relationship between a physician and his patient."[65] As Ziegler notes, "Sermon literature of the period is saturated with allusions to the role of Christ and his ministers as physicians."[66] Yet I would add that this venerable set of meta- phors is also destabilized by a contradiction. The "medical model" is premised on "the belief in the existence of a perfect analytical similarity of body and soul," as Ziegler notes. But this a similarity is constantly undercut by Christian (especially Pauline) traditions of starkly opposing flesh to spirit, body to soul, and outward (*homo exterior*) to inward man (*homo interior*), as in 2 Corinthians 4:16: "though our outward man is corrupted, yet the inward man is renewed day by day." At its foundation, the "medical model" is on unsteady ground, always about to be knocked off balance by the changeable relation of body and soul.

This changeability gives rise to the heterogeneous, even contradictory, ways that bodies and souls refer to one another in homiletic literature. A diseased body often signifies a corrupted soul, and yet sometimes bodily corruption expresses spiritual exaltation. Healing may bespeak the soul's reconciliation to God, but sickness can also be the means to such reconciliation. This undecidability is apparent even in the decrees of the Fourth Lateran Council, which elsewhere draw a sharp opposition between "physicians of the body" (*medicis corporum*) and "physicians of the soul" (*medicos . . . animarum*)—"since the soul is much more precious than the body."[67] Nonetheless the same document relies on metaphors of bodily healing when it sets out to explain the proper workings of confession:

> The priest shall be discerning and prudent, so that like a skilled doctor he may pour wine and oil over the wounds of the injured one [*ut more periti medici superinfundat vinum et oleum vulneribus sauciati*]. Let him carefully inquire about the circumstances of both the sinner and the sin, so that he may prudently discern what sort of advice he ought to give and what remedy [*remedium*] to apply, using various means to heal the sick person [*diversis experimentis utendo ad sanandum aegrotum*].[68]

Here, the priest is instructed to model himself on the medical doctor, as soul is analogized to body. In the space of just two of the council's canons, then, the "medical model" shows its protean significance: the medical body is an apt metaphor for the care of souls even as that same body is the soul's competitor at the bedside of the sick. Such figural dynamism is in fact what gives medical similes their power in pastoral discourse. Rather than a routine equation between fleshly and spiritual levels, these analogies generate constant uncertainty about how literal and figurative levels interact, and thus the need for further spiritual discourse and reflection.[69]

Beyond this ceaseless work of saying both yes and no to the body, medicine's role in homiletic literature was also destabilized by the rhetorical friction between *exempla* and *similitudo*. Various late medieval preachers' manuals note the distinction: "*exemplum* is a narrative [*historia*] whilst *similitudo* is demonstrated by the thing itself."[70] Isidore of Seville, in a much-cited definition, explains *similitudo* as "that by which the description of some less known thing is made clear by something better known which is similar to it."[71] The similitude's analogical mapping between familiar and unfamiliar things operates very differently than narrative does. Analogy elaborates correspondences between vehicle and tenor, while the exemplum sets terms into narrative relation, contiguous in a shared matrix of causality. A story is likely to flatten out metaphor's two distinct planes, of materiality and spirituality, entangling them in a single network of forces—so that in a narrative portrayal of a miraculous cure, for instance, physicians and clerics might compete rather than signifying one another. Just as no settled decision can be reached about whether bodies are like or unlike souls, there can be no conclusion as to whether similitude or narrative best portrays their relation. The tensions among these possibilities gave the "medical model" much of its power as an instrument of pastoral discourse in the later Middle Ages.

The macaronic sermon collection in Oxford, Bodleian Library, Bodley MS 649 (which contains the elaborate conceit on fevers discussed above) is characteristic of late medieval preaching in its mixture of technical and colloquial accounts of medicine. Further engagement with *phisik*'s technicalities is evident in, for instance, the collection's references to "long-term illnesses, which according to the physicians are called chronic illnesses [*secundam phisicam vocantur morbi cronici*]"; to the "radical moisture [*humidi radicalis*]" thought to be slowly consumed as fuel for bodily life, here attributed to Aristotle; and in another extended nosological conceit, which moralizes the *corporales infirmates* suffered by Adam after his fall—the "swelling dropsy [*bolling dropesy*]," the "shivering palsy [*chyvringe palsy*]," and "a sorry blindness [*sory blindnes*]."[72] Following this account of Adam's illnesses, the "art of a good doctor [*Ars boni medici*]" is described: "first, to touch the pulse and the veins of the sick one [*tangere puus et infirmi venas*] to understand the distemper from which he suffers. Then he will prescribe a diet for him according to his sickness [*dietam suam secundum infirmitatem*]. Then he will make him an ointment of such flowers and herbs and lay it to his sore, and make him well [*and lay to his sore, et facere ipsum sanum*]. And in [the event] that the ulcer begin to infect all [*ulcus incipiat to infestre omnem*] to give him a preservative or a recipe that will drive it down again. Thus a doctor [*medicum*] must do."[73] The procedures of this medical art are then moralized through an extended analogy to "our artful doctor Christ [*artificiosus medicus noster Christus*]."[74]

However, in addition to such learned *similitudines*, sickness and healing also appear in the same sermon collection in less erudite iterations, in exemplary stories. In one, drawn from the *Gesta Romanorum*, two brothers contend over which of them truly possesses their father's magic ring, which is set with a "precious stone that has the power of curing the sick from his illness [*virtutem relevandi infirmos a sua infirmitate*]."[75] A sick man is brought before them both. The illegitimate ring has no effect on him, but "as soon as the true ring with the precious stone touched him he was cured [*sanabatur*]." Here, the sick body is a medium for registering causal force. The ring's stone is subsequently allegorized as Christ (*Christus est lapis*).[76] Another story, likewise drawn from the *Gesta Romanorum* (although referred to Jerome), tells of a "certain old man" in the desert one summer collecting herbs to cure the daughter of a noble lord in his care. As the man explains, "through foul fetid waters and corruption" the daughter has become "infected" and a "foul leper" (*inficitur and is become a foule lepur*).[77] In the moralization that follows, the daughter is glossed as the soul and the old man is the collective "you" addressed by the sermon, who are instructed, "while it is summer, while it is the time of grace and your life lasts in the body, seek the health-giving herbs [*salubres herbas*] of confession, contrition, and satisfaction, for without these herbs this lady cannot be saved [*sanari*]."[78] These two exempla show the mixing of narrative and allegorical logics that helps define healing's role in homiletic literature. In the context of the sermon collection, they also demonstrate the cheek-by-jowl juxtaposition of "unrealistic" models of bodily change alongside evocations of learned medicine.

Certain exempla circulating in late medieval England seem to thematize the interpretive difficulties that the unstable correlations of body and soul might pose for the individual Christian. For instance, a story in a Middle English sermon for Pentecost (in London, British Library, Additional MS 34888) stages their divergence with gentle irony: "*Bonus Theobaldus* was often ill. When he passed a year without being ill, he began to weep, believing that God had abandoned him."[79] For the devout Theobald, the commonsensical association of health and well-being is inverted. God's favor is manifest in bodily affliction, and his acceptance of this difficult truth marks his virtue. The exemplum occurs in the portion of the sermon describing "semiplenum gaudium," or the earthly state of being "half-full" of spiritual grace, in anticipation of the full joy to be found in heaven. It is preceded by various biblical citations warning against the satisfactions of present pleasures. Health, then, represents the joys of this world, and Theobald's unwillingness to value it shows his exemplary virtue. Part of the story's elegance, however, is that health also occupies its conventional place as a reward. *Bonus Theobaldus* cannot recognize the reward for his goodness on account of his goodness. The model of purifying, penitential sickness is crossed with the motif of virtue's health to stage the tensions between this life and the next that is the sermon's message.

A similar story, from the popular Middle English festial of John Mirk, reimagines corporeality's polysemousness in terms of one man's confusion. A devout man becomes ill and prays to Saint Thomas for help. He is cured according to the familiar intercessionary model—"and anon he was helyd." "But aftyr," the man begins to worry:

> he thoght that God send hym that sekenes for gret encrese of soule mede, and yede ageyne to Saynt Thomas prayng hym, yf hit wer more helpe to his soule to be secke then to be hoole, that he most be seke ageyne. Then anon the sekenes toke hym ageyn, and he thonkyd God and Saynt Thomas.[80]

> [he speculated that God had sent him that illness for the great increase of his soul's reward, and he went again to Saint Thomas, asking him that if it were more help to his soul to be sick than to be healthy, then he must be sick again. Then immediately the sickness seized him again, and he thanked God and Saint Thomas.]

Like the story of *Bonus Theobaldus*, this exemplum sets forth two models for understanding the relation of body and soul. The first emphasizes the etiology of the cure: Saint Thomas's miraculous power to heal is demonstrated. In the second, the stress falls on the divine etiology of sickness and its opportunity for "encrese of soule mede." The saint's again striking the man with disease confirms that it is "more helpe to his soule to be secke then to be hoole." The audience moves with the petitioner across different models of body-soul relation, progressing from the desirability of bodily health to a more perfect wish for spiritual health. The quick denouement, with the man's prayers of thanksgiving for the illness that "anon" afflicts him, confirms that the exemplum's transvaluation of health and illness has been recognized. *Sekenes* and "soule mede" become neatly identified.

Uncertainty about the moral and penitential status of sickness is the topic of advice in the *Ancrene Wisse*, a Middle English guide for anchoresses. The text explains,

> Secnesse is a brune hat forte tholien, ah na thing ne clenseth gold as hit deth the sawle. Secnesse thet Godd send—nawt thet sum lecheth thurh hire ahne dusischipe vor mani maketh hire sec thuruh hire fol herdischipe, auh this miscwemeth God.[81]

> [Sickness is a burning that causes powerful suffering, and no thing purifies gold as sickness does the soul—that is, sickness that God sends, not the sickness that some catch through their own ignorance, for many make themselves sick by their foolish feats of hardship, and this displeases God.]

An anchoress needs to understand the etiology of her illness, whether God has sent it to her or she has made herself sick through overzealous feats of asceticism. In other words, what kind of exemplum does she find herself living out? The former possibility implies a penitential model of infirmity, in which, like *Bonus Theobaldus* and the petitioner to Saint Thomas, the anchoress should recognize God's favor in the purifying force of suffering. The latter possibility suggests the dangers of actively pursuing the first, when penitential enthusiasm crosses over to pride. Illness, in this scenario, is the consequence of behavior not pleasing to God and thus resumes something of its status as punishment. The passage from the *Ancrene Wisse* continues, "Secnesse maketh mon to understonden hwet he is, to cnawen him seolven [Sickness compels man to understand what he is, and to know himself]." The anchoress is encouraged to parse the forces that shape her body and to distinguish her own agency from God's. As the body becomes the topic of reflective scrutiny, it becomes the medium for understanding "hwet" she is—how materialized, how produced and self-produced. The trickiness of distinguishing the two trains of causation in this scenario, God's gift of purgative suffering and the anchoress's mistaken enthusiasm for hardship, suggests the fineness of the etiological discernment necessary to interpret and embody sickness properly.

The variability and ambivalence expressed in medieval depictions of infirmity help to correct historiographic misperceptions of the period. In *longue durée* histories of the body, medieval culture is frequently accused of yoking disease and disfigurement unequivocally to divine punishment. However, in recent years revisionary scholarship has challenged the thesis that medieval infirmity was necessarily negative.[82] For instance, Irina Metzler's influential *Disability in Medieval Europe: Thinking About Physical Impairment in the High Middle Ages, c. 1100–c. 1400* debunks any monologic equivalence between impairment and sin. Drawing on the variousness of infirmity's causes in the Bible, Metzler argues for the "complexity, and ambiguity, of medieval attitudes towards sin and physical illness and impairment."[83] Similar developments have taken place in the study of medieval leprosy. While historians of the nineteenth and twentieth centuries often linked medieval leprosy unequivocally to ideas of contagion, punishment, and ostracism, a recent generation of medievalists has shown the insufficiency of these earlier accounts. Since the 1990s, revisionary scholars including François-Olivier Touati, Luke Demaitre, and Carole Rawcliffe have placed leprosy's negative associations within more complex and complete historical frameworks, demonstrating the changeability of the disease's significance across contexts.[84] Certainly, illness-as-punishment was a widespread plot device, but it did not apply to every scenario. It was rather a narrative habit, a ready-to-hand plot structure, that circulated alongside many other models of endowing bodies with significance.

The high stakes of interpreting body and soul properly are on display in the final passus of Langland's *Piers Plowman*. Throughout, the poem has employed the language of medicine, frequently as a *similitudo* for spiritual care and occasionally as a dangerously materialist craft to be regarded with suspicion.[85] This changeability in medicine's portrayal is bound up with the poem's profound ambivalence about the legitimacy of bodily need and the status of material *lifelode*. From Hunger to Hawkyn, Langland's engagements with corporeality both draw on metaphors that assume the analytical similarity of body and soul and then turn against that similarity as a source of dangerous confusion. Under the pressure of physical appetite, metaphors of body and soul become entangled; vehicle and tenor will not remain in straightforward signifying relation. Instead, both semantic levels crowd violently onto the poem's literal level, with body and soul seeming to compete.

Something of this dynamic is evident in the poem's final passus. As the army of Antichrist rages, Conscience calls up Kynde (Nature), who sweeps in with a battery of infirmities (in the words of the B-Text), "feveres and fluxes / Coughes and cardiacles [heart ailments], crampes and toothaches, / Rewmes and radegundes and roynouse scalles [Colds and running sores and unwholesome scabs], / Biles and bocches and brennynge agues [Boils and ulcers and burning fevers], / Frenesies and foul yveles [Frenzies and foul diseases]."[86] Elde (Old Age) is also summoned, who sends Life running "to Phisik after helpe."[87] In a neat bit of satire, Phisik proves vulnerable to Elde despite "dyas and drogges [remedies and drugs]": Elde "hitte / A phisicien with a furred hood, that fel in a palsie, / And there dyed that doctour er thre days after."[88] The joke is on Will too, who also receives a blow from Elde and cries out for vengeance. Will's injuries—he is struck bald, his teeth are beaten out of his mouth, and he becomes sexually impotent—are both comic and poignant. "Will" is here not the personification of a mental faculty but a personal name, attached to a body in time. Kynde advises him to retreat to the Barn of Unity. His bodily suffering evidently serves a positive, penitential function, but its harshness presages problems to come. His outrage testifies to his ongoing confusion here at the poem's end about what it means to suffer physically—a problem that eludes the sharp division of the battle lines.

The scene then shifts to the Barn of Unity, where bodily suffering has a different meaning. Those in the barn have been wounded by Hypocrisy, not by the plagues unleashed by Kynde in the midst of battle. But the ostensible shift from bodily harms (like those Will suffers from Elde) to spiritual harms (inflicted by the army of Antichrist) is belied by the continuities of one scene to the next, especially the atmosphere of besieged disorder. The battlefield and the barn share an ambience of mingled physical and spiritual disaster. Conscience calls for a *leche* to care for the barn's wounded. The initial physician, Shrift, at first appears successful, both in caring for those who need it and in making good on the system of salvific medical metaphors that the poem has relied on over the course of the visions. But soon enough, the system comes under strain, as Sire Leef-to-lyve-in-lecherie requests a surgeon that "softe kan handle" and "fairer . . . plastreth."[89] The literal body becomes more and more materially prominent, as Sire Leef complains that fasting on Fridays will be the death of him, and Peace reports that someone like the new *surgien* "salvede so oure wommen til some were with childe."[90] At last, Friar Flatterer so salves and plasters Contrition that "contricion he lafte, / That is the soverayneste salve for alle kynne [all kinds of] synnes."[91] With this line, salve negates "the soverayneste salve," and Contrition is made to contradict himself. The difficulty of keeping bodily and spiritual registers apart means that the Barn of Unity is no stronghold against attack, and Conscience abandons it, setting off to find Piers Plowman. For Langland, the restless incongruities of the "medical model" in late medieval pastoralia echo the Christian subject's interminable relation to sin and the demands of the body.

The Bodies That Exempla Make

At the climax of "Merelaus the Emperour," a story from the *Gesta Romano-rum*, four men stand before the good and faithful empress they have wronged. She is at this point in disguise, hiding in a convent where she has acquired a reputation as a great healer. Ignorant of her true identity, her several erstwhile persecutors have come in hopes of a cure. The brother of the emperor, who abandoned her naked in a forest, has become a "foul lypre [leper]"; the knight who framed her for murder is now "def and blynde"; the servant who betrayed her is "haltyng [lame]"; and the ship's captain who abducted her is "halfe out of mynde."[92] The narration emphasizes the connection between each man's crime and his ailment by listing them in tidy juxtaposition. Infirmity is the shorthand in which the diegetic universe inscribes the men's pasts on their persons: what had been their actions in the plot—their attempts at rape, incrimination, and betrayal—are recoded in their flesh.

This bodily disfigurement takes place by means of a causal force that the narration leaves unspecified. Despite the vaguely Christian setting (the empress is in a convent), it is not God per se who inscribes their respective illnesses on their bodies. Instead, infirmity and disfigurement seem simply to happen, and, in happening, they register the distinctive logic of the exemplary plot. The plots of exempla are generally concerned to make each element—their sparsely realized characters and quickly sketched settings and props—subject to their general ordering function. This underexplained, force-saturated atmosphere might even be identified with the story form's *chronotope*, or (in the words of Mikhail Bakhtin) "the intrinsic connectedness of [its] temporal and spatial relationships."[93] According to Bakhtin, distinctive conjugations of time and space give narrative genres their particularity, and exempla invite us to extend Bakhtin's notion to include factors like the connectedness of one event to another. In "Merelaus the Emperour," the circuit of translation that runs from the men's transgressions to their suffering bodies and finally to their confessions manifests the plot's centripetal energy of totalization. It is this sequence of transgression and correction, deceit and revelation, that makes the plot's ordering power apprehensible.

Among the four stricken men, it is the brother of the emperor who receives the greatest narrative attention. He is the character who betrays the empress first, the story's archvillain. As the men stand before the empress, the grotesqueness of his leprosy is vividly described, with worms that "sprunge out at the visage on ech syde [sprung out of his face on each side]."[94] The disguised empress announces that before she can cure him, he must make a public confession. His stricken body is made to function like a riddle, only to be healed by the translation of symptoms into self-narration. Initially the brother confesses only partially, leaving out any mention of the empress or his mistreatment of her. She appeals to the emperor, "'Sir, if I putte medecyne to him, it is but veyn that I do, for he is not yit fully confessid.'"[95] The emperor then turns to his sick brother and demands incredulously, "'Seist thou not wele [Do you not well see], that thou art a lothly lypr [loathsome leper]? Wolt [Will] thou not telle all forth, that thou may be maade hoole [healthy] and cleene?'"[96]

The two rulers in the story, empress and emperor, serve as mouthpieces for what could be termed the plot's sovereign imperative, namely, that all of its components finally speak the same authorized version of events. The emperor's words to his brother are especially striking in this regard. He demands that his brother "see well" that he is a leper and on the basis of such chastened self-perception "telle all forth" and confess what the story requires—a reiteration and admission of what has happened, of what the tale has already told. This imperative insists on a detour through the brother's self-consciousness, to translate symptoms into voice. The plot, we might say, is hungry to get inside the emperor's wicked brother. His most notable quality throughout the story has been his dishonesty—or, to put it in positive terms, the free play between his appearance and his self-knowledge, his disclosures and his desires. His constant deceptions have created the figure of a subjectivity in hiding, menacingly concealed beneath appearances. The brother's refusal of frank confession is a refusal of the exemplum's narrative imperative, that all of its elements finally wear the mark of the plot's telos.

The pulse of silence before the brother's full confession is the point of greatest torsion in the narrative workings of "Merelaus the Emperor." The centripetal energy of the exemplum's plot, which tends to swallow up narrative elements into its momentum, here strains against the brother's dishonesty, this figure of privacy that holds back, briefly, from the exemplary imperative to open revelation. He is where the exemplum ciphers its resistance to its own totalizing, self-indicating cohesion. His deceptiveness throughout the tale exemplifies the provisional freedom that different facets of narrative enjoy, and his initial refusal to confess, even as his body is being consumed, temporarily slips the narrative logic to which he is finally subjected. And in this torsion, this grinding of narrative dynamics, the brother barely holds his bodily coherence. The corporeal locus of his identity—his *visage*, or literally his *seen-ness*—is being devoured by worms. The force of plot against character assumes fleshly palpability. Simultaneously, of course, the brother's disfiguring leprosy can be understood to figure forth his true character, disclosing as symptoms his unconfessed actions. His body stages at once defacement and revelation, disfiguration and figuration. This is in part, I think, what exempla are designed to do—to show the aesthetics of emplotment acting on bodies as personae are made to suffer and embody ideological imperatives. Soon enough the brother confesses, his illness disappears, and the sovereignty of empress and narrative order are reconfirmed.

Exemplary illness is a long-standing technique of narrative meaning-making, which generates its significance in historically and discursively specific contexts. These contexts, as it turns out, could vary wildly. The collection of which "Merelaus the Emperour" is a part is known as the *Gesta Romanorum*, compiled around 1300, perhaps in England and almost certainly as a resource for preachers. The collection survives in well over two hundred manuscript versions, including at least thirty-six from medieval England.[97] Four are in Middle English. Perhaps the most unusual feature of the *Gesta Romanorum* is its elaborately allegorizing morals, a point I have left aside until now. In the case of "Merelaus the Emperour," the moral explains that the emperor represents "our lord ihesu crist," the empress, "the sowle of man," and the emperor's brother, mankind as such.[98] These moralizations—which were in many cases superadded to preexisting stories compiled from other sources[99]—introduces the logic of *similitudo*. Rather than transforming the causal entailment of plot into a precept operative for other scenes of practical deliberation (as exempla typically do), these allegorizing morals jump to a different ontological plane, that of the universalized Christian's spiritual struggle, and they try to locate the tale's governing logic there. Such interpretive paratext cuts against the tales' power of narrative meaning-making by abandoning the link between emplotment and *telos*. Some manuscripts of the *Gesta Romanorum*, like Cambridge, Cambridge University Library MS Kk.1.6, contain no moralizations. In the version of "Merelaus the Emperour" included in Hoccleve's *Series*, the moralization is first forgotten and then added, as though to emphasize its contingent relation to the tale. The same exemplum, then, could signify in exceedingly various ways depending on its hermeneutic frame.

Even apart from its setting within the *Gesta Romanorum*, the basic plot of "Merelaus the Emperour" was subject to numerous acts of reimagination during the Middle Ages. Its analogues include a closely related tradition of Marian miracles (recorded most influentially by Vincent of Beauvais) as well as a portion of Nicholas Trivet's chronicle of world history, which was the source for Chaucer's "Man of Law's Tale" and Gower's "Tale of Constance." A version of the story appears in the Middle English exemplum collection the *Alphabet of Tales*. In these several versions, there is no allegorizing moral. The manuscript London, British Library, Harley MS 7333 (the basis for the edition of "Merelaus the Emperour" quoted here) contains its Middle English translation of the *Gesta Romanorum* alongside imperfect versions of Chaucer's *Canterbury Tales* and Gower's *Confessio Amantis*. Thus, as it happens, the single manuscript includes "Merelaus" together with its analogues the "Man of Law's Tale" and the "Tale of Constance." Manly and Rickert describe Harley 7333 as a "library of secular literature," which suggests that readers of this manuscript would have approached interpreting "Merelaus the Emperour" very differently than if they had heard it incorporated into a sermon or found it among pastoralia.[100] Within these frameworks of contextual reinvention, it is not possible to know just what the story meant in the later Middle Ages. Certainly its durable plot, with its mechanics of exemplary infirmity and healing, served a varied range of rhetorical ends.

Another narrative from the *Gesta Romanorum*, "Bononius the Emperour," likewise entails the coordination of symptoms and speech in a contest over who controls the causal logic of emplotment. "Bononius" is a tale of "thre lechis [physicians]" in Rome who grow jealous of their emperor's favorite doctor, Averoys, who is "sotill in crafte, and a good practiser."[101] (*Averoys* is presumably a variation on "Averroes," the Latinized name of Ibn Rushd [d. 1198], the Andalusian physician, philosopher, and Aristotelian commentator.) The plot of "Bononius" revolves around the scandal of characters who usurp the power to make someone sick, a power that in other stories belongs to the unfolding of the plot. Here it is achieved by speech acts internal to the story. The ringleader of the "thre lechis," in a scheme to get rid of their rival and master Averoys, alights on what he thinks is the perfect crime. "'And we shul distroy him withoute any hurt,'" he remarks to his two co-conspirators and then continues:

> "Somday we shul passe oute of this cite to visite seke men of his
> cure, and I shal stond in his wey, and that fer from the citee, by the
> space of a myle. And whan he comyth to me-ward, I shal lifte up
> myn hond, and make upon me the signe of the crosse, and I shal
> sey, Allas! allas! maister, what eileth the, thou art lepre? And oon
> of you shal stond fro me the space of ii. or iii. myle; and when he

comyth to him, he shall afferme my word, and sey as I seid. And
the thrid of us shall be thre or four myle beyonde; and when he
seth him nye, he shal begynne to go, and make lamentacion, and
seyn, oute, alas! my maistre is ymade lepre. And when he seth us
alle accorde in oon, he shall trow in us, and then for drede he shal
bycome lepre; for so a lepre may be made."[102]

["One day, we will leave the city to visit sick men in his care, and
I will stand along his path a mile outside the city. And when he
comes toward me, I will lift up my hand and make the sign of the
cross, and I will say, 'Alas, alas, what is wrong with you, sir? Are you
a leper?' And one of you will stand two or three miles from me, and
when he comes upon him, he will affirm my words and say as I said.
And the third of us will be three or four miles beyond, and when he
sees him nigh, he shall begin to make lamentation and say, 'Alas, my
master is made leprous.' And when he sees us all agree together, he
will believe us, and then for dread he will become leprous—for so a
leper may be made."]

Leprosy, the physician claims, can be *made*, through words and their reception. Ignoring the material causes of leprosy except as a screen for his malicious plan, the jealous doctor focuses on the disease's production through
language—which is the same power that the exemplum itself usually commands. In "Merelaus the Emperour," the brother's leprosy operates as a narrative reality principle that curtails the character's self-fashioning through
rhetoric and deception. At the start of "Bononius the Emperour," by contrast,
rhetoric and deception are held to produce corporeal reality.

As Averoys rides out, he meets the first conspirator. "'Maister, what eileth
you?'" the scheming physician asks. "'Nought but good,'" Averoys replies,
"'what, whi seist thou so? what seest thou in me?'"[103] In this series of phrases,
Averoys slips from confident assertion to an admission of his dependence
on another's perspective: "'what seest thou in me?'" This is the condition of
the symptomatic subject, to have one's physical form expressing something
beyond the ambit of one's own awareness. Like Chaucer's Summoner, whose
scabbed face is reflected back to him in the fear of children, Averoys cannot
quite dismiss this perspective that sees what lies outside his first-person point
of view. "'Forsoth I se thou art lepre,'" the conspirator replies. Although Averoys calls the man a liar and rides on with a show of bravado, "Nevertheles he

dradde moche of the forseid word, and gretly dullid therwith [Nevertheless he felt much dread because of the exchange, and he greatly deadened on account of it].” Meeting the second conspirator, who laments his condition, Averoys repeats his panicked, poignant question, “‘what seest thou in me?’” and the conspirator replies, “‘thou art a grete lepre.’” After hearing the third conspirator’s pitying salutation, Averoys “thought, that hit myght not be fals, that thre had so affermed; and toke so grete drede, that, he becom a foule lepre.”[104]

It would be possible, with the system of Joannitian non-naturals, to offer a medicalized explanation for this infection. Humoral theory linked dread to black bile, and a predominance of the melancholic humor could contribute to leprosy. But the story of “Bononius the Emperour” does not encourage materialist explanations for the physicians’ success, and the instantaneous effects of their diagnosis eschew verisimilitude. Instead, the narrative’s rhetorical energy is invested in the dialogue between the three jealous physicians and Averoys. The story stages the volatility of the exemplary body, its tremulous sensitivity to redefinition by the ordering operations of the story. For Averoys, the accord of three opinions rises to the level of truth—“hit myght not be fals, that thre had so affermed”—and this shared judgment transforms Averoys. This version of bodily change undercuts the moral authority of nature on display in “Merelaus the Emperor” and many other exemplary stories, where bodily change exposes human deception. It is the jealous physicians’ seizing control over bodily change—their usurpation of the diffuse “way of happening” that typically causes sickness and healing in exempla—for which the story ultimately punishes them.

The conclusion of “Bononius the Emperour” reinstitutes a properly “natural” (though not naturalistic) causality for disease by reasserting the sovereign monopoly on violence. Averoys, drawing on his medical know-how, heals himself in a bath of goat’s blood, and his surprisingly quick recovery allows him to conclude that “‘I was not smyten with lepre naturelly.’”[105] In punishment, the emperor orders the conspirators “to be drawe to the gybet [gibbet], atte the tailles of the hors, & so made hem to be hongid.”[106] Such public, juridical violence stands as the inverted image of the physicians’ machinations to destroy Averoys “withoute any hurt.” The propriety of the emperor’s justice is confirmed by the once-again trustworthy voice of social consensus (now that the *lechis’* false diagnostic accord has been exposed): “And all men hily [highly] commendid the emperour, that he had yoven [given] so just a dome [judgment].” *Dome* is a Middle English word that denotes a medical opinion as well as a legal ruling and act of justice, and the story would seem to restore the distinctiveness of these meanings.[107] The emperor is aligned with the exemplum's own controlling power to make norms palpable on characters' bodies, while the physicians ought to be subject to those norms and to issue their own *domes* in conformity with the diegetic world. And yet at the same time, the jealous conspirators have shown the power of language to remake the bodies that ought to testify to the naturalized causal order of narrative.

The *Gesta Romanorum*'s moralization of "Bononius the Emperor" is a freewheeling turn through the *similitudines* that yoke physical and spiritual care. The physician Averoys is "a discrete confessour," who has to "deme [judge] thi lyfe, and to considre the uryne of contricion, and by that he moste [must] ordeine for medicynes of penaunce."[108] But then again, Averoys bathing in goat's blood is like each Christian—"so let us fill oure hertes with good and meritory dedis or werkis, and let us be bathid therin."[109] The emplotted logic of the story is here discarded for a series of allegorical riffs upon the flexible analogy of body and soul. Indeed, the fundamental polysemousness of exemplary bodies in stories like "Merelaus" and "Bononius" suggest that, at their bedrock, such tales are not about teaching a particular content but are aesthetic forms allowing audiences to watch and experience the causal interplay between bodies and norms.

This chapter has focused on the narrative logic of exempla, which are forms of etiological thought that mediate between the causal logic emplotted in concrete events and the general precepts pertaining both to narrative and to the audience's world. The dense interpretive webs in which late medieval bodies took on significance meant that narrative exemplification always operated in generative interaction with other semantic codes and rhetorical procedures. In stories from the *Gesta Romanorum* like "Merelaus" and "Bononius," narrative and allegorical logics unfolded alongside one another, in partial complementarity and partial contradiction. Similarly, the works discussed in the next four chapters all deploy plural etiological and interpretive systems for understanding bodily change, and all make their meaning amid the friction of these systems' differing claims.

PART III

Emplotting *Phisik*

Chapter 5

The Metaphysics of *Phisik*
in the "Knight's Tale"

At a crucial turning point in Geoffrey Chaucer's "Knight's Tale," the narration erupts into the language of medicine. In this first of the Canterbury tales, the sudden density of physiological terms occurs just when the fates of the cousins Arcite and Palamon are pulling irrevocably apart. Prior to the tale's climactic tournament, the near perfect sameness of the Theban knights, especially in their competing claims to the maiden Emelye, has constituted the narrative's central conundrum. Chaucer altered his source, Giovanni Boccaccio's *Teseida*, to heighten the cousins' similarity and so to cast their equality as the main obstacle to the romance's narrative closure.[1] The apparent arbitrariness of any choice between them concentrates interpretive attention on the tale's resolution. Not just the knights' respective fates but also the ordering operations of the narrative world hang in the balance, awaiting disclosure. *Phisik*, when it obtrudes into the narration, serves to mark the harrowing materialization of Arcite's person and to task readers with unraveling the causes behind his broken form.

The urgency of understanding *why* Arcite dies is heightened by another set of changes that Chaucer rang on his sources. He multiplies the entities that make things happen. Causation is rendered more multifarious and more mysterious than it is in the *Teseida*—shared out among psychological compulsion, knightly prowess, empathic responsiveness, political calculation, planetary influence, meddling pagan deities, benevolent providence, chance, fate, literary tradition, and narratorial whim. These are forces with decidedly different ontologies, which exert influence from incommensurate levels or modes of being. To interpret Arcite's injury, to give an account of why it happens and what it means, demands that readers adjudicate among these heterogeneous operative powers. The tale culminates in an etiological puzzle.

When narrative closure does arrive, its meaning and suitability remain open to debate. At least since Charles Muscatine's 1950 essay "Form, Texture, and Meaning in Chaucer's *Knight's Tale*," the task of determining the relative claims of "noble designs and chaos" has been recognized as central to the tale's interpretation.[2] Questions of whether the diegetic world and the literary work are harmonious are posed in miniature with respect to Theseus's famous speech of consolation after Arcite's death, which centers on the "Firste Moevere of the cause above," a transcendent deity who gives order to the universe.[3] The Athenians listening to Theseus's consolation, like Chaucer's readers, face the riddle of why things happen as they do—why Arcite lies "in his colde grave / Allone, withouten any compaignye" and Palamon is "lyvynge in blisse, in richesse, and in heele [health]" (2778–79, 3102). The duke's oration, which seeks to resolve all intermediary causes to an absolute cause, and "every part" to its "hool [whole]" (3006), does not so much explain the narrative convolutions that have preceded it as dismiss their salience. Some critics have followed Muscatine in seeing Theseus's speech as a hard-fought achievement of moral and metaphysical integration.[4] Others have argued that the duke's account is undermined by his own will to power and by the forces of violence and chance at work in the world of the tale.[5] From either vantage, Arcite's death sends a current of etiological retrospection—*why?*—back through the rest of the narrative. Arcite's deathbed questions become those of the audience as well: "'What is this world? What asketh men to have?'" (2777). Not unlike the grief-stricken Athenian mourners, readers find themselves asking Arcite, "'Why woldestow be deed? [Why would you be dead?]'" (2835). These queries turn out to be at once etiological and hermeneutic, moral and cosmological.

This chapter argues that Arcite's body is at the center of the tale's thinking against totality, which is to say, its efforts to imagine and represent what is not whole (what is fragmentary or in a state of becoming) as well as what escapes incorporation into unity (what is wasted, lost, or errant). I do not go so far as to claim that the "Knight's Tale" endorses chaos over design—but that, as all its best readers have observed, it is deeply ambivalent about its own structures of coherence and evolves a host of literary means for disturbing them. That Arcite's death poses serious philosophical problems for the tale's resolution is acknowledged by the cosmic sweep and grandeur of Theseus's speech; its weightiness implies the heft of the events it is balanced against. The pages that follow seek to give an account of the several aesthetic, discursive, and narrative disruptions that are routed through Arcite's body over the course of the tale.

One of these disruptions takes place through the language of medicine.[6] When he is dying, Arcite is exposed as being made of material stuffs and shot through with the physical forces of the universe. Described in the terms of learned medicine, he disaggregates into a melee of subpersonal causes. *Phisik* in the Middle Ages exercised what might be termed a strategic materialism, a pragmatically physicalizing regard trained on the material world, on palpable effects, and on the biological life of individual bodies. Only in satire would medicine avow such materialism as doctrine, and medical writers readily admitted their art's subordination to the divine matters of theology and the *scientia* of natural philosophy.[7] And yet, when Theseus offers his Neoplatonic theodicy as counterpoint to Arcite's medicalized death, the duke implicitly invites his audience to think of *phisik* as a kind of metaphysics—one that the duke is intent to argue against. The stridency of Theseus's consolation speech has a consolidating effect, acting to amalgamate as one threat all of the tale's shadowy alternatives to monotheistic order. This means that a cosmology of medicine becomes imaginable. The milieu of pagan Greece, I will contend, is a part of this. It functions as a thought experiment at the unraveling edge of totality—a cosmos of squabbling forces unsupervised by any sovereign deity and a form of life without afterlife, which is to say, for which death is annihilation. Paganism's metaphysical conditions correspond to the practical domain of the medical art, concerned as it is with proximate causes and mortal bodies. In the "Knight's Tale," the materialist specters of untotality are made to circulate around and through Arcite's medicalized body.

"No aspect of *The Knight's Tale* is so difficult to interpret as the circumstances of Arcite's death," writes Edward Schweitzer. "It is, in fact, Arcite's death and the manner of its presentation that above all make the meaning of the whole elusive."[8] The possibility that Arcite's flesh might short-circuit what Schweitzer calls "the meaning of the whole" has consequences, I argue, for the narrative poetics of the whole first fragment of the *Canterbury Tales*. If Theseus posits a stability within and beyond the flux of creaturely life, which operates as its law, Arcite's corporeality asks about a different cosmos, one of perpetual loss and becoming. This cosmos is in some ways quite close to the vision that Lee Patterson has located (in a historical register) in the *Thebanness* of the poem, or the "self-destructive rivalry that gives full rein to the violence of the appetitive self" and the "fatal recursiveness that undermines all progressivity."[9] Chaucer's metaphysics of *phisik* locates a similar energy of dissolution in the natural world. In its strongest version, this vision threatens to dissolve the forms of totality from within, whether those forms are metaphysical or literary. As the "Knight's Tale" wends to its conclusion, it will itself come to function as a rebel component in the larger social, philosophical, and literary whole in which it participates. Ultimately I argue that, as Fragment I of the *Canterbury Tales* continues, the Miller appears as a second Arcite, only this time the power of mutability that Theseus's consolation has sought to subordinate, that of counterfactual emergence, breaks forth.

Phisik's Body

The "Knight's Tale" initially gives the impression that it will resolve itself within the balanced architectural framework built to cordon Palamon and Arcite's violence—and also within the decorum and conventions of historical romance. With much pomp, the knights' two armies clash on the field of the new Athenian stadium, and Arcite ekes out a victory. Watching the scene, Theseus declares, "'Hoo! namoore, for it is doon! / I wol be trewe juge, and no partie [partisan]. / Arcite of Thebes shal have Emelie'" (2656–58). Yet the pronouncement of this "trewe juge" turns out to be false. Just as Arcite rides forward to encounter Emelye, the scene shudders with a chthonic interruption: "out of the ground a furie infernal sterte" (2684). Bursting from the earth, the "myracle," as it is called, punctures the edifice of the stadium and obviates the careful rules made so that the combatants "shal nat dye" (2675, 2541). Arcite's horse takes fright and shakes its rider violently. He lies momentarily motionless as though dead, blackened with the "blood yronnen in his face," before being carried to Theseus's palace, "alwey criynge after Emelye" (2693, 2699).

When the narration returns to Arcite, it is within a radically different lexical framework. Just as a "furie infernal" starts from the tournament grounds, so an unexpected register of language burst into the courtly romance—the technical language of medieval medicine:

Swelleth the brest of Arcite, and the soore
Encreesseth at his herte moore and moore.
The clothered blood, for any lechecraft,
Corrupteth, and is in his bouk ylaft,
That neither veyne-blood, ne ventusynge,

Ne drynke of herbes may ben his helpynge.
The vertu expulsif, or animal,
Fro thilke vertu cleped natural
Ne may the venym voyden ne expelle.
The pipes of his longes gonne to swelle,
And every lacerte in his brest adoun
Is shent with venym and corrupcioun.
Hym gayneth neither, for to gete his lif,
Vomyt upward, ne dounward laxatif. (2743–56)

[Arcite's chest swells, and the injury (or pain) at his heart increases
more and more. In spite of any medical skill, the clotted blood
turns fetid and remains in his torso, so that neither bloodletting
nor cupping nor herbal remedy can help him. The expulsive, or
animal, power, which derives from that power called natural, may
not remove the poison nor expel it. The pipes of his lungs began
to swell, and every muscle down his chest is clogged with poison
and corruption. Neither purgatives nor laxatives help him maintain
his life.]

In these lines, the language of *phisik* ostentatiously draws attention to itself.
A handful of words have here their earliest recorded uses. *Ventosinge, expulsif,
animal* (adj.), *expellen, lacerte*, and the compound *veyne-blood* each appears for
the first time, and all but one has its next documented appearance in medical
or scientific writing.[10] This is markedly technical vocabulary, and in shifting
abruptly from the idiom of classicized romance to that of learned medicine,
Chaucer would have been aware of giving his readers pause. The passage's
insistent technicalism is also evident in the constraint it puts on terms of more
general usage. *Blood, soore, herte*, and *vertu* are all richly polysemous, and by
this point in the "Knight's Tale" the narration has employed them repeatedly,
layering upon each a diegetically specific resonance. Yet at Arcite's sickbed, the
words signify narrowly, their semantic resonance muffled. Despite its lexical
novelty, the passage manages to be strikingly repetitive. Within the span of
fourteen lines, *swelle, brest, soore, vertu, venym*, and *corrupteth* all repeat, either
nearly or exactly. The lines' choppy negations and alien, insistent lexicon create something of a formal correlative for Arcite's clogged and failing body.

The passage stands out for additional examination because it departs
sharply from Boccaccio's portrayal of the same scene. In the *Teseida*, no similar

scientific terminology appears, yet Boccaccio does include a bedside physician, "the great Idmon of Epidaurus [*il grande Itmon venire / d'Epidauria*]."[11] Examining Arcita, Idmon declares straightaway that the patient is as good as dead, and a doctor is useless ("il vostro Arcita è morto veramente, / né luogo ci ha di medico valore").[12] The great physician invokes the work of medical science only in its loftiest, most aureate terms, under the names of Asclepius and Apollo, even though these healing deities are unable to help. The effect of Boccaccio's passage, then, is to exempt Arcita from medical technicalities and to uphold the tragic nobility of his impending death. The "Knight's Tale," by contrast, mires Arcite in the crisscrossing forces of the material world. Ever attuned to the language of craft and profession, Chaucer nonetheless excises the figure of the medical doctor who might have grounded the passage's technical terminology in the social life of discourse. Instead, it seems to arise out of the corrupting body itself.[13]

The medical description also transforms how readers see Arcite. The young Theban knight is the focus of the scene, but it is not he who acts. The grammatical subjects of the sentences are all *within* Arcite or *part* of him—"the brest of Arcite," "the soore," "the clothered blood," "the vertu expulsif," "The pipes of his longes," "vomyt [purgative medicine]," and "laxatif." The passage insists on the subhuman granularity of life. This is pitched battle, but it takes place not among combatants but between the body's impulse to circulate its fluids and a counterprocess of coagulation, as the thickening blood gathers in the knight's chest. In the vocabulary of *phisik*, this is *vertu* versus *corrupcioun*. Each of these terms is mentioned twice in Arcite's medical description, and both will be reinvoked in Theseus's final speech of consolation. Despite their ethical valence in other contexts, *vertu* and *corrupcioun* are here pointedly naturalistic. In medieval pathology, corruption was among the most common causes of disease, and it referred to the morbid state of a substance, often a humor, transformed by an imbalance of its qualities or some tainting admixture. Faith Wallis explains that the concept's "core metaphor is one of putrefaction: an internal disease is visualized as a collection of rotting organic matter that needs to be diverted away from important organs and then evacuated, or as an internal wound that is suppurating with diseased matter."[14] Just so, Arcite bleeds internally, and his unevacuated blood begins to rot. Here, then, what was a component of the physical creature undergoes a toxic change, in a process that exemplifies the disquieting partibility and mutability of the physical self. To be a living creature, subject to the explanations of *phisik*, means being made out of matter that can turn venomous, rebel against the organism that contains and regulates it. The subject's embodied agency is dependent on other scales of inhuman powers.

Vertu is a word of sprawling semantic range in Middle English; indeed, the *Middle English Dictionary* lists nineteen definitions.[15] In Arcite's medical description, however, it is perhaps the most constrained of terms. It is crabbed round with the signs of Latinate translation, nigglingly specified, and then portrayed as drastically unsuccessful: "The vertu expulsif, or animal, / Fro thilke vertu cleped natural / Ne may the venym voyden ne expelle" (2749–51). The tripartite Galenic scheme of *virtutes* undergirds this reference, which was known through its inclusion in the Joannitian scheme of naturals, non-naturals, and contra-naturals. The *res naturales* were the vital components of living creatures, and they included the *virtutues* together with the body's elements, mixtures of qualities, humors, members, faculties, and spirits. The virtues were divided into three—*virtus naturalis, spiritualis,* and *animalis*— and they carried out the major functions of life: the natural virtue was responsible for nutrition, growth, and reproduction; the spiritual virtue handled respiration, heat, and emotion; and the animal virtue was in control of sensation, voluntary motion, and cognition.[16] In the description of Arcite in the "Knight's Tale," the lines' attempt to allude to a hierarchy of causation—with the "vertu expulsif, or animal" deriving from the "vertu cleped natural"—is somewhat confused in terms of physiological theory, but it succeeds in evoking a complex hierarchy of forces operative within the embodied self. As the Joannitian scheme implies, the body is a composite thing that sustains life by means of an intricate series of microevents.

In this sickbed scene, Chaucer chooses to present Arcite's fate in the framework of what might be called *phisik*'s body. This body—trafficked by humors, responsive to innumerable contingent factors, ceaselessly calibrating its qualities of heat and moisture—came to be newly remarked, understood, and written about in the late fourteenth century when the "Knight's Tale" was composed, as previous chapters have detailed. The dissemination of medical knowledge took place at widely varying degrees of intellectual sophistication, but all of it centered on the model of a dynamic body strafed with causal forces and ceaselessly recalibrating itself. Avicenna's *Canon* gives a paradigmatic account of *phisik*'s body in its discussion of complexion: "The complexion is that quality which results from the mutual interaction and interpassion of the four contrary primary qualities [heat, cold, wetness, dryness] residing within the elements. These elements are so minutely intermingled as to lie in very intimate relationship to one another. Their opposite powers alternately conquer and become conquered until a quality is reached which is uniform throughout the whole; this is the complexion."[17] It is embodiment conceived in these terms, as the medium of "interaction and interpassion" and of inhuman conquest, that the "Knight's Tale" invokes in its rendering of Arcite's interior. His constituent substances evidently play out their drama without any supervising intelligence. As Joel Kaye has brilliantly shown, this aspect of Galenism undergirded intellectual optimism about the possibility of self-ordering systems in the late thirteenth and early fourteenth centuries: "Within the working whole, faith in the systematic process of interior self-ordering replaces the need for an external orderer or overarching ordering intelligence."[18] The "Knight's Tale," however, invokes *phisik*'s teeming and dynamic body without any confidence in the outcome. The scene of Arcite's suppurating wound dramatizes the chaotic underside of physiology's recalibrations, where the interplay of physical powers gradually render life impossible. The forces of life and morbidity churn beneath the threshold of awareness, and they redound catastrophically on the experience of the human subject.

The perspective from which the sickbed passage is narrated is a peculiar one. Arcite's body becomes the space through which the narrating vantage moves—to his chest, at his heart, in his torso, lungs, muscles, upward, downward, throughout "thilke regioun" entirely "tobrosten" (2757). The shift to the present tense effects immediacy and vividness, but here it also makes the passage's words seem performative, as if they were accomplishing the decomposition they describe. The unsettling descriptive style arguably links Arcite's sickbed to another crucial episode in the tale, the elaborate ekphrasis of the temple-wall paintings, which constitutes much of the tale's third section. V. A. Kolve describes these ekphrastic passages as "modally indeterminate, spatially unfixed, and devoid of any clear structure."[19] The paintings, he continues, "can be imagined in their parts but not as wholes."[20] Kolve's characterization captures the effects of Arcite's medicalization too, which decomposes the knight within an indeterminately focalized gaze, seemingly produced out of Arcite's permeable body. The temple paintings, as Kolve notes, "combine mythographic and astrological traditions" and "emphasize malign planetary influence above all else."[21] These paintings too, then, are about the causal forces that impinge on and undergird human life. From planets to the medical "naturals," causal power gathers at scales above and below the human and disturbs the regularities of narration. The curiously untotalizable quality of Arcite's wounded body and of the temples' picture planes, which are (as

Kolve says) imaginable as parts but not wholes, result from the verses' efforts to represent the teeming forces of human determination, natural and supernatural respectively.

An earlier episode in the tale foreshadows the scientific register in which Arcite's final injuries will be described.[22] It takes place when Arcite is exiled from Athens and his beloved Emelye. He cannot eat or sleep. He cries and moans through the night, and over the course of "a yeer or two" his appearance changes: "lene he wex and drye as is a shaft; / His eyen holwe and grisly to biholde, / His hewe falow and pale as asshen colde [He grew lean and dry as a stick; his eyes were sunken and terrible to behold, and his hue was sickly yellow and pale as cold ashes]" (1381, 1362–64). The narrator reports that Arcite seems to be suffering not only from lovesickness but also mania:

> he ferde
> Nat oonly lik the loveris maladye
> Of Hereos, but rather lyk manye,
> Engendred of humour malencolik
> Biforen, in his celle fantastik. (1372–76)

[He behaved not only like he had the lovers' malady called *Hereos*, but rather like he had mania, engendered by the melancholic humor in the imaginative chamber (of his brain).]

The double diagnosis of "Hereos" and "manye [mania]," together with the etiology of black bile in the imaginative cell of the brain, functions to cast his love into a material, physiological register. The medicalization appears to be a deliberate stylistic choice: Chaucer adapts the parallel passage in the *Teseida* (IV.26–28) by adding the disease names and the humoral explication.[23] The pathologization of love is conventional in chivalric romance,[24] so, unlike Arcite's jarring medicalization after the tournament, these details of pathology do not interrupt the style of the tale. However, they do help establish *phisik* as an idiom for heteronomy. During his lovesickness, those elements of self that would seem to give consistency to Arcite's character, "Bothe habit and eek disposicioun," are turned "al up so doun [entirely upside-down]" (1379, 1378)—a metaphor of reversal that is literalized more than a thousand lines later, when Arcite's horse shies before the "furie," and "pighte hym on the pomel of his heed [pitched him onto the crown of his head]" (2689). Further foreshadowing occurs in the comparison of Arcite's pallor to "asshen colde," previewing the moment when his corpse is incinerated, "brent [burned] to asshen colde" (2957). Like Arcite's early exclamations that Emelye's "fresshe beautee sleeth me sodeynly" and that he is "but deed" without her mercy (1118, 1122), the account of his lovesickness becomes lit up with retrospective significance only after Arcite's fate is revealed and the puzzle of the story's end demands rereading and reinterpretation.

In this initial episode of lovesickness, Arcite finds a way to reclaim his physiologically alienated body. He is urged by Mercury in a dream to return to Athens, and his first action thereafter is to find a mirror:

> And with that word he caughte a greet mirour,
> And saugh that chaunged was al his colour,
> And saugh his visage al in another kynde.
> And right anon it ran hym in his mynde,
> That, sith his face was so disfigured
> Of maladye the which he hadde endured,
> He myghte wel, if that he bar hym lowe,
> Lyve in Atthenes everemoore unknowe,
> And seen his lady wel ny day by day. (1399–1407)

> [And with that word, he grabbed a large mirror and saw that his complexion was entirely changed and saw that his face was all of another nature. And immediately it came into his mind that since his face was so disfigured by the malady that he had endured, he might well live forever unrecognized in Athens if he conducted himself humbly, and he might see his lady nearly every day.]

When Arcite looks at himself, he is able to take possession of the alien physical thing he has become, this figure of changed *colour* and "visage al in another kynde." His face's disfigurement, he realizes, allows for self-refashioning, which he carries out under the name Philostratus. In what reads like a restaging of the Lacanian mirror stage, the reflected image brings Arcite back to an agential relation to his body. Before this, physical changes were merely happening *to* him, thanks to a physiological Real of humors and cranial cavities insusceptible to his first-person knowledge. With his glance in the mirror, Arcite becomes able "To maken vertu of necessitee," as Theseus would say: he assumes as chosen the thing he is compelled to be (3042).

But the sequence also illustrates the strangeness of the subjectivity that Arcite then plays out. His erstwhile appearance, his previous complexion, his own "habit" and "disposicioun" have all disappeared under the effects of the "loveris maladye." The fictional and provisional nature of his new identity is registered in his adoption of the pseudonym Philostratus. Neither Philostratus nor Arcite seems to be grounded on anything permanent. It is the face of someone else, "al in another kynde," that looks back from the mirror. Arcite's self-canceling reclamation of his symptomatic body prefigures his gesture of sacrifice on his deathbed, when he briefly covers over the brute unchosenness of his death with the decision to give Emelye to Palamon, in an act following what Louise O. Fradenburg has called "the logic of sacrifice," or the pattern of "renunciation which seeks to recuperate loss by making us choose it."[25]

The medical description of Arcite's body shows him to be a composite system undone by his parts in riot. The burden of the remainder of the present chapter is to give an account of how his flesh, or *phisik*'s body, matters to the tale's several competing etiological imaginaries.

The Aesthetic Logic of Causation

During Arcite's medicalization, the "Knight's Tale" briefly trades the stylistics of agency for those of physical causality. This lexical eruption of *phisik* can in fact be fit within a broader consideration of how the tale portrays the forces that make things happen. What might be called its aesthetic logic of causation undergoes a general shift between its first and second half. During the first two of the four parts of the "Knight's Tale" (lines 859–1880), human bodies seem to make good vehicles for causal efficacy, and the narration savors their iconographic resources. The scenes are distinguished by their gestural lucidity. Theseus listening to the beseeching widows, Emelye gathering flowers, Palamon peering through the prison bars, Hippolyta and Emelye appealing to Theseus for pity—all are sharply delineated tableaux where feelings and intentions flow into expressive action. This is not to say that agency in the first half of the tale is unproblematic but that the doings of human figures remain at the aesthetic heart of these scenes.[26]

It is in the third and fourth parts of the tale, when the pluralization of causal factors picks up steam and the pagan gods begin to crowd the plot, that bodies are abandoned as the figures of effective action. Instead, efficacy shifts to a different scale—as it does at Arcite's sickbed. Gestural acuity grows

muddled, and causal forces, depersonalized. A change in the aesthetic logic of
causality is evident, for instance, in the contrast between Palamon and Arcite's
secret duel in the grove and the knights' subsequent stadium warfare. In the
grove, the figures of the two knights stand forth in sharp relief. Their battle is
carefully anticipated in the plot, with a charmingly improbable sequence of
Palamon happening to overhear Arcite's love lament. As they fight, each strikes
and is struck in turn, laboring on and on in a kind of emblem of chivalric exertion. They enact their (formally identical) individualities, each upheld against
the other: "'Heere cometh my mortal enemy! / Withoute faille, he moot be
deed, or I'" (1643–44).

In the narrative span between grove and stadium, however, gestural vividness dissipates. The final tournament has none of the stark clarity of the
knights' duel. When Palamon and Arcite return to Athens, each with his
hundred knights, the mass of combatants acts to diffuse the human body's
salience. The tournament is almost eerily dull, its narration riddled with
impersonal constructions:

> In gooth the sharpe spore into the syde.
> Ther seen men who kan juste and who kan ryde;
> Ther shyveren shaftes upon sheeldes thikke;
> He feeleth thurgh the herte-spoon the prikke.
> Up spryngen speres twenty foot on highte;
> Out goon the swerdes as the silver brighte;
> The helmes they tohewen and toshrede;
> Out brest the blood with stierne stremes rede. (2603–10)

> [In goes the sharp spur to the flank. There, men were seen who
> could ride and joust. There, shafts shattered against thick shields.
> Someone felt a wound through the breastbone. Up sprang spears
> twenty feet high; out came swords bright as silver; they hewed and
> shredded helmets; out burst blood in red streams.]

Action and suffering are transferred to objects—to spears, spurs, shields,
swords, and helmets. Blood streams and bones burst, but they belong to no
one in particular. Who feels the "prikke" of the weapon in his chest? The pronoun's referent is general, displacing the individuating force of bodily pain.
Even Arcite's victory and Palamon's defeat is likewise diffused through a multitude of actors:

> The stronge kyng Emetreus gan hente
> This Palamon, as he faught with Arcite,
> And made his swerd depe in his flessh to byte,
> And by the force of twenty is he take
> Unyolden, and ydrawen to the stake. (2638–42)

[The strong king Emetreus seized Palamon as he fought Arcite and made his sword bite deeply into his flesh, and by the force of twenty he is taken, unyielding, and drawn to the stake.]

The narration refracts Arcite's would-be moment of triumph into "the force of twenty" and a passive construction ("is he take"). The repetition of the third-person masculine pronoun encourages confusion: Is it Palamon who is making his sword bite deep into Arcite's flesh, or Emetreus who sinks his blade into Palamon? The event is marked as the fulfillment of narrative necessity—for "Som tyme an ende ther is of every dede" (2636)—but it scatters the satisfactions of resolution into a blur of agents.

When eventive clarity does occur, it does not transpire through the actions of any human figure. Victorious, Arcite lifts his helmet and rides forth toward Emelye, seeming for a fleeting instant to restore gestural clarity to the scene. Then: "Out of the ground a furie infernal sterte, / From Pluto sent at requeste of Saturne" (2684–85). There is no further description. The fury has no determinate shape, and no one in the scene seems to see it except Arcite's horse. By contrast, in the *Teseida*, Erinys storms forth from the underworld with serpent tresses, ornamental hydras, and a whip of snakes, inciting horror in the spectators as she passes.[27] Chaucer's version strips the plot's inflection point of figuration so it is as though pure necessity erupts. The fury's only qualifiers are the causal chain of which it is a part: it came from the underworld ("infernal"), "From Pluto sent at requeste of Saturne"—and, we might continue—in the interests of Venus, in answer to Palamon's prayer, which he offered for the love of Emelye, whom he saw while imprisoned by Theseus. Readers are returned to the tangled etiological chain that knots Arcite's fate to the tale's disorganized cosmos.[28]

The poem's most prominent means of complexifying causation is its pantheon of pagan gods, which become an increasingly active presence in the poem's second half. Up until then, the narrator has left it pointedly unspecified why things happen as they do. Turning points in the plot have been padded round with decidedly unexplanatory explanations: it is "by aventure or cas [by chance or accident]" that Palamon first sees Emelye (1074); Palamon comes to the secluded grove "by aventure or destynee— / As, whan a thyng is shapen, it shal be [by chance or destiny, that is, as when a thing is ordained, it shall be]" (1465–66). Similar examples abound. These references to chance and providence are vaguely Boethian, and they skittishly register the pressures of external determination, whether cosmic or metafictional; after all, the telling is unspooling according to what "olde bookes seyn [say]" (1463). When the Greek characters comment on causal determination, it is often in terms of the gods. When Palamon complains, "'I moot been in prisoun thurgh Saturne, / And eek thurgh Juno, jalous and eek wood [I must be in prison because of Saturn and also Juno, who is jealous and crazy]'" (1328–29), readers are free to interpret his explanation as a sign of his pagan worldview rather than a statement of narrative fact. Indeed, when Arcite names first Fortune and then Saturn to explain his and Palamon's predicament— "Fortune hath yeven [given] us this adversitee. / Som wikke aspect or disposicioun / Of Saturne, by som constellacioun, / Hath yeven us this" (1086–89)—the interchangeability of the two powers suggests that the pagan gods are just culturally specific versions of the familiar medieval figure of Fortune.

Medieval thinkers understood the classical pantheon to index problems in causal understanding.[29] According to the Christian explanatory framework developed by the Church Fathers, paganism hypostatized as deities forces that had no actual autonomy. Cultural processes of mystification—explainable via euhemerism, natural symbolism, and moral allegory—resulted in the portrayal of causes in pseudo-divine form. In a memorable passage of the *City of God*, Augustine ridicules the animistic proliferation that was supposedly proper to a Roman wedding night, when the gods Jugantinus, Domitius, Manturna, Virgenensis, Subigus, Prema, Pertunda, Venus, and Priapus all had their parts to play. "Why fill the bedchamber with a swarm of deities when even the wedding attendants have departed?" Augustine asks mockingly. "Let the husband himself have something to do."[30] This is pantheon as farce: the conjugal sex act dissipates into an infinite regress of shared-out efficacy. The ubiquitous medieval personification of Fortune shares something of the logic of the pagan gods, which helps explain Arcite's easy reference to both. In Boethius's *De consolatione philosophiae*, which was at the root of the medieval tradition, Fortune's ontological status is decidedly subordinate to that of Lady Philosophy and Boethius's narrator. She appears only *within* their dialogue, not as a figure endowed with the trappings of diegetic being in her own right. One of Lady Philosophy's lessons, after all, is that Fortune is a fiction, a certain figural by-product of humans' limited perspective on the cosmos. She *seems* like she makes things happen, but she does not. She is a reflex of the contingent order of events and our place in them.

Yet if the gods and Fortune are fictions, medieval thinkers could not simply dismiss them as false. Their figures bubble up from real conundrums in etiological knowledge. Though certain truths were effectively settled by Christianity—Fortune is an illusion; Christendom knows only the one triune God—the pagan pantheon had an ongoing epistemic role to play. Natural philosophy used the gods to organize discussion of humoral complexions and planetary influences, forces that were thought to have real if not absolutely determining power.[31] This scientific role, moreover, was indistinguishable from the gods' general allegorical function. In the classicizing literature of the high and late Middle Ages, the gods served as speculative instruments, figural props for abstract thought and experimental theory. Like allegorical personifications generally, they gave provisional being and agency to secondary causes, to accidents and qualities, and to motive forces that did not stand forth for regular observation. This is clear in the pioneering philosophical allegories of the twelfth century like Bernard Silvestris's *Cosmographia* and Alan of Lille's *De Planctu Naturae*. Chaucer is heir to this tradition, as dream visions like the *House of Fame* and the *Parliament of Fowls* attest. In each of these works, an unsystematized field of ontologically varied beings generates the world in which action happens. This heterogeneity of entities calls for interpretation, but dream visions do not demand a painstaking calculus of real efficacy. Their setting in a dreamer's psyche, or in another world, frames and compartmentalizes whatever bizarre models of causation unfold. By contrast, the diegetic actuality of Arcite's death in the "Knight's Tale" enforces a reality principle. This is a pagan world, yes, but something irrevocable has happened in it, and the tale encourages us to puzzle over why.

Chaucer makes the gods a diegetic problem, then, by giving them real and direct narrative force. He amplifies their role over and above the one they play in the *Teseida*, for instance, making a visitation from Mercury the catalyst for Arcite's return to Athens (1384–93) and promoting Saturn, who is nowhere mentioned in Boccaccio's poem, to the foremost instigator of Arcite's death. When Venus and Mars are said to be squabbling in the heavens (2438–42), their discord is narrated with just as much diegetic actuality as the bickering of Arcite and Palamon. In other words, by the end of the tale's third part, the gods have jumped discursive levels, asserting their existence not just in the minds and culture of the Greeks but in the tale's diegetic reality. Nowhere is this clearer than in Saturn's mythography. The powers of Venus, Diana, and Mars are catalogued in their respective temple paintings, so that although these gods' attributes occupy a large section of the poem, their mythography still appears as a cultural production. After all, Theseus has paid every "portreyour" and "kervere of ymages" to decorate the temples (1899). Saturn, however, dispenses with the frame of the cultural artifact and speaks his own mythography directly:

> "Myn is the drenchyng in the see so wan;
> Myn is the prison in the derke cote;
> Myn is the stranglyng and hangyng by the throte,
> The murmure and the cherles rebellyng,
> The groynynge, and the pryvee empoysonyng;
> I do vengeance and pleyn correccioun,
> Whil I dwelle in the signe of the leoun." (2456–62)

> ["Mine is the drowning in the sea so dark; mine is the prison in the
> dark chamber; mine is the strangling and the hanging by the throat,
> the muttering and the peasants' rebellion, the grumbling, and the
> secret poisoning; I effect vengeance and punishment while I dwell
> in the sign of Leo."]

Saturn uses the first-person pronoun with relish in this initial and most extensive scene of the gods' diegetic action. He moves from self-predication to the promise of action: he will arrange for Venus to have her way as well as Mars. He will send the fury. The unambiguously direct presence of the gods functions to pluralize causation in the tale and to do so with decidedly dark implications.

I thus disagree with Jill Mann's account of the pagan gods in the "Knight's Tale," which reduces them to their astrological role. "Saturn does not," she writes, "act as a free agent; he acts as a planet," and she continues, "the other 'gods' too act not with divine freedom, but in accordance with their planetary natures."[32] On Mann's reading, the planetary deities are constrained by a higher organizing power: "The forces [that Palamon and Arcite] activate wear to them the personal aspect of gods, but their power resides in their impersonal role as planets—planets whose movements and influences are determined not by themselves, but by the First Mover. . . . Identifying the planetary gods as 'hidden causes' of the catastrophe does not, that is, involve identifying them as its *ultimate* causes."[33] However, it is not only for Arcite and Palamon that the gods wear a "personal aspect"; they appear as such to readers as well. Chaucer does add extensive astrological material in the process of adapting the *Teseida*, but the effect is not to reduce the gods to planets.[34] Rather, the astrological additions compound the difficulty of figuring out the mode of the deities' effectivity. Part of what is unsettling is precisely the overlay of their "personal aspect" and their astrological and complexional roles. This is not to say they are portrayed as ultimate causes, each omnipotent and absolute, but neither are they shown to participate in an orderly etiological hierarchy. Instead, Mars, Venus, Diana, Saturn, Juno, Mercury, and Jupiter create what Piero Boitani calls "a truly medieval ambiguity," in which "gods *and* planets define a field of force."[35]

The ambiguity of the gods in the "Knight's Tale" partakes of a longstanding hesitation in medieval thought, between the essentially fictional status of the classical deities and what was thought to be the scientifically explicable influence of the planets on bodily dispositions and events.[36] The gods' ontological wavering—their flickering between mythic, mythographic, characterological, and planetary modes—*is* their narrative purpose in the tale. Their commingling of metaphysics and physics, theology and natural philosophy, caprice and order, personality and impersonality, and interiority and exteriority exemplifies the tale's cultivation of etiological complexity. The pantheon gives figural shape and personality to certain ambiguities of causation, and their interpretive consequences cannot be cordoned off from the tale's ultimate meaning. They are also the most important of Chaucer's tactics for turning the tale's aesthetic logic of causation away from human agency.

Death

Though Chaucer augments the direct agency of the gods throughout the "Knight's Tale," at particular points he prunes away references to the pantheon and to the afterlife. This careful management of the presence of the supernatural in the tale indicates Chaucer's concern to control precisely what resources of transcendence and divinity his pagan world would contain. Most famously, Chaucer eliminates the ascent of Arcita through the heavenly spheres in Boccaccio's *Teseida*, which he had likely already used in his account of Troilus's death. The effect is to leave the reader with no report of Arcite's continued existence after he dies. The excision places new emphasis on creaturely life, as the horizon that these narrative selves do not, apparently, extend beyond. As

I have argued elsewhere (about the *Book of the Duchess*), Chaucer experiments with portraying death as absolute loss in part by using pagan settings and by suppressing mention of the afterlife.[37]

Another place where Boccaccio's references to divinity are cut follows just after Arcite's sickbed medicalization. Once readers are told that neither purgatives nor laxatives help Arcite, the narrator tries to hurry the scene along:

> Al is tobrosten thilke regioun;
> Nature hath now no dominacioun.
> And certeinly, ther Nature wol nat wirche,
> Fare wel phisik! Go ber the man to chirche!
> This al and som, that Arcita moot dye. (2757–61)

> [That region (of his body) is entirely crushed. Nature now has
> no dominion, and certainly where Nature will not work, farewell
> *phisik*! Go bear the man to church! This is the sum of it, that Arcite
> must die.]

The repetition of *nature* may have been suggested to Chaucer by the comment of the physician Idmon of Epidaurus in the *Teseida*. Delivering up his dire prognosis, the doctor remarks, "Only Jove can save his life, if he should so will, for he is greater than nature and can accomplish much more than nature is able to do. But leaving miracles in their place, I say that Asclepius would avail neither much nor little to restore his health [*Giove potrebbe in vita solamente / servarlo, se volesse, ch'è maggiore / che la natura e puote adoperare / assai più che natura non può fare. // Ma lasciando i miracoli in lor loco, / dico che Esculapio non varrebbe / per sanità di lui molto né poco*]."[38] In the "Knight's Tale," there is no reference to Jove's miraculous powers or to any authority higher than nature itself. The *miracoli* that Boccaccio mentions are reserved to describe Saturn's commission of the "furie infernal" to unhorse Arcite: "a myracle ther bifel anon" (2675). Here, divine intervention effects destruction rather than healing.

The glib tone and speed of the narrator's lines as he bids *phisik* farewell jar against the detailed physical description preceding. The particularized *res naturales* become the abstraction *nature*; a chipper proverb inflects the failures of medicine; and with a flourish of conclusiveness, it is announced, "This al and som, that Arcita moot dye." By this point, readers are familiar with the narrator's performances of hurrying the plot along, which have peppered the telling from the start ("And certes, if it nere to long to heere, / I wolde have toold" [875–76], etc.). Yet in these lines, the haste to conclude is aligned with death. Arcite's perishing will be the means to narrative closure since (as Theseus remarks) "Ye woot yourself she may nat wedden two / Atones" (1835–36). The proverbial "Go ber the man to chirche!" speeds over-hastily to Arcite's tomb, before the knight has even made his parting speech. The word *chirche*, for its part, contributes to the lines' indelicacy. In the tale's pagan setting, *chirche* refers simply to a religious building[39]—in other words, to a place that precisely cannot be assumed to guarantee the soul's fortunes after death. The narrator's refusal to speculate about miracles and the afterlife and his brusque hurrying to death continue the materializing effects of the medical passage that has come just before.

The meaning of *nature* as it is used in these lines declaring Arcite's death ("Nature hath now no dominacioun," "Nature wol nat wirche") is something like "life-force." The *Middle English Dictionary* gives this definition: "restorative powers of the body, bodily processes; regulatory processes expelling poison, excess humors, etc., from the body; vital forces, healing powers, powers of growth; state of bodily equilibrium, proportion, health; ability to reproduce."[40] This sense is closely related to the *res naturales* as a set of vital parts and powers. But the other primary definition of *nature*—that of the created universe, the made world—lurks as the underside of *nature*'s meaning in the passage.[41] It is precisely Arcite's dying, as nature loses dominion and fails to work, that proves he belongs to nature, in the sense that he belongs to the mutable and corruptible world. In death nature extends its *dominacioun* over him, rather than relinquishing it. It is in this sense, of the created and corruptible world, that Theseus will use *nature* when he invokes it in his consolation.

It is a fragile gesture of self-possession on Arcite's part that instigates the tale's transition from the narrator's bathetic commentary to Arcite's moving deathbed speech. The narrator reports, "This al and som, that Arcita moot dye; / *For which* he sendeth after Emelye, / And Palamon" (2761–63, emphasis added). Arcite calls for Emelye and Palamon *because* he is dying: the hypotactic conjunction reveals that he too knows what the narration has elaborated from its materializing perspective. Similar to when he peered into the mirror and made his estranged physiology the grounds for his action, here he attempts the agential reclamation of his broken body. Chaucer distills the thirty-two lines that Arcite speaks in the "Knight's Tale" from hundreds that are exchanged in the parallel scene in Book X of the *Teseida*. Most of this highly condensed discourse is concerned with Arcite's self-sacrifice, as he disavows his primary role in the narrative to that point, his claim to Emelye. Instead, he conforms his intentions to the new exigencies of the plot. In giving up this own claim, Arcite sanctions what will be the explicit aim of Theseus's consolation speech, to effect the marriage of Palamon and Emelye, and thus Arcite legitimates the romance's generically mandated ending. His gesture of sacrificing his own now impossible desire shows him making "vertu of necessitee," as Theseus will soon enjoin everyone to do in the face of death. Yet Arcite's speech is also roiled by contrary impulses. The luminousness of his words comes from the desires they constrain and suppress, which still manage to disturb the verses' rhetoric.

In his address to Emelye, Arcite flits among the several forms of self-overthrow that he has suffered: "Allas, the deeth! Allas, myn Emelye! / Allas, departynge of oure compaignye! / Allas, myn hertes queene! Allas, my wyf, / Myn hertes lady, endere of my lyf!" (2773–76). In this conventional but also unbearably concentrated bit of love lament, the exclamatory anaphora yokes the nouns in paradoxical equivalence; Emelye is made parallel to Arcite's death and to her own *departynge*, at once herself and her absence. Only at the end of a circuitous and tenuous causal chain could Emelye be identified as the actual *endere* of Arcite's life, so the epithet seems to testify instead to the intensity of Arcite's romantic suffering and, more profoundly, to his wish to locate his death in Emelye, a re-siting that would give it a meaning it lacks in its emplotment, where it is the outcome of the gods' squabble, the fury's upstart, the horse's fright, and his blood's putrefaction.

From this series of exclamations, Arcite breaks into the most philosophical words of his dying speech: "What is this world? What asketh men to have? / Now with his love, now in his colde grave / Allone, withouten any compaignye" (2777–79). The first-person pronouns of the preceding lines fall away, as though signaling the existential universality of his questions and perhaps also the limits of what Arcite can bear to say. He seems not quite able to place himself, his *I*, in the cold grave. The line's yoking of contraries echoes an earlier antithesis to form a despairing chiasmus: "Allas, the deeth! Allas, myn Emelye! . . . Now with his love, now in his colde grave" (2773, 2778). The repetition of the deictic terms *now* and *his*—"Now with his love, now in his colde grave"—cipher two, mutually exclusive meanings in the line. The obvious sense depends on *his* having a constant referent and *now* shifting: someone is living and then dead, with his beloved and then alone. But the latent significance emerges when *now*'s referent stays constant and *his* shifts between two figures: now someone is with his love, and now, at the same moment, someone else is in his grave. Between the two clauses there might even be suppressed hypotaxis—he is now with his love *because* he, the other he, is dead. This secondary meaning helps explain the line's haunting power, as Arcite wonders what the world is and what form his tragedy truly takes.

Once Arcite's speech concludes, he dies—but slowly. The slow-motion intensity of the account as it moves across Arcite's body links it to his preceding medicalization:

> For from his feet up to his brest was come
> The coold of deeth, that hadde hym overcome,
> And yet mooreover, for in his armes two
> The vital strengthe is lost and al ago.
> Oonly the intellect, withouten moore,
> That dwelled in his herte syk and soore,
> Gan faillen whan the herte felte deeth.
> Dusked his eyen two, and failled breeth,
> But on his lady yet caste he his ye. (2799–2807)

[From his feet up to his breast came the cold of death, which had overcome him, and furthermore, in his two arms the vital strength is lost and all gone. Only the intellect alone, which dwelled in his sick and sore heart, began to fail when the heart felt death. His two eyes grew dark, and his breath failed, but upon his lady yet he cast his eye.]

The description traces the graded transition from person to cadaver. Chaucer seems concerned to bring his readers as close as possible to the point where the body is saturated with physical determination, when agency constricts to infinitesimal smallness and vanishes, and the corpse comes into view. To do so, the passage draws on two sources. It echoes the death lyrics that were part of the *ars moriendi*, or the "art of dying"—a discourse minutely attuned to the stages of agency's dissipation as the end of life drew near.[42] The passage also calls on medical and scientific vocabulary. The unusual adjective *vital* has here its first recorded use, and its early meaning in Middle English was physiological, naming and specifying the forces that sustained an organism's life.[43] In Galenic medicine, it was the *spiritus vitalis*, seated in the heart, that controlled respiration, heat, and to some degree motion and emotion.[44] The vital spirit was one of the three *spiritus* that, like the *virtutues*, helped constitute the body's *res naturales*. Here it is "lost and al ago" (2802), as Arcite's faculties withdraw to the beleaguered organ that is closest to his corrupted wound ("the

soore / Encreeseth at his herte moore and moore" [2743–44]). The narration
draws the reader to the very brink of where Arcite as subject ceases to be.

The narrator then carelessly leaps the gap between life and death that the
previous lines so assiduously trace:

> His spirit chaunged hous and wente ther,
> As I cam nevere, I kan nat tellen wher.
> Therfore I stynte; I nam no divinistre;
> Of soules fynde I nat in this registre,
> Ne me ne list thilke opinions to telle
> Of hem, though that they writen wher they dwelle.
> Arcite is coold, ther Mars his soule gye! (2809–15)

> [His spirit changed house and went where I never came, so I cannot
> tell where. Therefore I stop; I am no diviner; I find nothing of souls
> in this volume, nor would I wish to tell such opinions of them,
> though it had been written where they dwell. Arcite is cold, thus
> may Mars guide his soul!]

The grave's creeping chill is suddenly an accomplished fact—"Arcite is
coold"—and the invocation of Mars sounds glib. These lines replace Boccaccio's famous account of Arcita's soul posthumously ascending through the
heavens and looking back to laugh at earthly vanity.[45] Here the narrator protests against the idea that he would have anything to say about souls like
Arcite's. The result is to continue the materialization of Arcite's person by dis-
allowing any report of the afterlife. His death functions as a kind of oblivion.

Together, the medical objectification of Arcite, the narrator's flippancy,
and the easy excision of the soul's fate threaten to ironize the scene of Arcite's
death. Yet the lyrical and existential force of Arcite's final words stands up dis-
sonantly against these elements. In contrast to the consistently tragic gravitas
of Arcite's death in Boccaccio's *Teseida*, facilitated by Arcita's role as protagonist and by the poem's decorum and unified tone, here the scene's cumulative
effect is fragmented and uncertain. It is met by the reader not with mourning
and cathartic affect but with the question *why?* and the interpretive energies
that this question incites. Charles Muscatine expresses unease concerning
Chaucer's representation of Arcite's death, urging the critic "not to convert
a deftly administered antidote for tragedy into an actively satiric strain. This
would be to mistake Chaucer's balance for buffoonery."[46] Muscatine's assertion

that "balance" is the net effect of the death's patchwork depiction is, I think, wishful thinking, but the effect is not "buffoonery" either. It rather creates a kind of interpretive irritation, an infelicity around which hermeneutic energy and anxiety circle. Muscatine writes of the narrator's flippancy, "Were the narrator's comments to be read as a satiric comment on Arcite's death, the whole noble fabric of the speech, and of the poem too, would crumble."[47] Indeed, it is telling that the satisfaction of the plot's major point of suspense—which knight will win Emelye?—appears here only in the form of stylistic and hermeneutic *dis*satisfaction. The mutual implication of completion and incompletion in Arcite's death does in fact menace the "whole noble fabric," or what Schweitzer calls "the meaning of the whole,"[48] by disrupting the tale's approach to formal and moral coherence.

"Firste Moevere of the Cause Above"

The existential tumult and philosophical uncertainties that burst from Arcite in the midst of his farewells to Emelye are what Theseus tries to lay to rest two hundred lines later. Arcite's questions "What is this world? What asketh men to have?" find collective expression in the Greeks' extravagant grief, which Theseus seems to regard as a potential source of saturnine chaos. As many critics have observed, the duke's defining commitment throughout the tale is to the imposition of order.[49] The new Athenian stadium that he builds to contain Arcite and Palamon's quarrel, for instance, is constructed so as to balance contending aesthetic, social, and cosmological factors.[50] Accordingly, Theseus brings his talent for order to Arcite's seemingly capricious fate. His consolation seeks to spin a line of reasoning that, like Ariadne's thread, would lead out of the maze of tangled efficient causes to a totalizing perspective.

Yet Theseus does not so much discover the logic inhering in the swarming circumstances of the "Knight's Tale" as dismiss their relevance. Adapting a version of Boethian providence, Theseus redescribes the arbitrariness of Arcite's fate as a mere trick of perspective, which can be corrected by shifting one's interpretation from the immanent realm to the transcendent. The first thirty lines (2987–3016) and a later six (3035–40) of Theseus's speech are Chaucer's Boethian additions to the material from the *Teseida* that is used for the rest of the oration. The adaptation of Lady Philosophy's lessons from *De consolatione philosophiae* gives the duke's remarks a greater philosophical ambition and explanatory scope than they possess in Boccaccio's version. But what Theseus does not say is also striking. Despite the tale's demonstrated interest in *phisik*, none of Lady Philosophy's metaphorics of healing make their way into Theseus's consolation—none of her concern that "lyghtere medicynes" must precede "myghtyere remedies," or her worries that her interlocutor "is fallen into a litargye [lethargy], whiche that is a comune seknesse to hertes that been desceyved" (in the words of the *Boece*, Chaucer's prose translation of Boethius's *De consolatione*).[51] Instead, Theseus reaches straight for cosmology.

To frame the pagan gods with metaphysical optimism and to delimit Saturn's orbit "that hath so wyde for to turne" (2454), Theseus calls on the furthest limit of the celestial spheres, the Prime Mover, from whom the order and movement of the cosmos supposedly emerge. At stake in Arcite's death, Theseus seems to think, is the relation between *physis* and metaphysics—that is, between the flux of generation and corruption and the stability that can be discerned within that flux as its law. The source of such natural stability, he says, is "the Firste Moevere of the cause above," who binds "with that faire cheyne of love" the components of the material universe, "the fyr, the eyr, the water, and the lond / In certeyn boundes, that they may nat flee" (2987–93). This image of striving matter yoked in chains of form is a philosophical commonplace, and one that is elaborated in Boethius's *De consolatione*. For instance, Lady Philosophy praises the creator who "byndest the elementis by nombres proporcionables, that the coolde thinges mowen accorde with the hote thinges, and the drye thinges with the moyste."[52] This familiar image is notable for implying that even the smallest building blocks of the universe, prior to and against their ordering, are charged with the impulse to flight, to escape into particularized and unchecked motion.

As the *Boece*'s Lady Philosophy explains, the order of causes "constreyneth by his propre stablete the moevable thingis, or elles [else] thei scholden fleten folyly [move madly]."[53] Crazed and swarming motion defines the counter-physics to which Philosophy gestures, a physics of particularity in which each entity moves according to its own singular impulses. Lady Philosophy warns that if love's bridle is loosed, "alle thynges that now loven hem togidres wolden make batayle contynuely, and stryven to fordo the fassoun of this world [undo the disposition of the world]."[54] These are images of metaphysical strife, in which matter's impulses become rebellion against what *is*, or "the fassoun of this world." When Theseus in his speech shifts from the topic of the elements to "al that is engendred in this place," his remarks emphasize the parallels between elemental motion and organismal desires for self-preservation. Living things "may not pace [step]" beyond their allotted duration of life (2997–98). The ordaining of "certeyne dayes and duracioun" is like the "certeyn boundes" that hold the elements (2996, 2993). And yet the wish to step past death, the desire to live, is precisely why mourning is so extravagant and why Theseus's stern consolation is necessary.

Theseus's Boethian images, in spite of themselves, testify to an alternative cosmic energy below the evident order, for which the "faire cheyne of love" acts as constraint. On his account, this is the drive toward impulsive and atomized motion, which, unbound, would result in a frenzy of spontaneous, ephemeral becoming. It is also a version of the primitive desire for life that arises from all creatures' "love of hire [their] lyvynges," as the *Boece* has it—a hunger for vitality that is inherent in the very "bygynnynges of nature."[55] When, in the course of Boethius's dialogue, Lady Philosophy explains this self-preservative "naturel entencioun of things," she uses it to support her claim that "desiren alle thinges oon [all things desire unity]," insofar as they wish to preserve their own identities.[56] But Arcite's body realizes a different vision of what "naturel entencioun" generates, namely, the teeming interpenetration of natural desires at various scales, which cannot be stabilized into unity. From the planetary deities wrangling in the heavens to the body's cavity churning with *vertu* and *corrupcioun*, this nature is not *oon* but a flurry of impulses, which evokes, in the register of physics, the Thebanness that Lee Patterson finds haunting the "Knight's Tale"—a "self-destructive rivalry that gives full rein to the violence of the appetitive self" and ends in "endless repetition."[57]

The structure of Theseus's remarks has the effect of allying the figure of Arcite with these unfree elements and "al that is engendred." As he goes on, Theseus returns to some of the language of Arcite's jarringly physicalized death, redeploying *nature* and the root *corruptio* (each used twice in quick succession in the deathbed scene).[58] Theseus says:

Wel may men knowe, but it be a fool,
That every part dirryveth from his hool,
For nature hath nat taken his bigynnyng
Of no partie or cantel of a thyng,
But of a thyng that parfit is and stable,
Descendynge so til it be corrumpable. (3005–10)

[Well may men know, unless they are fools, that every part derives from its whole, so nature has not taken its beginning from any part or portion of a thing, but from a thing that is perfect and stable, descending until it became corruptible.]

On Arcite's deathbed, *nature* names the vital powers of the organism to maintain itself, eventually overwhelmed by morbid corruption: "Nature hath now no dominacioun. / And certeinly, ther Nature wol nat wirche, / Fare wel phisik! Go ber the man to chirche!" (2758–60). Then, in Theseus's speech, nature and corruption become two aspects of a single whole, *parfit* and *stable*, which is these forces' origin and ultimate identity. Although nature is a realm of change and death, it issues from "Juppiter, the kyng, / That is prince and cause of alle thyng" (3035–36). As a result, stability subtends creaturely annihilation, for "speces of thynges and progressiouns / Shullen enduren by successiouns [species of things and natural processes shall endure by succession]" (3013–14). Across these two passages, then, *nature* is translated from an organismal power to a super-individual constancy. Similarly, Arcite's bodily *vertu*, which struggled to purge his swelling chest, is transposed into Theseus's proverb, "Thanne is it wysdom, as it thynketh me, / To maken vertu of necessitee, / And take it weel that we may not eschue [escape]" (3041–43). *Vertu* is made to mean the subjective endorsement of death's necessity instead of, as at Arcite's sickbed, the physiological push back against it.

It should be emphasized that none of Theseus's cosmological formulations would have sounded unfamiliar to Chaucer's audiences. The idea that natural forms endure by mutability, or that nature binds the elements, was perfectly commonplace. What is unusual in the "Knight's Tale" is the peculiar moral and metaphysical power that accrues to Arcite's body and the thwarted particularities he is made to represent. Whoever "gruccheth ought [complains at all], he dooth folye," Theseus warns, "And rebel is to hym that al may gye [and is a rebel to him who guides everything]" (3045–46). The "contrarie" of the duke's lesson, Theseus insists, "is wilfulnesse" (3057). The direct target of the duke's admonishments are the Greek mourners, especially Palamon and Emelye:

> "Why grucchen we, why have we hevynesse,
> That goode Arcite, of chivalrie flour,
> Departed is with duetee and honour
> Out of this foule prisoun of this lyf?
> Why grucchen heere his cosyn and his wyf
> Of his welfare, that loved hem so weel?" (3058–63)

["Why do we complain, why do we have sorrow that good Arcite, chivalry's flower, has departed with all proper honor, out of the foul prison of this life? Why do his cousin and his wife complain about his welfare, him who loved them so well?"]

To Theseus, the mourners' wild grief seems to signal their solidarity with the perished Arcite and with the counterfactual future, the lost potentiality, that he now emblematizes. The fleeing elements, the creaturely desire to overstep one's allotted span of life, and the "grucching" of the mourners are so many cases of rebellion. The tale has shown the crowd's sorrow to be paralyzing to the social order, almost dionysian in its excess. Taken to its limit—which crucially the "Knight's Tale" does not do, though Theseus worries about it— solidarity with the dead Arcite would yield a vision of existence that rejects the Prime Mover's pretensions to totality and instead confines reality's horizon to the struggle among particular and perishable things. Lee Patterson has argued that for Chaucer, "Thebanness stands as the other that Boethianism suppresses."[59] Those two opposed ethos, I have been suggesting, also appear in the poem as cosmologies. A metaphysics of *phisik* is discernible beneath nature's ordained harmony. It entails an untotalized plurality of forces, bodies dissolving into their own dynamic constituents, and the utter urgency of preserving life. For Theseus's Boethianism, this eternal flux is the suppressed ground for his fantasy of sovereign providence and neoplatonic emanation.

My impression is that Chaucer intended Theseus's speech to have an air of monotheistic plausibility about it, which he expected to cast a soothing glow over the story's close. Yet he would have been aware that it hardly addressed all the questions raised by preceding events, except to dismiss their relevance. Its comparison with the rest of the tale produces an interpretive conundrum, as readers decide how to resolve the misfit between the two parts, the intricate tangle of causes and the blanket guarantee of the Prime Mover's benevolence. As though to avoid precisely such appraisal, Theseus tries to elide the necessity of his moralizing:

Ther nedeth noght noon auctoritee t'allegge,
For it is preeved by experience,
But that me list declaren my sentence.
Thanne may men by this ordre wel discerne
That thilke Moevere stable is and eterne. (3000–3004)

[One need not cite authorities, for this is proved by experience; I just wish to declare my understanding. Then men may well discern by this order that the Mover is stable and eternal.]

The duke claims that his oration is just a reiteration of experience properly understood. The direct referent of the "it" ("it is preeved by experience") is the remark about creaturely life and its limit to "certeyne dayes and duracioun," which immediately precedes it. Yet the "ordre" discernible in the experience of Arcite's death is precisely what makes Theseus's consolation so difficult to find consoling. One cousin has died and the other has not, according to apparently disarrayed and arbitrary circumstances. Arcite's last words, which are starkly juxtaposed against his medicalization, suggest the moral obscurity of his fate. As Muscatine writes, "in a literature in which the advent of death is one of the most powerful instruments of moral exemplum, Chaucer goes far out of his way to stifle any such construction."[60] The tale unravels, rather than stitches up, its causal coherence at the point of Arcite's fate. Chaucer has written what is in some sense an anti-exemplum, in which the suffering body serves not to ground causal structures and manifest moral meaning but to destabilize them. By overlaying a medicalized death, a character's disappearance, the fragmentation of narratorial tone, and the disruption of metaphysical order, the "Knight's Tale" leads the reader to confront the resistance of part to whole in literary as well as cosmic terms.

Theseus's euphemization of Arcite's death as a kind of cosmic recycling in his consolation speech—"convertynge al unto his [its] propre welle [source] / From which it is dirryved" (3037–38)—is jarring in its refusal to acknowledge the resistance of the microcosm to its dissolution. This resistance inheres not only in the struggles of the organism but in the sympathetic recognition of our own perceptions, which do not see Arcite as just a bit of the physical world. This perceptual resistance rhymes with tensions inherent in the experience of literary character, an experience drawn taut between the impression of a self-animating individual and the character's existence within a literary artifact. Much of the interpretive drama surrounding Arcite's death is created by playing between these registers of heteronomy: Arcite appears as both physical matter and a self-moving agent; he is both a piece of literary totality and an animate individual. His material embodiment, which is emphasized in a manner difficult to assimilate to the style or sense of the tale, takes on metafictional resonance. All of Athens grinds to a halt in mourning him, as does the plot.

Like the Athenian women who ask, "'Why woldestow be deed?'" the story at first seems itself unable to move past the question (2835). The friction between narrative subordination and *in*subordination comes to the surface as stylistic dissonance and as the emphatic materiality of his death. The grief of the Athenians at Arcite's end insists that this is no mere formal matter: "Infinite been the sorwes and the teeres" (2827).

The action of the "Knight's Tale" begins with unburied bodies: the women of Thebes waylay Theseus on his journey back to Athens with their spectacular grief, and Theseus agrees to overthrow Creon, who does "'the dede bodyes vileynye'" in allowing them "'neither to been yburyed nor ybrent'" (942, 946). These unburied bodies and the mourning they incite are associated with the dangerously recursive patterns of Theban violence, and in answering the women's complaint, Theseus intends to bury the dead and continue home. The problem with burying these bodies, however, is that the attempt produces *more* bodies, a "taas [heap] of bodyes dede" (1005). It is from these corpses that Arcite and Palamon emerge into the story: "in the taas they founde, / Thurghgirt with many a grevous blody wounde, / Two yonge knyghtes liggynge by and by," who are "nat fully quyke, ne fully dede" (1009–11, 1015). "Torn" "out of the taas," the twin cousins produce the story's central symmetry and conflict, its violence, and finally another corpse (1020). Try as he might to bury the dead, Theseus always winds up with a disruptive corporeal remainder.

Even after Arcite dies, his body continues to manifest the resistance of his character to the forward motion of the plot. The presence of his corpse has to be addressed before the "Knight's Tale" can reach its happy conclusion. Theseus decides that "He wolde make a fyr in which the office / Funeral he myghte al accomplice" (2863–64). The dead body, uncanny image of the living, is to be physically reduced to blank, inert matter, literalizing the mandate of the Prime Mover—"convertynge al unto his propre welle / From which it is dirryved" (3037–38). Arcite's funeral is characterized by lavish material and rhetorical expenditure, and it is no wonder: the funeral promises to return to social and literary totality the possibility of forgetting its own production. It is a cathartic ritual around which Theseus's Athenian order reconstitutes itself. At the level of style, the lines depicting the funeral are decadent with rhetorical flourish, pursuing description on and on under *praeteritio*'s coy prohibition. The catalogue of material objects that the Athenians throw onto the pyre evokes a fever of sacrifice. The narrator claims that he will not speak of

what jeweles men in the fyre caste,
Whan that the fyr was greet and brente faste;
Ne how somme caste hir sheeld, and somme hir spere,
And of hire vestimentz, whiche that they were,
And coppes fulle of wyn, and milk, and blood,
Into the fyr, that brente as it were wood. (2945–50)

[what jewels men cast in the fire, when the fire was large and burned
fast; nor how some cast in their shields and some their spears, and
their clothes, which they wore, and cups full of wine and milk and
blood, into the fire, that burned as though it were mad.]

Like the classical grove of trees chopped down for kindling, which are enumerated by their many mellifluous names (2921–23), all of these specific and
individuated objects of the mourners are thrown into the flames. Jewels, weapons, and clothing are palpable, tactile objects, taken from close to the body;
they are signifiers of personal identity, as the chivalric pageantry prior to the
tournament makes clear. The mourners both participate sympathetically in
Arcite's annihilation, casting in these extensions of themselves, and forget him
in the ocular proof that all materials, all objects, all bodies are reduced to
"asshen cold" (2957). The cups of milk and blood poured onto the fire represent almost a pure bodily materiality, which the fire devours "as it were wood
[mad]" (2950). The funeral constitutes a kind of metabolic action on the part
of the social, cosmic, and narrative orders. It marks and produces the disappearance of the individual who, for obscure reasons, could not be made a part
of their forms.

Yet even when Theseus has managed to reduce Arcite's body to ashes, the
Theban knight arguably continues to linger. The body—the injured body, the
medical body, the dying and dead body—remains stylistically and interpre-
tively unresolved to the orderly cosmological and literary whole. The reader's
why? continues to vibrate through the story, adding an uneasy irony to even
the cheerily pat romance ending: "For now is Palamon in alle wele, / Lyvynge
in blisse, in richesse, and in heele [health]" (3101–2). Readers now know very
well the answer to the narrator's early teasing query, "Who hath the worse,
Arcite or Palamoun?" (1348)—but we do not know why. Such narrative closure hums with the possibility that events might just as well have been otherwise, creating a sort of nervous energy of contingency that has no outlet in
the poem.

The Poetics of *Phisik*'s Metaphysics

Both the "Knight's Tale" and the framework of the *Canterbury Tales* portray ontological heterogeneity. In the edifice of the *Tales*, readers are asked to sort the variable degrees of reality that belong to the pilgrims and to the characters within their tales respectively and to track the constant affective and rhetorical crossings between these levels, most obviously in acts of *quyting*. Inscribing himself within the text and encouraging his readers to "Turne over the leef and chese another tale" (3177), Chaucer foregrounds the interplay between fictional entities and the audience, the author, and the material object of the text. Ontological complexity becomes a theme within the compositional and interpretive matrix that Chaucer develops across the *Canterbury Tales*. Incorporated into this framework, the "Knight's Tale" shares in and refracts this attention to ontological variability. In the tale, the actions of characters, the meddling of the pagan gods, the effects of physical forces, and the providential control of the Prime Mover are ontologically heterogeneous and create a pervasive etiological uncertainty about what causes what.

Necessity and ontological constraint are preoccupations of Chaucer's other philosophical romance, *Troilus and Criseyde*, which relies for its tragic power on the structural analogy between literary narrative and the Boethian cosmos. The Boethian struggle to recognize two incommensurate perspectives simultaneously—that of the human subject in the flux of time and that of the Prime Mover, who comprehends the course of events as a completed form—echoes readers' oscillating experience of literary events. This is particularly easy to recognize with the character of Criseyde. She flickers between the mimetic illusion that her narrative personage is an animate agent, free to influence the flow of events, and readers' knowledge that she is a structural component in a finished narrative totality. In literary tradition, Criseyde's very name is synonymous with erotic betrayal—even as her name, in the course of Chaucer's narrative, also designates a seemingly spontaneous and self-moving intelligence.[61] Parallels and echoes between the determined nature of literary character and the fatedness of human action make for moments of queasy shifting across ontological modes—as when Criseyde foresees her literary fate within a text that is part of that very heritage: "'thise bokes wol me shende [ruin]. / O, rolled shal I ben on many a tonge!'" (V.1060–61).

Scholars generally agree that the *Troilus* and the "Knight's Tale" were written in close succession, and their shared formal and thematic preoccupations show Chaucer thinking through closely related problems. In the

"Knight's Tale," the linked philosophical and literary levels familiar from the *Troilus* are figured through the dying body of Arcite. His heteronomy is represented in physiological, medical terms. In the process, the "Knight's Tale" elaborates the structural analogy between literary character and embodiment. Physiologized subjectivity revolves around the condition of having simultaneously an active and passive relation with one's own flesh: I at once possess my body and coincide with it; I use it and suffer it. Literary character operates somewhat similarly, mediating self-animation and formal determination. Literary characters "act" according to a mimesis of agency that is limited by the narrative medium in which they have existence. If *Troilus and Criseyde* explored this through Boethian meditation and a generic mixture of tragedy and romance, the "Knight's Tale" adds the further scrim of *phisik* and cosmologized materiality.

Both *Troilus and Criseyde* and the "Knight's Tale" culminate with spectacular gestures of closure that do not entirely resolve the questions raised by their respective narratives. Rosemarie P. McGerr observes of the *Troilus*'s "almost parodic 'piling on' of traditional medieval closure devices" that in effect the end protests too much.[62] While the "Knight's Tale" is not quite so baroque in its concluding flourishes, it too wraps up with an abruptly happy ending:

> And thus with alle blisse and melodye
> Hath Palamon ywedded Emelye.
> And God, that al this wyde world hath wroght,
> Sende hym his love that hath it deere aboght;
> For now is Palamon in alle wele,
> Lyvynge in blisse, in richesse, and in heele,
> And Emelye hym loveth so tendrely,
> And he hire serveth so gentilly,
> That nevere was ther no word hem bitwene
> Of jalousie or any oother teene.
> Thus endeth Palamon and Emelye;
> And God save al this faire compaignye! Amen. (3097–3108)

[And thus with all bliss and melody has Palamon wedded Emelye, and God, who made all this wide world, send him his love who has it dearly bought, for now is Palamon in complete happiness, living in bliss, in wealth, and in health, and Emelye loves him so tenderly, and he serves her so nobly, that there was never a word between

them of jealousy or other vexation. Thus, end Palamon and Emelye.
And God save this fair company! Amen.]

In these lines' celebration of the dyadic bliss of Palamon and Emelye, there is
no mention of Arcite's starkly different fate. Acknowledgement of the absent
knight would interrupt the closure of wedded bliss by demonstrating its par-
tialness, by pointing to its outside. The laughter of Arcita looking down from
the celestial spheres in the *Teseida* is absent from the "Knight's Tale," but the
specter of that ironic vantage nonetheless hovers over the conclusion. Because
the afterlife has been pared away from Chaucer's version, Arcite's imagined
perspective remains only counterfactual, but his absence is real.

It is probable that the narrative of the "Knight's Tale" originally stood on
its own as a complete composition before being incorporated, with relatively
little revision, into the Canterbury frame.[63] Chaucer's fitting of "al the love
of Palamon and Arcite"[64] into the *Tales'* structure would have entailed his
coming to see what had been an independent work now, newly, as a component element, a part. This incorporation also brought with it the task of
reimagining the tale as interpreted by an especially diverse range of listeners;
it meant hearing it with churl's ears, as it were. The "Miller's Tale," after all,
echoes and parodies many aspects of the "Knight's Tale," and its composition
seems to have been a process of rewriting the philosophical romance from the
standpoint of fabliau. The Miller's ribald Oxford story would have been written, as Helen Cooper puts it, "not only after Chaucer had decided to compose
a story-collection, but when he realized how the sequence of tales could be
articulated internally, through the parallelism of adjacent stories, and externally, through the dramatic exchange of the pilgrims."[65] Creating the "Miller's
Tale" alongside the preexisting "Knight's Tale" would likely have been Chaucer's first working-through of how the tale-telling contest would redound on
individual narratives.

The Miller, I want to argue in closing, can be read as another version of
Arcite. Against the force of formal and cosmic totalization that the "Knight's
Tale" ultimately endorses (even while troubling it), the Miller enacts the
power of appetitive, counterfactual emergence. If Arcite's body comes to mark
the dangerous place where elements might (but do not) "flee" their "certeyn
boundes," where "moevable thingis" could "fleten folyly," and a creature might
surpass its "duracioun" and "fordo the fassoun of this world"— the Miller
actually realizes these impulses, not so much in his personality or identity but
in the role he plays in altering the operations of the tale-telling frame.[66]

The Miller is initially slotted within an encompassing formal and social order, which pervades the hierarchical presentation of the "faire compaignye" through the lens of estates satire. The Host then settles on a game of chance to determine who will tell the first tale. "'Now drawth cut, er [before] that we ferrer twynne [go],'" he enjoins; "'He which that hath the shorteste shal bigynne'" (835–36). With a show of inclusiveness, the Host calls the Prioress, the Clerk, and "every man" to lots (841). After "every wight" (842) draws a straw, lo and behold, it is the Knight, first described among the pilgrims and highest in the secular ranks, who pulls the shortest straw: "Were it by aventure, or sort, or cas, / The sothe is this: the cut fil to the Knyght" (844–45). The narrator's triple invocation of chance, luck, and destiny is soon be echoed in all of the unexplanatory explanations made *within* the "Knight's Tale," to festoon those unlikely coincidences upon which the romance plot depends: "And so bifel, by aventure or cas," "Were it by aventure or destynee," "by som cas, syn Fortune is chaungeable," and so on (1074, 1465, 1242). These narratorial nods to chance contribute to the impression of obscure, unlocalizable order running through the tale's events; with the drawing of lots, that order is also made responsible for the tale's being told in the first place. Chaucer's treble qualification, "by aventure, or sort, or cas," has the air of a wink and nudge to his readers, but it is difficult to say for certain what is being acknowledged. Certainly, that the game is fixed—but by whom? By Harry Bailey, with his domineering sense of occasion? Or by the poet-narrator, coyly fashioning his masterpiece? Or is it simply the opaque imperative of what exists, "the fassoun of this world," which can never be fully articulated by etiological explanation, and which finally goes under the name of *necessite*? This undecidability is precisely the point, and following on from this destined chance, the "Knight's Tale" upholds the indistinction between hegemonic order and contingent chance.

After the Knight has finished speaking, the Host's invitation to the Monk to tell the second story, "to quite with [to answer] the Knyghtes tale," dispenses with the artifice of happenstance altogether (3119). As the reigning *governour* of the game, the Host now sees to its ordering directly (813). Significantly, *governour* is the title with which Theseus is introduced at the start of the "Knight's Tale" ("Of Atthenes he was lord and governour" [861]). In the General Prologue Harry Bailey has warned of penalties for "whoso be rebel to my juggement"—not unlike Theseus's admonitions against anyone who is "rebel is to hym that al may gye [guide]" (833, 3046). Theseus and the Host are figures of authority who also function as mouthpieces for a much broader, more diffuse web of ordering force. The Host's call to the Monk to be the next tale-teller is a crucial moment in the *Canterbury Tales*, when the work is poised on the edge of sequentiality. The hinge between first and second tales is another first for the work, the inaugural instance of relation *among* tales. It is at this tipping point of structuration, on the threshold of series, that the Miller drunkenly roars out, "'I kan a noble tale for the nones [occasion], / With which I wol now quite [match, answer] the Knyghtes tale'" (3126–27). With these words, the Miller concretizes what circulated as unrealized possibility in the "Knight's Tale," namely, that the amoral powers of vitality embodied in Arcite might act as *rebel* to those totalizing forms—social, cosmic, and literary—that governed him.

Soon enough, the Miller's rebel energies of interruption and "grucching" come to be recognizable as elements of a self-contradictory masculinity not able to sustain the project of the *Tales*. The first fragment, of course, runs aground a little way into the "Cook's Tale." From Miller to Reeve, and Reeve to Cook, the tales descend into an increasingly appetitive register, until finally, it would seem, no further composition is possible. Yet if the Miller's farcical reincarnation of Arcite does not provide a key to the totality of the *Canterbury Tales*, the odd couple of Arcite and the Miller do cipher between them, I think, the transition from Chaucer's philosophical romances to his final compositional project. The *Canterbury Tales* shifts away from the melancholy imperative that narrative necessity *must hold*, whatever the sympathies of poet or reader—an imperative that has ruled both *Troilus and Criseyde* and the "Knight's Tale." The Miller wrenches the pilgrimage away from the duty to make aesthetic *vertu* from what has been deemed *necessite*. In spite of the machinations of "aventure, or sort, or cas" the encompassing frame shudders a little and changes when the Miller wedges his tale into it. In the "Knight's Tale," such disruptions are effected only retrospectively or counterfactually, as readers trace interpretive paths back from Arcite's corpse through the tale's warren of forces and causes, seeking to understand how the knight's markedly material body fits and fails to fit the narrative world. Against Theseus's injunction to "maken vertu of necessitee" (3042), another energy, another vitality, strains against what *necessite* names, and in the *Canterbury Tales* it is tale-telling that is made, newly, the occasion for its coming into being.

Chapter 6

Desire and Defacement
in the *Testament of Cresseid*

In Robert Henryson's *Testament of Cresseid*, leprosy is the occasion for a complex experiment in the poetics of legible embodiment.[1] The Middle Scots rhyme-royal composition, written late in the fifteenth century, invents a new episode within the sequence of events narrated in Geoffrey Chaucer's *Troilus and Criseyde*.[2] After her acquiescence to Diomede but before Troilus's death, Criseyde—or Cresseid, as her name is spelled in Henryson's poem—contracts leprosy. This startling and apparently original plot twist in the matter of Troy effects a shift in the story's narrative mode, from romance to exemplum, which brings with it a corresponding change in the narrative's logic of bodily signification. Love lyric and romance, those genres of *fin' amor* that animate so much of Chaucer's *Troilus*, link the beautiful body of the beloved to aesthetic, semantic, and spiritual plenitude. Yet the bitter conclusion of Troilus and Criseyde's affair delegitimates beauty's body. By the end of Chaucer's poem, Criseyde's figure is where what is *fair* and what is *trew* have torn asunder. The *Testament* answers the devastation of that finale by offering in place of beauty's discredited ideal a new model of legible embodiment. Punishment overcodes loveliness, as exemplum replaces romance. When illness disfigures her, Cresseid's corporeality seems again to be invested with trustworthy meaning. Like the decipherable faces imagined by physiognomic treatises or the punitive illnesses recounted in exempla, Cresseid's leprosy seems to act as a simple index of her inner person, a true image of her falseness.

However, the legibility of justice on Cresseid's body is disrupted by two factors. The first is a fundamental incoherence in the *Testament*'s plot. Though her leprosy is narrated straightforwardly as a penalty for her faults, those faults

are not those that the poem ends by condemning, namely, the "greit unstabilnes" and "fals deceptioun" that have undermined her love affair with Troilus.[3] Instead, Cresseid's infection is the outcome of a judicial decision by the
planetary gods, who descend from the sky to castigate her for blasphemy.
The discrepancy between these two wrongdoings, blasphemy and romantic
betrayal, disturbs the logic of the would-be exemplum. The knot between
action and consequence is undone, and the question of exactly *why* Cresseid
contracts leprosy becomes an open one. Do the gods really cause her illness?
Are they mere allegories of natural forces, or agents of an absent monotheistic
power? Is her leprosy sexually transmitted, humorally induced, or psychosomatic? Is it the outcome of punishment, conscience, or misfortune? As in
Chaucer's "Knight's Tale" (the topic of the previous chapter), the proliferating
explanations for bodily devastation destabilize the story's moral logic, and etiological imagination leads to interpretive speculation.

Through the intricacies of its frame narrative, the *Testament* suggests still
another possible cause for Cresseid's leprosy: readerly desire. In an echo of
Chaucer's dream poems, the *Testament* commences by recounting the physical
vulnerabilities and erotic frustrations of the narrator, who reads first Chaucer's
Troilus and then "ane uther quair [another book]" containing the story of
Cresseid's fate (61). The frame mediates between the status of Cresseid's leprosy as something given—historically occurring and naturally caused—and
the contrary possibility that it is invented, dreamed up, and "fenyeit of the
new [devised anew]" (66). This opening sequence comes to act as a causal
genesis and etiological explanation for Cresseid's *tragedie*. Through a variety
of hermeneutic cues, readers are directed to reflect on how the persona of
the reader-poet might be understood to determine and invent Cresseid's fate.
Readers' corporeal desires impinge on literary tradition, the poem suggests,
and the bodies in Troy register the appetites brought to bear on vernacular
poetry.

If the incoherence of exemplary justice is one source of disorder in the
Testament's poetics of legible embodiment, another disturbance emerges from
the aesthetic and emotional power of Cresseid's leprous body. As fiercely as
the *Testament* tries to leave behind the discredited corporeality of courtly love,
Cresseid's flesh remains a locus of desire beyond the operations of punishment
and unmasking. Her leprous form conducts a subterranean current of fascination over the course of the poem, which scrambles crime-and-punishment
linearity and gives way to a flickering simultaneity of past and present, beauty
and disgrace, and figuration and disfiguration. These effects ultimately connect

Cresseid to medieval traditions of devotional and hagiographic writing about leprosy, in which the disease's symptoms have the power to *undo* the signifying function of flesh. Such effects might have remained mere stylistic whispers were it not for the poem's arresting "non-recognition scene," when Troilus and Cresseid meet a final time and fail to recognize one another.[4] Troilus's emotional convulsions on seeing Cresseid, though he does not know who she is, hint at a corporeality whose affective powers might overwhelm both erotic possession and narrative justice.

Misalignments of Justice

The fact that the cause and meaning of leprosy in the *Testament of Cresseid* are matters of debate might seem at first glance surprising. The scene of Cresseid contracting the disease seems to be written so as to display the neat mechanics of its exemplary justice. She falls ill just after accusing the gods Venus and Cupid of betraying their promise that she would always be the "flour of luif [love] in Troy" (128). She is at this point at her father's home, where she has fled after being cast off in disgrace by Diomede. "'O fals Cupide, is nane [none] to wyte [blame] bot thow, / And thy mother, of lufe the blind goddes!'" she declares reproachfully (134–35). As soon as the words are out of her mouth, she falls into a swoon, and the seven planetary deities assemble nearby. The gods fall into a makeshift court to try her on charges of blasphemy. Responsibility for her sentencing falls to Saturn and Cynthia, and the pair settle on the penalty of leprosy:

> For the dispyte to Cupide scho had done
> And to Venus, oppin and manifest,
> In all hir lyfe with pane to be opprest,
> And torment sair with seiknes incurabill,
> And to all lovers be abhominabill. (304–8)

> [For the injury to Cupid and Venus that she had done, patent and evident, in all her life with pain to be oppressed and tormented harshly with incurable sickness and to all lovers to be abominable.]

The verdict articulates Cresseid's crime (*dispyte*, or blasphemy) and her punishment ("seiknes incurabill," or leprosy). When she wakes and looks in the mirror, her exclamations confirm the court's rationale: "'Lo, quhat it is,' quod sche, / 'With fraward langage for to mufe [incite] and steir [provoke] / Our craibit [ireful] goddis; and sa [thus] is sene on me! / My blaspheming now have I bocht full deir'" (351–54). Her leprosy thus appears to be "what dream historians call an 'apport,' an artifact from the dream that guarantees its authenticity."[5] The punishment's grim reality in waking life confirms the dream's ontological standing and the punitive logic by which it has operated.

The legalism of the whole proceeding is notable.[6] It is called a *parliament*, a term for "the highest court in the land," and Mercury is elected *foirspeikar*, a chairman and advocate for the plaintiff (266).[7] Cupid addresses the gathered pantheon to explain his legal rationale: "quha [whoever] will blaspheme the name / Of his awin [own] god, outher [either] in word or deid, / To all goddis he dois baith lak [insult] and schame / And suld have bitter panis to his meid [reward]" (274–77). He then details Cresseid's offenses, her false claim against Venus and Cupid and the "sclander and defame injurious" of her calling Venus blind (281–84). It is for these harms to divine majesty that Cupid seeks redress (304–8). "Lawfullie" Saturn then imposes Cresseid's illness, and the "frostie wand" that he touches to her body is similar to the staff borne by officers in a Scottish court of justice (311–12).[8] Cynthia reads aloud a legal document, "ane bill," containing the "sentence diffintyve [final sentence]" that condemns her (332–33). Together, these judicial details give procedural rigor to the scene of Cresseid's infection, articulating her violent transformation through the intricate formulae of justice. Such legal ceremony does not necessarily legitimate the gods' moral authority, but it gives exaggerated clarity and the imprimatur of institutional order to the events leading up to her leprosy.

It is remarkable, then, that the remainder of the *Testament* undercuts the relevance of this scene and its intricate juridical logic. For instance, in the complaint that Cresseid makes on her first night in the leprosarium where she has gone to live (408–69), she attributes her disease to fortune's vicissitudes and time's inevitable corruption, with no mention of her blasphemy or the gods' punishment. In her self-excoriating lament after encountering Troilus a final time (546–74), Cresseid blames herself for her infidelity, not for her attacks on Cupid and Venus; addressing Troilus in his absence, she cries, "All faith and lufe I promissit to the / Was in the self fickill and frivolous: / O fals Cresseid and trew knicht Troilus!" (551–53). In these cases and others, blasphemy seems completely forgotten. The moralization offered in the poem's last stanza likewise reiterates Cresseid's romantic faithlessness, without any mention of her impiety:

Now, worthie wemen, in this ballet schort,
Maid for your worschip and instructioun,
Of cheritie, I monische and exhort,
Ming not your lufe with fals deceptioun:
Beir in your mynd this sore conclusioun
Of fair Cresseid, as I have said befoir. (610–15)

[Now, worthy women, in this short ballad made for your virtue and
instruction, I admonish and exhort you, for charity, do not mix
your love with false deception. Bear in mind this painful end of fair
Cresseid, as I have said before.]

Indeed, readers do not have to wait until they reach the finale of the *Testament*
to feel that the charge of blasphemy is out of step with the dynamics of the
poem. The opening frame narrative goes to considerable lengths to evoke the
tragic disappointments and frustrations of Chaucer's *Troilus* and to leverage
those dissatisfactions for its own literary appeal. Subsequent sections of this
chapter will argue for the entanglement of readerly desire and exemplary justice in the poem's frame, but suffice it to say for now, Cupid's charge of blasphemy departs from the expectations that the *Testament* has raised. Cresseid's
blasphemy and the court of the gods act like a tidy exemplum that has become
lodged somehow within the plot of a completely different story.

Literary critics have often managed the disparities among the meanings
for Cresseid's leprosy in the *Testament* by fitting them into a plot of moral
progress. According to this line of thinking, Cresseid, and the poem along
with her, gradually ascend from a false account of her disease's causes to a true
one, as she comes to recognize that Troilus's heartbreak is her leprosy's proper
significance. "From whatever point of view the *Testament* is considered," writes
John MacQueen in a representative formulation, "Cresseid's leprosy is to be
regarded as punishment for her 'brukkilnes,' her lightness in love."[9] Lee Patterson gives a stringent articulation when he claims that Cresseid's dream should
be dismissed simply because the gods "do *not* punish her for wantonness nor,
most significantly, for her betrayal of Troilus. To any reader of Chaucer (which
includes Henryson's narrator), Cresseid is worth bothering about because she
both created and destroyed a romance of almost transcendent beauty. . . .
Even her later collapse into promiscuity is secondary to her fundamental failure of *trouthe*."[10] MacQueen and Patterson seem certain that they know why,
really, Cresseid has to suffer, and on their accounts, the poem wends its way to

agreement with them, culminating in the final stanza's admonishment, "Ming not your lufe with fals deceptioun" (613).

Yet arguments like these often ignore more fundamental questions that their claims raise—for instance, in Patterson's case, questions about the criteria by which he distinguishes Cresseid's "fundamental" faults from her "secondary" ones, or how he can be sure that "Cresseid's past crime" is "far more serious than blasphemy."[11] What are the grounds of these moral distinctions? Can we be certain the poem shares them? Patterson cannot rely on normative frameworks of Christian virtue since those have little to say about betraying a love affair. His reading instead elevates "any reader of Chaucer" to the position of moral authority. He conflates what this posited reader thinks—that "Cresseid is worth bothering about because she both created and destroyed a romance of almost transcendent beauty"—with what he calls the "real Absolutes" that the *Testament* defends.[12] This conflation allows Cresseid's leprosy to appear as intertextual justice, and it casts the duration of her disease in the poem as a moral journey that gradually brings her into alignment with the viewpoint of the Chaucerian reader. But this attribution of the moral high ground to (implicitly masculine) readers ignores the vexed ethical relationship between literary tradition and literary characters that Henryson, like Chaucer before him, insists on raising.

Patterson's reading, now many decades old, is still worth engaging because it succumbs so vigorously to one of the *Testament*'s great temptations—the inducement to make its exemplary plot cohere, against the evidence of the text and on the strength of readers' own desires for justice, for psychological consistency, for a plot of moral redemption, or simply for Cresseid.[13] One of the primary functions of the court of the gods is, I think, to interrupt the production of such coherence. It would have been a simple matter for Henryson to have portrayed the gods' censuring Cresseid for her betrayal of Troilus, a crime that falls under Cupid's jurisdiction. But the poem instead stages the trial of a different crime. The scene occupies more than a third of the length of the poem, and the mythographic portraits constitute a set piece of aureate poetic finesse. It assumes real poetic gravity in the unfolding of the *Testament*, and all subsequent narrative events depend on this one. Moreover, as Steven Kruger has observed, the initial images of Cresseid's dream evoke "the love and harmony that bind the cosmos" and thus associate Cresseid's *extasie* "with divinely inspired experience."[14] Even if the gods are always available to suspicion in medieval Christian culture, they here seem to enjoy supernatural warrant. Cupid's *parliament* thus creates a genuine conundrum in the body of the poem.

Giving the court of the gods its due weight in interpretation does not mean accepting blasphemy as the true significance of Cresseid's leprosy, which my own reading does not. But it does entail allowing the episode, with its elaborately wrought legal detail and its strong claim to being the origin of Cresseid's disease, to interrupt the etiological coherence that seems to emerge elsewhere in the poem. The trial's peculiar combination of clarity (in its legalistic detail and punitive logic) and confusion (in its relation to the rest of the text) suggest that the operations of justice in Henryson's narrative might not be as straightforward as they seem. At the point where the *Testament* appears to bind its exemplary justice to Cresseid's own actions, it falters. Like Arcite's injury in the "Knight's Tale," it unravels the plot's moral coherence. What Cresseid is guilty of and why she is struck with leprosy never quite come into focus over the course of the *Testament*. These misalignments make the work a failed exemplum but a powerful framework for revealing the assumptions, desires, and narrative operations that go into the exemplum's literary project.

The Narrator's Body

In the course of the *Testament of Cresseid*, the authorial activity of the narrator is mentioned exactly twice, in the first stanza and in the last. The opening lines deliver a fully embodied voice, whose poetic authority and corporeal vulnerability are entwined:

> Ane doolie sessoun to ane cairfull dyte
> Suld correspond and be equivalent:
> Richt sa it wes quhen I began to wryte
> This tragedie; the wedder richt fervent,
> Quhen Aries, in middis of the Lent,
> Schouris of haill gart fra the north discend,
> That scantlie fra the cauld I micht defend. (1–7)

[A dismal season to a woeful poem should correspond and be equivalent. Just so it was when I began to write this tragedy. The weather was very turbulent when Aries in the midst of Lent made showers of hail fall from the north, so that scantily could I defend myself from the cold.]

The *Testament* unspools from a stylistic axiom: the season ought to match the poem. Before it is anything else, the narration is a normative claim about literary composition, enjoining correspondence. That this project of correlation runs throughout the *Testament* is suggested by what follows: *just so*, even as it ought to be, it was when I began to write this tragedy. The deictic "this" bridges the past of composition with the artifactual present of the text and marks the weather as hovering both inside and outside the poem. It is undecidable whether the hailstorm induces the poet-narrator to write the "cairfull dyte" or if his meteorological description follows from the genre—in which case, it would be the text's inaugural poetic shaping of the quasi-natural world. As in a dream vision, the interplay between the passivity of Henryson's narrator and his slyly admitted authorship puts the status of the poem's natural forces in question.

Much of the frame narrative is dedicated to recounting the narrator's exposure to the weather and, more broadly, to his material world. He reports that despite the storm, "within myne oratur [private chapel] / I stude," preparing to pray to Venus, "luifis [love's] quene" (8–9, 22). He hopes Venus will "mak grene," or revivify, his "faidit [withered] hart" (24). These devotions to Venus, coming fast on the mention of Lent ("in middis of the Lent" [5]), place the narrator in the emphatically literary milieu that the narrators of Chaucer's dream poems also inhabit, where classicizing ardor mingles with Christian colloquialisms. The narrator's supplications are interrupted by the bitter winds, which "fra Pole Artick come quhisling loud and schill, / And causit me remufe aganis my will [from the Arctic Pole came whistling loud and shrill and caused me to remove against my will]" (20–21). Under duress he retires to his hearth, lamenting, "I thocht to pray hir hie magnificence; / Bot for greit cald as than I lattit [prevented] was" (26–27). Venus in this opening sequence wavers between planet and goddess, as "hir bemis" (15) stream from the night sky even while the narrator seeks to pray to her. The planetary deity's ontological doubling foreshadows the interpretive difficulty that readers face later in the poem in trying the unknot the tangled influence of the gods in Cresseid's leprosy.

Venus is here described in an astronomical configuration that is impossible—rising in the east with "Hir goldin face, in oppositioun / Of God Phebus, direct discending doun" (13–14). On the basis of the astronomical knowledge that Henryson demonstrates elsewhere, Denton Fox concludes that the poet stages this heavenly contradiction to imply the planets' "impossibly great malevolence."[15] If Fox is right, then the planetary alignment portends at once the narrator's exposure of Venus's dire influence and, at the same time, the writer's ability to reconfigure the natural world according to his own literary imperatives. The impossibly ill-omened sky forms a kind of emblem for the duality of the narrator's status, divided between his exaggerated vulnerability and his authorial power to shape nature. This mixture of weakness and outsize power, of impingement and overreaching, is characteristic of how Henryson portrays the post-Chaucerian literary endeavor of his poem.

The physical cold that menaces the narrator's person seems to come from within and without at once. "Thocht lufe be hait [Though love is hot]," he remarks, "yit in ane man of age / It kendillis nocht sa sone [soon] as in youtheid, / Of quhome [In whom] the blude is flowing in ane rage; / And in the auld [old] the curage doif and deid [vigor is faint and dead]" (29–32). The narrator parrots Galenic humoral theory, according to which the body grows older and drier as it ages. Continuing this materialist account of himself, the narrator declares the "fyre outward" as the "best remeid [remedy]" for his cooling passion, a solution that helps "be [by] phisike quhair [where] that nature faillit" (33–34). Denton Fox suggests that Henryson is here "ironically perverting the common doctrine that the ailments of love can be cured only by the loved one."[16] The narrator's invocation of "phisike," then, expresses a masculinist fantasy, a vision of bachelor self-sufficiency mixed with bathos: the solitary old man has no need of a lady's favors, thanks to the fire's heat. It is in the midst of these creature comforts that the narrator soon sets about reading Chaucer's *Troilus and Criseyde*. If this is the persona that mediates readers' access to Cresseid's *tragedie*, then it associates that access with a contingent, corporeal, and self-concerned perspective.[17]

The opening of the *Testament* evokes the genre of the dream poem: a beleaguered first-person narrator, sleepless one seasonally appropriate night, pulls a book from the shelf and starts to read.[18] Though these initial expectations are never answered with the narrator's actual dream, the genre cues help to orient readers' interpretations. For instance, the *Testament* shares with dream poetry a concern with its narrator's physiology. In a commonplace inherited from Macrobius's commentary on the *Dream of Scipio*, dream visions often begin with a catalogue of dream types and their causes, including somatic etiologies. Causation was important because it was thought to determine a dream's nature, whether revelation or symptom, deception or truth. Steven Kruger has persuasively shown that in the later Middle Ages a "'somatizing' of dream theory" took place, as new protocols of interpretation came to insist that the "dreamer has a body that plays an important part in determining the content and form of his or her dreams."[19] Accordingly, late medieval dream poems tend to play on the fact that the meaning of the recounted vision is bound up with the embodied subjectivity of the author. The Black Knight in Chaucer's *Book of the Duchess* may be a symptom of the narrator's melancholy, and in the *House of Fame*, the narrator's admission that "folkys complexions / Make hem [them] dreme" directs hermeneutic attention to his own body.[20] Scholars have long noticed the physiological and psychosomatic dimensions of Cresseid's dream later in the *Testament*,[21] but Henryson plays with the bodily determinations of experience much earlier in the poem. Cresseid's *tragedie* is what occupies the structural position of the dream, and the *Testament* thus cannily argues that the narrator's role is like that of a dreamer, who is both the passive receiver and the active creator of the story he experiences. A similar doubleness has already been staged in the opening lines' oscillation between suffering and composing the natural world. Readers are encouraged to wonder what consequences the narrator's querulous masculinity might have for the fabulation of Cresseid's story.

It is notable that the narrator describes himself trying to pray in an *oratur* before arctic blasts drive him fireside (8). Later in the *Testament*, Cresseid's angry accusations of Cupid and Venus, the ensuing parliament of the gods, and her waking recognition of her leprosy all take place in "ane secreit orature" (120). These two characters' botched prayers in their respective oratories constitute one in a web of similarities that link them. The narrator and Cresseid also share physiological traits, like the "preponderance of cold and dry qualities";[22] both are associated with carnality;[23] and Amber Dunai points out their shared exclusion from the religion of love.[24] Like the Black Knight in the *Book of the Duchess*, Cresseid can be read as a psychosomatic phantasm of the narrator, through which he rejects his own vulnerabilities by attempting to exteriorize and judge them.[25] For both the narrator and Cresseid, the *oratur* is a space of would-be retreat and divine petition that comes to be the setting for physical vulnerability and exclusion from Venus's graces. The word also has strong Chaucerian associations, recalling the temples of Venus, Mars, and Diana in the "Knight's Tale"—"thise oratories thre."[26] Like Chaucer's pagan oratories, those in Henryson's poem raise the murky question of the gods' powers—whether those of Venus, to whom the narrator prays, or of the vindictive Cupid, who prosecutes Cresseid. Should they be read allegorically or literally, naturally or supernaturally? What sort of reality principle governs the poem? The "Knight's Tale" acts as an important intertext for the *Testament*,[27] in part because in both works the gods' vivid presence brings with it causal and moral confusion, which in turn allows for surprising interpretive dynamism.

Just as it does in the "Knight's Tale," the *oratur* in Henryson's poem names a crucible of disordered and overdetermined forces.

The frame narrative, then, is a device that allows readers to take some distance from the perspective of the aggressively vulnerable narrator. Henryson's aim, on this reading, is to cast the practices of post-Chaucerian vernacular reading—and, as I argue in the next section, vernacular authorship—under the same etiological scrutiny as dreams. Poetic fabulation here replaces oneiric fabulation, and the quasi-passivity of the dreamer is replaced by the quasi-passivity of the reader-writer, whose unsatisfied desires goad the production of new works. Suspended between physical impingement and creative potency, the narrator has the effect of spurring readers to recognize their own desires for Cresseid's leprosy and to regard the moral ground of those desires as contingent and personal, not absolute. The frame's effect is not, as Derek Pearsall has rightly recognized, one of "systematic irony," such that all the values and assumptions in the rest of the poem are subverted.[28] Instead, as with dream poetry generally, the frame encourages open-ended reflection on the relationship between what occurs in the enframed world and the bodies, desires, and circumstances that lie outside it, as its oblique reflection and cause.

The Narrator's Book

Fleeing from the icy blasts rattling the *oratur* and fussily warming himself by the fire, the narrator introduces Chaucer's romance:

> I mend the fyre and beikit me about,
> Than tuik ane drink, my spreitis to comfort,
> And armit me weill fra the cauld thairout.
> To cut the winter nicht and mak it schort
> I tuik ane quair—and left all uther sport—
> Writtin be worthie Chaucer glorious
> Of fair Creisseid and worthie Troylus. (36–42)

> [I stoked the fire and warmed myself all around, then took a drink
> to comfort my spirits, and I fortified myself well against the cold
> outside. To cut the winter night and make it short, I took a book,
> and abandoned all other pastimes, written by worthy and renowned
> Chaucer about fair Cresseid and worthy Troilus.]

Like Chaucer's sleepless narrator in the *Book of the Duchess*, who chooses a *romaunce* to "drive the night away," as "better play / Then playe either at ches or tables," so too the *Testament* narrator chooses a *quair* over "uther sport" to pass the evening.[29] But the Chaucerian work proves cold comfort. The narrator's paraphrase covers only the events of Book V of the *Troilus*, concentrating mostly on Troilus's bereavement, his *wanhope*, *teiris*, and *pane*, how he "neir out of wit abraid [almost went out of his mind] / And weipit soir" and "sorrow can [did] oppres / His wofull hart in cair and hevines" (45–49, 55–56). The summary draws a stark visual contrast between the two lovers, recounting how Cresseid, "that lady bricht of hew," is received by Diomede, while Troilus suffers on, "with visage paill of hew" (44, 46). The narrator's prior complaints about his own "faidit hart of lufe" and his loss of erotic enjoyment associate him with Troilus—or at least make us suspect that he associates himself with Troilus's pitiable state. His one-note retelling, focalized only through Troilus, invites his audience to share in his identification with the spurned Trojan prince.

By means of this tendentious summary of *Troilus and Criseyde*, the *Testament* casts Chaucer's work not just as its literary source but as the source of its desire. The *Troilus* gives ennobling form to the dissatisfactions plaguing the cold and aging narrator. Troilus's guileless heartache dignifies the desires of the masculine subject, and the lost Cresseid seems to embody all that makes him vulnerable. The *Testament*'s selective paraphrase of the *Troilus* facilitates a circuit of identifications running among the discomforts of the narrator, the outsize suffering of Troilus, and the disappointments of those Chaucerian readers who are presumed to make up Henryson's audience. The poem's confidence in linking these three figures shows what a canny and opportunistic reader of Chaucer's text Henryson was. He took the measure of the longing that Book V of *Troilus and Criseyde* induces and decided that it could power his poem.

In Chaucer's text, this longing for Criseyde is focalized through both Troilus and Panadarus during their long vigil on the walls of Troy. Pandarus's growing hatred for his niece and Troilus's perduring love are, as E. Talbot Donaldson has observed, combined and mediated in readers' experiences.[30] The lover's gaze straining for some glimpse of Criseyde on the horizon is overlaid by the more aggressive wish to access her thoughts and feelings, a privilege that readers enjoyed at other points in Chaucer's story. Why hasn't she returned? What kind of account can she give for herself? Over the course of Book V, readers' curiosity is teased and thwarted, and their emotional disposition is tugged between Troilus's desperate affection and Pandarus's baffled fury.

Criseyde's ambiguous letters, Troilus's dream-image of her, and the brooch all act as polysemous traces that promise but revoke full disclosure. Like Criseyde's "slydynge of corage," the Chaucerian story slides over any moment that would bring its lost heroine fully into view, either for embracing or for interrogation.[31] Instead, over the course of Book V, she recedes into a cloud of signifiers.

It is at just this point in Chaucer's narrative that the *Testament* cuts off its retelling. Troilus remains caught in the sublunary cycles of hope and disappointment, turning round and round the absent figure of Criseyde. The Trojan knight's eventual death and ascent to the heavens are not mentioned in the *Testament*. Indeed, the dismissal of all earthly attachments that so bracingly marks the end of *Troilus and Criseyde* would have stopped Henryson's poem before it started. Troilus's celestial ascent and his laughter at the woe of the "wrecched world" implicitly chastise readers for those desires that until just that moment they had shared with him—but which now they hold on their own.[32] The *Testament*, by contrast, seeks to legitimate those thwarted desires and to make them its motor force. As in the *Book of the Duchess*, where Alcione's abrupt and comfortless death provokes the narrator's answering dream, so here the erotic, emotional, and epistemological frustrations of Book V seem to drive the fabulation of new satisfactions. Thus, just before his paraphrase of Book V would need to leap into the heavens, Henryson takes his leave of Chaucer in stanzas that are dense with literary self-consciousness:

> Of his [Troilus's] distres me neidis nocht reheirs,
> For worthie Chauceir in the samin buik,
> In gudelie termis and in joly veirs,
> Compylit hes his cairis, quha will luik.
> To brek my sleip ane uther quair I tuik,
> In quhilk I fand the fatall destenie
> Of fair Cresseid that endit wretchitlie.
>
> Quha wait gif all that Chauceir wrait was trew?
> Nor I wait nocht gif this narratioun
> Be authoreist, or fenyeit of the new
> Be sum poeit, throw his inventioun,
> Maid to report the lamentatioun
> And wofull end of this lustie Creisseid,
> And quhat distres scho thoillit, and quhat deid. (57–70)

[I do not need to rehearse Troilus's distress because worthy Chaucer, in the same book, in eloquent words and lively verse, has compiled his cares, whoever will look. To break my sleep, I took up another book in which I found the fated destiny of fair Cresseid, who ended wretchedly. Who knows if all that Chaucer wrote was true? Nor do I know if this narrative is authoritative or devised anew by some poet through his own invention, devised to tell the lament and sorrowful end of this delightful Cresseid and what distress she suffered and what death.]

These stanzas together constitute a complex structure of literary-theoretical self-comment, a kind of "literary manifesto," as MacQueen puts it.[33] Scholarly consensus is that this "uther quair" most likely never existed outside of the *Testament*'s diegesis and is instead an instance of the not uncommon topos of the imaginary authority.[34] That consensus has grown stronger following William Stephenson's identification of the acrostic "O FICTIO" running down the left side of the stanza that introduces the "uther quair."[35] The stanza is an account of the narrator's actions as a reader, as he takes a book from the shelf and simply discovers ("I fand [found]") Cresseid's "fatall destenie." His bumbling persona is here overwritten with the decidedly textual signature of literary invention—*o, fictio!*—an exclamation that applies as much to this avatar of readerly passivity as it does to Cresseid's fate. The narrator's voice, argues the acrostic, is formed according to an authorial agenda that is legible when the text is regarded not as a voice speaking but as a literary artifact. The device insists on the entanglements of authorial making and desirous reading—much as the *Testament*'s opening stanza does, where controlling the weather and suffering its effects are made indistinguishable.

After this winking introduction of the *uther quair*, the poem shifts into lines punctuated with terms from latinate literary theory (*authoreist, poeit, inventioun*), and the voice breaks momentarily away from the narrator's limited perspective. The theoretical idiom reintroduces the canny, authoritative tones not heard since the poem's first stanza, with its announcement of the *Testament*'s genre and its poetics of correspondence. Now the poem turns itself to questions of literary truth: "Quha wait gif all that Chauceir wrait was trew?" The precise meaning of the word *trew* here is open to question. The word and its ambiguities are central to *Troilus and Criseyde* and to the *Testament*, and more generally, as Richard Firth Green has shown, *treuth* is a word pulled among social, moral, epistemological, and ontological senses; the same range of denotations informed the Scots cognate of Henryson's day.[36] The narrator here seems to be querying Chaucer's historical accuracy, an established topos in writings on Troy.[37] Yet every other use of *trew* or *untrew* in the *Testament* derives from its more archaic sense, of faithfulness: for instance, "trew knicht Troylus," "trew lufe," "Als unconstant, and als untrew of fay [faith]," "Scho was untrew and wo is me thairfoir" (546, 564, 571, 602).[38] Like John Lydgate in the *Troy Book* before him, Henryson seems to impugn the veracity of Chaucer's poem by associating it with Cresseid's failures of personal *treuth*.[39]

What is most surprising about the *Testament*'s charge of poetic feigning is that it is not merely an out-turned allegation. It also refers directly to the *Testament*'s own narrative. While what Chaucer wrote may not be *trew*, the same goes for the "uther quair," which may be "fenyeit of the new / Be sum poeit, throw his inventioun" (66–67). This is an early use of *inventioun* to mean the "faculty of inventing or devising; power of mental creation or construction; inventiveness."[40] The stanza is a backhanded poetic vaunt, in which the *Testament* deauthorizes Chaucer in order to, as Nicholas Watson puts it, "legitimize the writing of fictions that are set in the waking world of history and 'unauthorized' except as products of the 'feigning' poetic imagination."[41] Inventing something new is the point, and the narrator's partial identification with this *poeit* entangles the story that follows in his masculine corporeality and fragilized feelings. No dream proves necessary for this feigning, but the dream-vision's generic trappings imply that historical fictions may also be influenced by contingent subjectivities and bodily circumstances. The stanzas disclose both poetic power and poetic weakness, and the admission lays the poet open to ethical culpability. The model of vernacular *inventioun* presented here is that of a Chaucerian reader who carries his emotionally charged reading on into his own book, in an only partly avowed process of second-order fabulation.

The next three stanzas constitute the last sustained appearance of the narratorial persona in the *Testament* (although his voice resurfaces in scattered moments). Here he continues his role as reader and paraphraser, recounting what befalls Cresseid in this "uther quair"—though, as I have argued, the preceding passage suggests that his passivity is a kind of disguise and his role should be regarded as creative and constitutive as well. The narrator first reports Diomede's rejection of Cresseid and her desolate wandering "up and doun, / And sum men sayis, into the court commoun" (76–77). Then, as though to dramatize the vanishing boundary between the inset text and the subjectivity of the reader, the narrator responds to Cresseid's misfortunes with two stanzas of histrionic and contradictory response—"famously queasy," as Derek Pearsall deems them:[42]

> O fair Creisseid, the flour and A per se
> Of Troy and Grece, how was thow fortunait
> To change in filth all thy feminitie,
> And be with fleschelie lust sa maculait,
> And go amang the Greikis air and lait,
> Sa giglotlike takand thy foull plesance!
> I have pietie thee suld fall sic mischance!
>
> Yit nevertheles, quhat ever men deme or say
> In scornefull langage of thy brukkilnes,
> I sall excuse als far furth as I may
> Thy womanheid, thy wisdome and fairnes,
> The quhilk fortoun hes put to sic distres
> As hir pleisit, and nathing throw the gilt
> Of the—throw wickit langage to be spilt! (78–91)

[O fair Cresseid, flower and foremost lady of Troy and Greece, how is it that you were destined to change into filth all of your femininity, and be with fleshly lust so defiled, and go among the Greeks early and late, so lewdly taking your foul pleasure?! I have pity that such misfortune should befall you. Yet nevertheless, whatever men judge or say scornfully about your frailty, I will excuse your womanhood, your wisdom, and your fairness to the utmost that I can, which Fortune has put to such distress as she likes to do, not at all through your own guilt—to be ruined by slander.]

The depiction of Cresseid's agency fluctuates wildly within these verses. The couplet *plesance/mischance*, for instance, is a morally incoherent one: *mischance* suggests pitiable circumstances into which Cresseid falls, while "foull plesance" makes her motive appetites the key to her calamitous state. All of the active verbs narrating Cresseid's "fleschelie lust" are framed as what she was *fortunait*, or destined by fortune, to do: fated to change her femininity, go among the Greeks, take her foul pleasure, and so on. Action and constraint, decision and necessity blur together, as the narrator lurches between judgment and exoneration. It is as though the narrator has not yet separated Cresseid off from himself as an independent figure; she is a transitional object, still caught in the motions of his affects. Denton Fox remarks of the rather unusual adjective *maculait* ("with fleschelie lust sa maculait") that "*maculatus* was frequently used of lepers, as in Leviticus 13:44."[43] Cresseid's imminent physical transformation, it seems, will *literalize* the narrator's flights of moralistic rhetoric.

Although the narrator's first-person pronouns subsequently disappear from the *Testament*, readers are meant to keep in mind his contingent, desiring personality, even as it becomes diffused into the diegesis. In the narrator's reactions to the "uther quair" Henryson has illustrated (as Pearsall puts it) "the vulgarity of the rush to judgment . . . where the male reader is the cuckold or rejected lover whose wounded pride is disguised as moral outrage and sweetened with false compassion."[44] Yet even as the poem exposes this vulgarity, it relies on those same affective hydraulics to make its literary endeavor go. The frame narrative grounds the *Testament* on the shifting sands of the narrator's persona—a self-involved, emphatically corporealized, and emotionally erratic reader-poet, who nonetheless embodies something powerful about the desires that Chaucer's *Troilus* can be understood to produce. The *Testament* endorses the narrator's reactions by giving us the story it does, but it also declines to make the emergence of that story unproblematic.

In light of the metafictional reading I have been advancing, which attends to the aggressive desires and poetic invention peeking out from the mask of readerly dullness, Mercury's role in the pantheon of the planetary gods is significant. He is another avatar of the author. He carries "buik in hand" and is ready "with pen and ink to report all"—"Lyke to ane poeit of the auld fassoun" (239, 242, 245). And he is not only a writer but a "Doctour in phisick," supposedly "Honest and gude, and not ane word culd lie" (250, 252). It is he who is elected spokesperson of the parliament (265–66). Here, then, is an archetype of authorship who is also an expert in bodies, one who presides over Cresseid's transformation. As Jill Mann remarks, "Henryson's poker-faced assurance that Mercury is 'Honest and gude, and not ane word culd lie'" functions to draw "attention to the lying nature of poetry."[45] In assigning Mercury the judicial role of *foirspeikar*, Henryson ciphers his shaping power over Cresseid's fate. Mercury also clarifies the likeness shared between the gods and the role of the poet. Both have power over "thing generabill [created things] / To reull [rule] and steir [control] be thair greit influence / Wedder [Weather] and wind, and coursis variabill [mutable]"—a power that Henryson claims in the poem's first stanza (148–50). But neither gods nor poets fully transcend their own mutability or the provincialism of judgment that goes with it.

Contraries and Correspondence

Critics have long noted a pattern of harsh oppositions woven through the imagery of the *Testament*. Kurt Wittig posits that "sustained thematic contrast is the source from which the immense tension of the *Testament* arises"; Douglas Gray draws attention to how the poem "holds contraries in tension"—"hot and cold, 'faded' and 'green,' age and youth, ugliness and beauty"; and Jill Mann argues that the "pattern of contrasts that runs through the whole of the poem" acts as a structuring force.[46] Yet this imagery of dyadic opposition, I suggest, is opposed to another of the poem's aesthetic commitments, namely, to the principle of correspondence. If contraries put harsh polarities into the same frame, correspondence mandates their resolution into a decorum of aesthetic accord and limpid expression. This tension between contrast and correspondence is never merely formal in the *Testament*; it rather answers to the poem's deepest undertakings. As we have seen, Henryson's work positions itself as the inheritor of Criseyde's doubleness and the ironic rift that her betrayal opens across the entirety of Chaucer's *Troilus*, revealing it to be filled with "ambages— / That is to seyn with double wordes slye, / Swich as men clepe a word with two visages."[47] The harsh contraries of the *Testament* thus reproduce the self-difference that *Troilus and Criseyde* stages, between its heroine's virtue and her "slydynge of corage," her lovability and her untruth. In the pattern of imagistic contrasts, Henryson distributes this two-facedness across the surface of his poem, and these are the disparities on which his own narrative poetics will go to work, starting with the rule that season and poem, and eventually body and character, "Suld correspond and be equivalent" (2).

The primary literary instrument of Henryson's poetics of correspondence is the narrative operations of the exemplum. The general procedure of exemplary stories is to make their diegetic components ring with plot, or to become saturated with a sense of causal entailment. In the case of exemplary bodies, characters' flesh is made to conform to, and therefore be expressive of, the governing forces of the diegetic world.[48] The *Testament of Cresseid* goes to work on its matrix of contrasts by means of the exemplum's narrative structure, which can be said to redistribute aesthetic oppositions into narrative time. The exemplum disciplines doubleness by means of change and revelation:

deceptions are unveiled, characters are punished, all becomes clear. At the end of Chaucer's poem, readers are left with Criseyde as an ironic and contradictory figure, one who evidently contains within herself the potential for tenderness and betrayal. The *Testament* subsequently attempts to disambiguate her, to eradicate what is desirable in her, and to make her "to all lovers be abhominabill" (308).

The planetary gods might be understood as exemplars—and enforcers—of this poetics of legible embodiment. In the succession of their elaborately conventional portraits, the well-established topoi of astrological allegory give voice to a universe of correspondences. Mars is martial; Phoebus beams with light; Mercury displays his traditional gifts for rhetoric and music. While some are portrayed in their beneficent aspect and some malevolently, they are united by the agreement between their respective identities and corporealities. According to astrological theory, Saturn is a cold and dry planet, whose influence is linked to the melancholic humor, and Henryson's portrait of the god emphasizes exactly these qualities in his physiognomy: "his lyre [complexion] was lyke the leid [lead]," he has "lippis bla and cheikis leine and thin," and "ice schoklis" hang from his hair (155, 159, 160).[49] He, together with the Moon, is charged with giving Cresseid her leprosy, and the assignment reflects the homologies between planet and disease: leprosy is a cold, dry affliction whose symptoms proceed from an excess of burnt black bile.[50] As John Trevisa relates in his translation of Bartholomaeus Anglicus's *De proprietatibus rerum*, "undir the mone [moon] is conteyned sikenesse, losse, fere and drede, harm and damage. Therefore aboute [with respect to] the chaunginge of mannes body the vertue [power] of the mone worchith [works] principally."[51] Cynthia's portrait emphasizes her resemblance to Saturn and also to the leprous symptoms that Cresseid soon bears: Cynthia is "of colour blak" and "haw [livid] as the leid [lead]," and she wears a gray dress "full of spottis blak" (255, 257, 260).

Though critics have puzzled over the ultimate significance of the gods' procession—one hundred lines of aureate description that stand out in a poem otherwise notable for its concision—the deities' portraits are distinctly appropriate to the scene they precede, that of Cresseid's infection, where she is made to embody the judgment against her. The fact that the *extasie* within which their judgment is framed is called a "doolie dreame" recalls, again, the poem's opening line, with its enjoining of correspondence between "doolie sessoun" and "cairfull dyte" (344, 1). The gods are depicted coming together for the judicial assembly that will make Cresseid "correspond and be equivalent" to her wrongdoings.

The *Testament* thus makes Cresseid's body the primary medium of its literary project. Her figure is where the conventions of the exemplum go to work on the legacy of romance and where her own doubleness, the simultaneity of her falseness and fairness, will be traded for *doolie* correspondence. This centrality of her body to the poem's literary and aesthetic undertakings is of course by no means inevitable. Though Criseyde receives intermittent physical description over the course of Chaucer's poem, her body is not the poem's primary way of invoking and imagining her. Yet the *Testament* adopts the beautiful body of Criseyde as the figure that concretizes the dangers of love lyric and romance that are dramatized by Chaucer's poem. In these literary traditions of idealization, the corporeality of the beloved is made to brim with aesthetic, affective, and even metaphysical significance. Chaucer invokes this convention in the *Troilus*'s first description of Criseyde:

> Nas non so fair, forpassynge every wight,
> So aungelik was hir natif beaute,
> That lik a thing inmortal semed she,
> As doth an hevenyssh perfit creature,
> That down were sent in scornynge of nature.[52]

> [There was none so fair, surpassing everyone, so angelic was her
> natural beauty that like an immortal thing she seemed, as does a
> heavenly perfect creature that was sent down in scorning of nature.]

Criseyde is so fair that she seems to transcend nature. In answer, Henryson's poem will bring the natural forces of corruption to bear on her body. Appropriately, then, Saturn begins his sentencing of Cresseid by "excluding" those physical qualities that have made her a courtly paragon: "Thy greit fairnes and all thy bewtie gay, / Thy wantoun blude, and eik thy goldin hair, / Heir I exclude fra the for evermair" (313–15). Cynthia declares, "Thy cristall ene mingit [mingled] with blude [blood] I mak, / Thy voice sa cleir unplesand hoir and hace [harsh and hoarse] / Thy lustie lyre [lovely skin] ovirspred with spottis blak, / And lumpis haw [purplish lumps] appeirand in thy face" (337–40).

As Cynthia and Saturn speak their judicial sentences over Cresseid, their words thrust her into fleshly visibility, figuring her as spectacle and disfiguring her before our eyes. As I have argued, the *Testament* cleverly draws its poetic energies from the presumed frustrations of Chaucerian readers. In Book V of the *Troilus*, the hero, tossing and turning sleeplessly, gives voice to his anxious curiosity and desire for Cresseid's body: "'Wher is myn owene lady, lief and deere? / Wher is hire white brest? Wher is it, where? / Wher ben hire armes and hire eyen cleere / That yesternyght this tyme with me were?'"[53] Readers are invited to share Troilus's restless ignorance and to speculate with him. Henryson, as though in rebuke of Criseyde's slow fade from the Chaucerian poem, brings her harshly into view. The scene of her infection is one of scopophilia and sadism, which makes a spectacle of its exemplary justice. It unveils the figure concealed by all of Chaucer's deflections and feints and sets about destroying it. Mirth changes into melancholy; moisture dries up; bodily heat cools; "play and wantones" become "greit diseis" (319–20). The direction of change is unvarying, oriented by decline, decay, and perishing.

And yet the aesthetic effect of this language of defacement is more complex than it first seems. It creates an undertow of memory in the poem. Insofar as Saturn's and Cynthia's phrasing is dominated by the rhythm of before and after, readers' efforts to picture Cresseid in the moment of her metamorphosis render "then" and "now" co-present on her figure. *Two* faces appear at once: one beautiful and one diseased, one courtly and one admonitory, one crystal-eyed and one bleary, overlapping one another. Nor is the simultaneity of Cresseid's beautiful and infected bodies restricted to the representation of her sentencing by the gods. Each time someone is shown reacting to Cresseid's appearance, the pattern recurs. When Calchas comes to see Cresseid after her dream, "He luikit on hir uglye lipper [leprous] face, / The quhylk [which] befor was quhite [white] as lillie flour" (372–73). Two faces again are conjured, one leprous and one lily pale. Similarly, when she goes to live in the lazar house,

> Sum knew hir weill, and sum had na knawledge
> Of hir becaus scho was sa deformait,
> With bylis blak ovirspred in hir visage,
> And hir fair colour faidit and alterait. (393–96)

> [Some knew her well, and some had no knowledge of her because she was so deformed, with black boils spread over her face and her fair complexion faded and changed.]

For the inhabitants of the leprosarium, she wavers in and out of recognizability, and her "fair colour" is recalled even as it is declared faded and changed. These details create the undertow of memory in the poem, pulling the reader back toward the idealized lady of Troilus's affection. This backward pull is an upshot of the poem's pursuit of correspondence: as the exemplary plot works to change Cresseid into a different kind of expressive body, a physiognomy of fault, what she *was* is continuously evoked as well. Indeed, throughout the *Testament* Cresseid is never merely ugly but always appears as beauty canceled, or partially canceled—still haunting its own ruin.

The *Testament*'s continued recourse to the word *fair* hints at the ongoing allure of Cresseid's flesh. Despite the gods' verdict and its terrible effects, the phrase *fair Cresseid* persists throughout Henryson's narration. It is the adjective used most frequently to describe her, from the first mention of her name to the last: "fair Creisseid and worthie Troylus," "fair Cresseid, that endit wretchitlie," "O fair Creisseid, the flour and A per se / Of Troy and Grece," "fair Cresseid, sumtyme his awin darling" (42, 63, 78–79, 504).[54] Saturn's choice of Cresseid's "greit fairnes" as the first attribute to strip from her seems, from one angle, to capture leprosy's violence: the punishment despoils what seems almost inalienable, a quality grafted onto her proper name. Cresseid's thrice-repeated lament near the end of the poem—"O fals Cresseid and trew knicht Troylus!" (546, 553, 560)—seems to confirm the efficacy of the exemplum's narrative mechanics; her epithet has been replaced by its moralized negation. Yet the persisting use of *fair* even after her infection also points to the difficulty of leaving beauty behind when imagining Cresseid. Immediately after Saturn carries out the judgment against her, the narrator asks, "On fair Cresseid quhy [why] hes thow na mercie?" and he mourns the "wraikfull [vengeful] sentence gevin on fair Cresseid" (325, 329). "Fair Cresseid" endures all the way to the *Testament*'s concluding moral: "Ming not your lufe with fals deceptioun: / Beir in your mynd this sore conclusioun / Of fair Cresseid" (613–15). One effect of the adjective's ongoing presence is irony, but it is not merely ironic. It also points to an imaginative problem. When we picture Cresseid, what do we see? Insofar as she has referential heft, or a substantial identity shaped by literary tradition, she is constituted by Chaucer's poem as well as Henryson's. The *Testament* makes her body the medium of literary continuity, the common object that binds "ane quair" and "ane uther" to form a shared diegetic world and narrative tradition (40, 61). Having been evoked and described according to the generic conventions of romance in *Troilus and Criseyde*, Cresseid remains ontologically bound up with them. If the *Testament* sets out to eradicate the germs of courtly love borne in her figure, it cannot help but disseminate them as well.

The tension between linear sequence and unstable simultaneity finds concentrated expression in the "complaynt of Creseyde," which elaborates the well-known poetic theme of *ubi sunt* (literally, "Where are they . . ."). The complaint bears its own title in the manuscripts and deviates from the rhyme-royal stanzas of the rest of the *Testament* in favor of the nine-line stanzas of Chaucer's *Anelida and Arcite*. Henryson clearly regards it as a lyric set piece. *Ubi sunt* complaints tend to be premised on a chastening then-and-now structure: the authority of last things and the triumph of mutability over mortal life determine the poem's content and form. Yet the lyric voice, in its memorial reflections, simultaneously resurrects what has passed. What is present and absent coexist side by side, each with its own imagistic power. Cresseid laments,

> "My cleir voice and courtlie carrolling,
> Quhair I was wont with ladyis for to sing,
> Is rawk as ruik, full hiddeous, hoir and hace;
> My plesand port, all utheris precelling,
> Of lustines I was hald maist conding—
> Now is deformit the figour of my face;
> To luik on it na leid now lyking hes." (443–49)

> ["My clear voice and courtly caroling, when I was accustomed to sing with other ladies, is raucous as a crow, most ghastly, hoarse and harsh. My pleasing bearing, surpassing all others, of attractiveness I was held most fitting—now is deformed the figure of my face. No man takes pleasure to look at it."]

The complaint sets up the grim contrasts between then and now that are to be expected of the genre and of Cresseid's *tragedie*, but it also serves as a catalogue of all the courtly pleasures that her person is meant to have condensed within her.

The stanza quoted above is the fifth in the complaint, although it is the first to take up the first-person voice and speak in Cresseid's *I*. Before this point, though it is unambiguous that Cresseid is the speaker, the complaint is in the second person, speaking *to* Cresseid, in apparent self-apostrophe: "Thy greit triumph and fame and hie honour / Quhair [When] thou was callit of eird-lye wichtis [worldly people] flour, / All is decayit" (434–36). The displacement from *I* to *thou* intensifies the violence of the complaint's images, as they are made to function as imperatives: "This lipper ludge tak for thy burelie bour /

And for thy bed tak now ane bunche of stro [Take this leper house in place of your fine bedroom, and for your bed now take this bunch of straw]" (438–39). This second-person address seems to hover outside of Cresseid, pitying, relishing, and haranguing, before it insinuates itself into her grammatical subject position. The start of the lament—"O sop of sorrow, sonkin in cair, / O cative Cresseid"—recalls the beginning of the narrator's lurid apostrophe to her more than three hundred lines before: "O fair Cresseid the flour and A per se / Of Troy and Grece" (407–8, 78–79). In light of this uneasy echo, the complaint's movement from second person to first seems to reflect the way the poem's moral mechanics gradually work their way into her person and become her voice.

Cresseid here comments on her own disfigurement, noting, "Now is deformit the figour of my face." In the small extravagance of specifying the *figour* of her face, the line evokes, however faintly, the process of literary figuration that must continuously produce her both as who she was in Chaucer's poem and as the cancellation of that person in Henryson's. An analogue for Cresseid's paradoxical doubleness can be found in the face of the goddess Venus in the *Testament*. Venus is described in the court of the gods, "cled in ane nyce array [showy outfit], / The ane half grene, the uther half sabill blak" (220–21). Her face figures forth the constant motions of variability: "in hir face semit greit variance, / Quhyles [Sometimes] perfyte treuth and quhyles inconstance" (223–24). Truth and inconstancy are then visualized crowding into monstrous co-presence:

> Under smyling scho was dissimulait,
> Provocative with blenkis amorous,
> And suddanely changit and alterait,
> Angrie as ony serpent vennemous,
> Richt pungitive with wordis odious;
> Thus variant scho was, quha list tak keip:
> With ane eye lauch, and with the uther weip. (225–31)

> [While smiling she was dissimulating, alluring with loving glances and then suddenly changed and altered, angry as any venomous serpent, very caustic with offensive words. Thus variable she was, whoever cares to take heed—with one eye to laugh and with the other to weep.]

Contraries collide with one another—just as they do in the figure of the leprous Cresseid. In the case of Venus, however, any pretension to linear sequence is absent: one eye laughs at the same time that the other weeps. The insistent anaphora in the following lines pushes the effect further: Venus is "Now hait, now cauld, now blyith, now full of wo, / Now grene as leif, now widderit and ago" (237–38). "Now" hovers between a succession of narrative moments—*now* and then *now* and then *now*—and the singular *now* of coming face-to-face with the self-undoing identity of mutability.

In holding together an array of contraries on her teeming surface, Henryson's Venus converges with the medieval iconography of Lady Fortune, who was often portrayed with a divided face, light and dark, a smile and a tear.[55] Several prominent descriptions in the *Testament* link Cresseid directly to the two goddesses. In Cresseid's self-accusing final lament to Troilus, she mourns, "Sa efflated [puffed up] I was in wantones, / And clam upon the fickill quheill [wheel] sa hie. / All faith and lufe I promissit to the / Was in the self fickill and frivolous" (549–52). The fickleness of Fortune's wheel and the fickleness of Cresseid's vows associate her actions with the goddess's. In her lament's final stanza, she describes herself in terms that echo Venus's "greit variance": "I knaw the greit unstabilnes, / Brukkill as glas, into [within] my self," she remarks (568–69). "She concludes by realizing it was she herself who acted in the manner of the fickle goddess," E. Duncan Aswell remarks.[56] Douglas Gray agrees: "Cresseid thus seems the victim of Fortune. . . . And yet, with a change of perspective, it would not be hard to see Cresseid not as the victim, but as the *figura* of such a goddess."[57]

However, as much as Cresseid resembles Venus and Fortune, the doubleness of her leprous face is distinct. Her leprosy translates the goddesses' two-facedness into a new medium, into flesh that suffers mutability rather than personifying it. Her body is where the *Testament* viciously disciplines feminine doubleness, whether it comes from Venus or from Chaucer's poem. Green and black, laughing and weeping, true and false, fair and foul: these are among the contraries that constitute an aesthetic problem for the *Testament* and upon which its exemplary plot and poetics of legible embodiment go to work. Soon enough, Cresseid is made "uglye" and "abhominabill," and thereby correspondent to her wrongdoing (372, 308). In professing her own falseness ("O fals Cresseid"), by the end of the poem she attains again to a kind of paradoxical truthfulness. The *Testament* and its heroine thus lay claim to precisely that quality that is put in doubt in Chaucer's poem: "Quha wait gif all that Chauceir wrait was trew?" (64). Cresseid's doubleness survives only in the melancholy intermingling of past and present, of her face and its *deformit* figure, which cannot be shaken loose from her portrayal in the *Testament*. There is no further narrative step. As soon as her self-accusation is complete, Cresseid begins preparing herself for her demise, and "incurabill" leprosy meets no miraculous cure (307). As the final line reads, "Sen scho is deid I speik of hir no moir" (616).

The *Testament*'s Leprosies

Three distinct traditions of writing about leprosy in the Middle Ages inform the representation of the disease in the *Testament of Cresseid*; these can be deemed the naturalistic, the moralistic, and the affective traditions. Scholars have long been aware of the medical accuracy of the portrayal of Cresseid's leprosy—in its humoral etiology, its astrological affinities, and its symptomology.[58] Saturn and Cynthia's sentencing issues in such a detailed clinical description that Fox speculates that Henryson was "probably relying on the medical works of his time."[59] Because the diagnosis of leprosy was a high-stakes endeavor for patient and examiner alike in the later Middle Ages, discussions of leprosy in medical treatises and encyclopedic works tend to describe the disease's symptoms at length.[60] Henryson draws on such clinically precise accounts of bodily signs to give Cresseid's leprosy its vividness and verisimilitude. In turn, the planetary figures of Saturn and the Moon are used to organize a series of references to the natural causes of the disease—humoral, astrological, and environmental. The naturalistic aspects of Henryson's portrayal seem to make leprosy an effect of lateral correspondences, of metonymically linked bodies, powers, substances, and processes.

By contrast, in the moralistic scheme of leprosy's representation, the disease functions as a stock metaphor for sin or sign of transgression. For instance, in the widespread story *Amis and Amiloun*, a voice from heaven tells Amiloun that if he enters combat under a false identity, then "Fouler mesel nas never non / In the world, than thou schal be! [Fouler leper was there never in the world than you will be!]"[61] Sure enough, after the battle, "Al so [Just as] that angel hadde hem told, / Fouler messel [leper] that nas non hold / In world than was he."[62] The romance here treats the disease as a straightforward index of wrongdoing. While medical accounts of leprosy tend to dwell on the body's surface and to connect it to a dense web of physical forces, moralistic portrayals rely on vertical rather than lateral modes of connection. Even if leprosy is not portrayed as the direct result of a transcendent power, its meaning comes from a different ontological level; the body is the vehicle, and the soul or will is the tenor of the metaphor. This passage from a fourteenth-century English homily is typical:

> For riht als leper mas bodi
> Ugli, and lathe, and unherly,
> Sua mas the filth of licheri,
> The sawel ful lath, gastelye,
> And the bolning of prive pride
> Es leper, that na man mai hide.[63]

> [For just as leprosy makes the body ugly, loathsome, and repulsive, so the filth of lechery makes the soul very loathsome spiritually, and the swelling of secret pride is leprosy, which no man may hide.]

Leprosy's moralistic tradition is closely allied with the practices of biblical commentary and their attendant labor of moving between literal and allegorical levels. If naturalistic traditions of the disease dwell with the material body and the forces that combine and interact to influence it, moralistic articulations make leprosy itself a sign with meaning in the ethical or spiritual sphere.

One of the distinctive aspects of the *Testament*'s portrayal of leprosy is its careful integration of punitive and naturalistic idioms. The lateral correspondences effected by the medical tradition are crossed with the vertical correspondences of the moralistic one, and it is striking how neatly the scene of Cresseid's infection interleaves the gods' juridical proceduralism with symptomatic precision, as when Cynthia reads the *bille* with the *sentence diffinityve* including reduced "heit of bodie," a voice "hoir and hace [harsh and hoarse]," and a complexion "ovirspred with spottis blak" (334, 338, 339). Modern readers have often failed to appreciate the distinctiveness of Henryson's handling of leprosy in the *Testament* because they have assumed he worked from a singular and totalized model of the disease. Such a one-size-fits-all notion of medieval leprosy has been overturned by historical scholarship over the last several decades.[64] The moralistic tradition of leprosy in the Middle Ages was in fact quite distinct from its medical portrayals, and Luke Demaitre has demonstrated, for instance, the *absence* of blame and moralism in medical works of the kind that Henryson is likely to have consulted.[65] Different discourses and traditions of *lepra* had their own integrity, and it was generic context or writers' interpretive cues that signaled which model of the disease was being invoked. Leprosy in the Middle Ages did not automatically signify punishment, though its narrative use as such was conventional; on its own, it did not point definitively to a certain etiology or meaning, though its overdetermined status meant that varying associations could easily be activated.[66]

As I have argued, the disjunction between Cresseid's conviction for blasphemy and the poem's passionate investment in her wronging Troilus creates a discrepancy in the *Testament*'s exemplary plot, one that does not allow the moralization of Cresseid's disease ever to come to rest. But this inconsistency occurs in the midst of a completely different set of effects. Henryson is masterful in overlaying causal systems in arrangements of mutual reinforcement and amplification, achieving what Jill Mann calls the poem's "sinister effect of claustrophobia."[67] With Cresseid's leprosy, the *Testament* overlays his exemplum's incoherence with the impression of what might be called hypercoherence, created by the tight, even suffocating integration of disparate etiological models. This impression is achieved most spectacularly in the gods' parliament, which skillfully harmonizes the naturalistic and moralistic traditions of leprosy—while at the same time acting as the *Testament*'s key episode of emplotted incoherence, out of sync with the expectations that the poem has raised. The juridical procedures of the pantheon fold together medicine's detailed attention to the symptomatic body and the interplay of natural causes with the exemplum's mechanisms of judgment and exegesis's transit from body to moralized meaning. This hypercoherence expresses something like the fantasy of physiognomic knowledge, that the natural body can be made to reveal moral character and so render the viewer invulnerable to the depths of intention and possibility in other people.[68]

One might observe, then, that the poet expends considerable energy to naturalize his poem—and Cresseid's leprosy especially—but also to denaturalize what appears as nature. From the explicitly poetic motive for the weather to the aureate brilliance of the mythographic planets, these are natural forces of a peculiarly artificed quality, not free from a questionable will to power, whether the narrator's, Cupid's, or Henryson's own. The mutual reinforcement of art and nature takes place through moments of hypercoherence, when natural causation, cosmic justice, and literary satisfaction draw into tighter and tighter alignment. Simultaneously, the artifice of this integration makes room for a critique of the poem's apparent reality principle. Cresseid's leprosy, the terrible necessity she is made to bear, emerges from the fictional depths of the *Testament*—from classical gods within a dream, within a *quair*, within the narrator's subjective mediation, within the writer's *tragedie* ("quhen I began to wryte / This tragedie," 4–5). Hypercoherence is recognizable not just as the sign of a justly ordered cosmos but as the outcome of human making; as the acrostic reads: *o, fictio* (57–63).

However, there is yet another tradition of medieval leprosy that can be seen to shape the *Testament*'s portrayal of Cresseid. In the *affective* articulations of the disease that appear in hagiographic, homiletic, and pastoral writings, the encounter with leprosy is the occasion for intense aesthetic and emotional reactions—disgust, fear, pity, and ecstatic love. In these evocations, leprosy makes ordinary experience and narrative time seize up; attention is gripped by what defies easy apprehension. One of the influential texts at the root of this tradition is the comparison of the Man of Sorrows to a leper in Isaiah 53. In the early Wycliffite version of this book of the Bible it reads, "Ther is not shap to hym ne fairnesse & wee seeyen hym & he was not of sighte & we desireden hym dispisid," or, in the later version, "we sien [saw] hym, and no biholdyng was."[69] Several verses later, this unrecognizability is equated with leprosy: "wee heelden [beheld] hym as leprous." The Man of Sorrows, it seems, is just on the edge of recognizability or, more radically, of perceptibility ("not of sighte"). His appearance *quasi leprosus* indexes an encounter that cannot quite be grasped, that recedes from the viewer.[70]

In the religious culture of the high Middle Ages—which placed new emphasis on the corporal works of mercy, saw the ascendance of the mendicant orders and new hospital orders, and concentrated devotion on the incarnation of Christ—the leprous body came to be regarded as the medium of perceptual, affective, and mystical transformation. This tradition emphasized not only leprosy's radical undoing of bodily form but the subjective undoing of those who encountered leprous bodies. What had been a hagiographical topos that emerged from Jesus' curing of leprosy in the Gospels became in the life of Saint Francis a fulcrum of personal conversion, as Francis's original disgust for the disease is made over into wonder, love, and a practice of caregiving. The visceral force demanded to reverse disgust into *caritas* is captured in Raymond of Capua's 1395 *Legenda* of Catherine of Siena. When Catherine uncovers the stinking ulcer of a patient, she is seized with repulsion. In response she rebukes herself and "bent over the sick woman and pressed her mouth and nose to the festering sore, and in that posture she remained a long time, until she felt that the power of the spirit had subdued the nausea of the flesh."[71] Disgust functions both as a feeling to be disciplined and as a kind of affective heat, which melts Catherine's self-possession and makes further spiritual transformation possible. Such affective encounters between the sick and the well thus present *two* disfigured bodies—one racked by the effects of disease, one by aesthetic and emotional reactions to the leprous body. Face-to-face, infected and affected mirror one another in a moment of physical undoing.[72] This tradition gives depth to the *Testament*'s ongoing aesthetic fascination with Cresseid's body, which is never only an object of disgust but also bears within it the remembered promise of enthralling love. Henryson's secular work thus gains resonance from what it shares with the pervasive religious traditions of leprosy, both affective and moralistic.[73] Nowhere is this more evident than in the final face-to-face meeting of Troilus and Cresseid.

At least since William Godwin—who in his 1803 *Life of Geoffrey Chaucer* claims that in "the half-recognition, half-ignorance, attributed to Troilus in his last encounter with Creseide, there is a felicity of conception that is impossible to be surpassed"—readers have noted an unsettling power in Troilus and Cresseid's ultimate meeting.[74] The scene's roiling failures of recognition link it to the medieval affective tradition of leprosy, and they crystallize the melancholy allure of Cresseid's figure throughout the *Testament*. Just as the Man of Sorrows *quasi leprosus* seems to escape visibility and to scramble distinctions between despised and desired, so in this scene Cresseid threatens to slip the logic of narrative punishment and to transfix readers' looks on the quavering simultaneity of her destruction and beauty. Not unlike how Catherine of Siena is shaken and undone by the sick body she nurses, so is Troilus shaken by the leprous Cresseid. The look shared between Troilus and Cresseid, I suggest, is one that escapes the *Testament*'s narrative logic of punishment and legible embodiment. Here, leprosy is not a complex of symptoms or an index of moral transgression but a means of confusing such correspondences. The long, dilated moment of the lovers' encounter vibrates with an intensity that the logic of the exemplary plot cannot contain.

The encounter takes place sometime after Cresseid has joined her lazar house, on a day when she accompanies the collective of lepers as they beg for alms. Troilus happens to ride by with a company of victorious Trojan knights. Hearing the lepers' cries, he takes pity on them and "neir by the place can pas [did pass] / Quhair [Where] Cresseid sat, not witting quhat [knowing who] scho was" (496–97). At this point, a new stanza begins:

Than upon him scho kest up baith hir ene,
And with ane blenk it come into his thocht
That he sumtime hir face befoir had sene,

Bot scho was in sic plye he knew hir nocht;
Yit than hir luik into his mynd it brocht
The sweit visage and amorous blenking
Of fair Cresseid, sumtyme his awin darling. (498–504)

[Then upon him she cast up both her eyes, and with a blink it
came into his thought that he had seen her face sometime before,
but she was in such a plight that he did not know her. Yet then her
look into his mind brought the sweet face and loving looks of fair
Cresseid, once his own darling.]

The several hundred lines leading to this episode have been confined to the
report of Cresseid's experiences, but here the focalization shifts surprisingly to
Troilus, to his pity and ignorance as he approaches the beggars. With the stanza's first line, the narrative perspective shuttles briefly back to Cresseid, as she
turns her eyes to him. Then, "with ane blenk"—though it is not clear whose,
Troilus's or Cresseid's—it comes into Troilus's thought that "he sumtyme hir
face befoir had sene" (500). The verses' delicate interweaving of sight lines
establishes the mutuality of the couple's seeing and their not seeing. Although
the passage follows Troilus's perceptions inward to his thoughts, the initial reciprocity of their looking suggests that Cresseid too may be shaken and moved.

The lines zigzag along with Troilus's hesitation: he knows her, yet he
doesn't know her. Simultaneously, the verses waver between two narrative vantages, between what the narration knows, that Cresseid is in "sic plye" that the
Trojan cannot recognize her, and, contrastingly, something like free indirect
discourse, colored with Troilus's affection and evident in the tenderness of the
phrase "fair Cresseid, sumtyme his awin darling." Her *luik* ("than hir luik into
his mynd it brocht")—which refers ambiguously to Cresseid's appearance and
to her active gazing—is what works on Troilus's consciousness, bringing her
vanished (and yet uncannily present) beauty into his awareness. The "amorous
blenking" of this remembered figure echoes the "blenk" that has led Troilus
to his sense of near-recognition four lines before. The flash of her eyes marks
the temporal distance between now and then and also signals the collapsing
of that distance, for in the midst of his memories it *is* Cresseid who gazes at
him. The word *sumtime* is repeated here—first referring to a point uncer-
tainly placed in time, shimmering between memory and fantasy ("his thocht
/ That he sumtime hir face befoir had sene"), and, second, naming a punctual
but definitely lost past ("sumtyme his awin darling"). These two senses of

sumtime, the spectral and memorial, overlay one another to create the tremulous, haunted temporality that surrounds the couple.

The feelings evoked by what Troilus sees and remembers affect him powerfully; he trembles, sweats, and nearly faints. In explanation of his strong reactions, the narrator launches into a wrongheaded citation of Aristotelian psychological theory. Or rather, the psychology is sound enough according to medieval understandings, but it hardly applies to the scene unfolding between the erstwhile lovers. Assuring the reader that Troilus's response to Cresseid's face "Na wonder was," the narration explains that because Troilus has the "idole" of Cresseid's face "Sa deip imprentit in the fantasy [imagination] / That it deludis the wittis outwardly," the knight supposedly sees her even where she is not: "And sa appeiris in forme and lyke estait / Within the mynd as it was figurait" (505–11). The explanation presumes Troilus to be overriding his perceptions with a powerful phantasm, "deip imprentit" in his psyche. But the narration's explanatory gloss occludes the subtlety and strangeness of Troilus's actual experience. It is not something merely internal to him, a mental *idole*, that makes Cresseid seem to him at once present and absent. It is her own corporeality, defaced but present.

The physiology of Troilus's displaced recognition dominates the following stanza, which describes how he embodies the semiconscious, subterranean apprehension of his former beloved. The *blenk* of an eye sends up "Ane spark of lufe," an impassioned glint that "kendlit all his bodie in ane fyre; / With hait fewir, ane sweit and trimbling" (512–14). His own complexion begins to change color, so affected is he by Cresseid's figure flickering in and out of reality: "Within ane quhyle he changit many hew [colors]" (517). Troilus's physical alteration renders him briefly symmetrical to Cresseid, with both of their features transformed. This echoes the affective tradition of leprosy, where one body's loss of form incites the other's quavering affective response.

Following this description comes one of the most puzzling lines in the whole *Testament*: "Within ane quhyle [a little while] he changit many hew; / And nevertheles not ane ane uther knew" (517–18). Not only does Troilus fail to recognize his disfigured once-beloved—explained by her radically altered condition—but Cresseid does not recognize Troilus. After Troilus rides away, another leper, standing at a distance, identifies the Trojan warrior easily (535–36). This detail undercuts any obvious explanation for Cresseid's ignorance, for instance that the knight's visor has concealed his face or that leprosy is taken to damage vision. Instead, Troilus's identity is uniquely concealed from Cresseid. The illogic of the couple's mutual nonrecognition signals the conflicting imperatives that govern their reunion. They must and must not know one another. The juxtaposition of the two identical words "ane ane" ("not ane ane uther knew") mirrors the simultaneous isolation and parallelism of the pair. As Troilus's psychosomatic responses attest, they viscerally register one another's presence but in a manner that escapes the normal circuits of identification. Troilus does not speak to Cresseid but rather throws a stash of riches in her lap and rides away unsteadily. The ironic repetition of her name in these concluding lines of the encounter marks the distance that the single word, "Cresseid," must encompass: "For knichtlie pietie and memoriall / Of fair Cresseid, ane gyrdill can he tak, / Ane purs of gold, and mony gay jowall, / And in the skirt of Cresseid doun can swak [did fling]" (519–22). The two Cresseids, the fair and the leprous, remain distinct in Troilus's consciousness until the very end of the story when he is told the news of her death. In the interval between their face-to-face meeting and the revelation of her fate, Troilus is still innocent of his part in the story's narrative economy, wherein his "wanhope" and "teiris" on the walls of Troy are compensated by the exemplary spectacle of Cresseid's punishment.

Cresseid, likewise, is momentarily oblivious to the final shame of her transformation. Once Troilus has departed, another leper tells her the name of the knight and she faints; upon reviving she seals her narrative arc with the repeated line "O fals Cresseid and trew knicht Troylus" (546, 553, 560). The refrain monumentalizes the couple in moralistic opposition, disregarding the exchange of glances that has shaken Troilus's body with an unplumbable eros and suspended recognition in merciful incompletion. Pinned down by their static and contrary epithets, divided forever on two sides of a judgment, the lovers within Cresseid's refrain are precisely unlike the susurrating interpenetration of perspectives, affects, and memories that characterizes their final meeting. The affective tradition of leprosy here acts not to theologize the couple but to undo the signifying logic of bodily form in favor of unstabilized feeling. Leprosy, while first and finally functioning as a vehicle of exemplary justice in the *Testament of Cresseid*, figures briefly in the lovers' last encounter as the means of aesthetic transport and an eros that has no other expression than the wordless exchange of looks.

PART IV

Personalizing *Phisik*

Chapter 7

Symptoms and the Signifying Condition
in Hoccleve's *Series*

The first stanza of Thomas Hoccleve's "My Compleinte" invites its readers to see the poet-narrator in a state of symptomatic self-loss. "Witnesse uppon the wilde infirmite / Wiche that I hadde," Hoccleve enjoins, "as many a man wel knewe, / And wiche me oute of mysilfe caste and threwe."[1] The lines refer to an episode of insanity that he suffered some five years before the events of the poem, the aftershocks of which are still with him. The "wilde infirmite," as he recounts it, was first and foremost an event of self-exile, which "caste and threwe" him out of himself and left only his symptomatic body behind. As he explains, "my witte were a pilgrim, / And wente fer from home" (C232–33). Because he can remember nothing of what happened during his madness, to describe it he has to rely on what other people tell him; if it is he who "hadde" his sickness, it is others who "knewe" it. In these opening lines, in a gesture of striking self-exposure, Hoccleve asks his audience to peer into this gap in his account of himself: "Witnesse." It is this bout of insanity that is turned round and round during the first two parts of Hoccleve's *Series*, the five-part composition, mostly of Middle English rhyme-royal stanzas, that is thought to be the poet's final work.[2]

Over the course of the *Series'* frame narrative, Hoccleve constantly recalibrates his poetic *I* in response to what exceeds and lies outside it. The most obvious exteriority is Hoccleve's audience, in its various avatars—the *prees*, or crowd, of London; God, to whom he prays; a *frende* who stops by Hoccleve's home; Duke Humphrey, ostensible patron of the *Series*; and a female readership reportedly angry about one of his prior compositions. Solicitous sensitivity to interpreters is entirely in keeping with Hoccleve's poetics. His work "is above all a poetry of address," as John Burrow remarks, and James Simpson observes that he "is extraordinarily sensitive to the conditions of discursive exchange."[3] But the *Series* does something distinctive insofar as it gives that exteriority other forms. The most important figuration of what lies outside Hoccleve's persona is his madness. For that interval of symptomatic self-loss, Hoccleve's physical body becomes something alien and inaccessible to him, more real than he is. It can be added back to his account of himself only retrospectively, on the basis of rumor and report. In the most original and moving parts of the *Series'* frame narrative, Hoccleve struggles in a tangle of bodily and interpretive vulnerabilities, anxiously animated by the sense that he cannot stop signifying beyond himself.

The composition of the "Compleinte" and "Dialoge" has been dated to between 1419 and 1421, although there is evidence that Hoccleve continued to tinker with them until his death in 1426.[4] They are notable for the specificity with which they particularize their protagonist, "Thomas Hoccleve," who works as a clerk in the office of the Privy Seal in London, just as the author Thomas Hoccleve in fact did. As A. L. Brown has observed, there is also biographical warrant for a period of unwellness in the author's life matching the one described in the *Series*.[5] The correspondence between actual circumstance and poetic persona would likely have been apparent and relevant to Hoccleve's early audiences. Thus, unlike Chaucer's "Knight's Tale" or Henryson's *Testament of Cresseid*, the events of the *Series'* frame-narrative do not take place in a legendary or fictional world. Instead, the text makes claims for the actuality of what it narrates, both through its verisimilar detail and by recounting the coming-to-be of the literary work itself. Of course, the autobiographical conflation of poet and narrator does not mean that what the *Series* recounts is true but rather that readers are constantly referred to the paradoxical figure of the poet-narrator, who flickers between his existence as an *effect* of the text, brought to life by his diegetic representation, and his role as textual cause and informing principle.[6] Scholars have sometimes drawn a sharp analytical distinction between the *Series'* narrating protagonist and its author, reserving "Thomas" for the character and "Hoccleve" for the historical individual. I have chosen not to do so. On my reading, the effect of the work depends on the unstable overlap between these categories as they constantly implicate one another.

It is a commonplace of scholarship on the *Series* to observe that the text is an account of its own origins. As Burrow remarks, "It not only describes the making of a book, but also *is* that book"; Simpson quips, "If ever there was

a poem whose composition is part of its own subject, it is Hoccleve's *Series*";
Ethan Knapp calls it a "self-referential meditation on writing"; "it dramatises
its narrator's attempt to overcome the challenges presented by material book
production," for David Watt; and A. C. Spearing deems it a work "of *méta-
écriture*, much concerned with the process of its own creation, an apparently
(and perhaps really) improvised textual performance that never allows us to
forget its textuality."[7] In this plot of bookish making, the poet-narrator gradually assembles both the materials and the authority to compose the *Series*.[8]
The present chapter joins the critical conversation on the *Series'* literary reflexivity by giving an account of what the work's fascinations with embodiment,
pathology, and symptoms have to do with writing. As Spearing has argued
at length, writers in the later Middle Ages were keenly aware of the implications of the writtenness of their texts: "When composed in writing, vernacular
poems, like Latin legal documents, do not *represent* speech, but take its place,
and thereby receive both the advantage of being carried down to posterity
and the disadvantages of the loss of a speaker's presence and of his ability to
adjust his words to their recipients."[9] The *Series* is a sustained meditation on
this textual condition, or the status of the literary work vis-à-vis a readership
that is anticipated but constitutively absent to the author. Yet unlike Spearing's
account, which follows a long tradition of contrasting writing to the responsive powers of the "speaker's presence," the *Series* makes its author's body the
problem. Even in face-to-face encounters, Hoccleve cannot make his flesh
signify properly, and as he struggles to explain himself, this somatic obscurity
seems to spread outward, infecting his every communication. At times, his
symptomatic embodiment seems almost like an allegory for the textual condition, though it is perhaps more accurate to call them two aspects of what it
means to Hoccleve to be a signifying creature.

If, in the two previous chapters, *plot* appeared as the literary form most
apt for thinking about etiology—which could orchestrate various systems of
causation into a single sequence of events and demand readerly puzzling over
which causes really made things happen—here, the crucial etiological form
is *narration*. In the *Series* (as in the *Book of Margery Kempe*, discussed in the
following chapter), the textual "speaking" that recounts events incorporates a
variety of idioms, subject positions, and signifying systems within itself. One
of the questions that the *Series* poses is what kind of cause lies at the root of the
text's polyvocal narration. Is it the scene of poetic authorship that the *Series*
cannily circles, where the masterful writer gathers up all sources and voices
into his own control? Or is it something closer to the scene of Hoccleve's

madness, where he is more medium than agent of signification? By the end of the *Series'* frame, Hoccleve seems to have assured us that the former answer is the right one. In a narrative arc that runs from "My Compleinte" through the "Dialogue," Hoccleve's poetic *I* travels a path of semiotic ascent, from symptom-ridden pathology to confident literary bravura. In what looks like a consolidating rebuke to his vulnerabilities, he attaches his achieved rhetorical mastery to Chaucer's legacy and stabilizes it against a trivialized audience of female readers. Yet, I suggest, the constitutive vulnerabilities of the expressive condition linger on—in the self's inability to master its own materiality and the signifier's incapacity to guarantee its own meaning.

"Wilde Infirmite"

From the start, "My Compleinte" establishes that one's continuity of self does not at its deepest level depend on self-consciousness or self-recollection. The common reference for the *I* rests instead on a viewpoint from outside, an external social regard turned on the apprehensible body. This is the first lesson of Hoccleve's madness. He has no firsthand knowledge of his insanity, when, as he says, the "substaunce of my memorie / Wente to pleie as for a certein space [interval]" (C50–51). But despite this absence from his memory, his madness is still part of the identity attached to him—"the wilde infirmite / Wiche that I hadde, as many a man wel knewe" (C40–41). Not self-consciousness but other people's knowledge binds Hoccleve's present to this body in the past.

It is this blind spot in his self-accounting that is bothering Hoccleve at the outset of the *Series*. To incorporate his madness into the identity he articulates for himself, to make it properly *his*, he initially has to rely on the reports of other people. These reports, as it turns out, are widespread: "It was so knowen to the peple and kouthe [familiar] / That counseil [secret] was it noon, ne not be might. / Howe it with me stood was in every mannes mouthe" (C43–45). The poem's most extended description of Hoccleve's madness dramatizes these epistemological conditions:

> Men seiden I loked as a wilde steer,
> And so my looke aboute I gan to throwe.
> Min heed to hie, anothir seide, I beer:
> "Full bukkissh is his brayn, wel may I trowe."
> And seide the thridde, "And apt is in the rowe

To site of hem that a resounless reed
Can geve: no sadnesse is in his heed."

Chaunged had I m[y] pas, somme seiden eke,
For here and there forthe stirte I as a roo,
Noon abood, noon areest, but al brainseke.
Another spake and of me seide also,
My feet weren ay wavynge to and fro,
Whanne that I stonde shulde and with men talke,
And that my yen soughten every halke. (C120–33)

[Men said I looked like a wild ox, just so I began to cast about
my look. I carried my head too high, another said: "His brain is
completely buck-like, well may I believe." And a third said, "And
he is apt to sit in the company of them who give reasonless advice:
no soundness is in his head." I had changed my pace, some said
also, for here and there I started as though I were a roe, not resting,
not stopping, but entirely brain-sick. Another spoke and said of me
additionally that my feet were always waving to and fro, when I was
supposed to be standing still and talking with other men, and that
my eyes sought every corner of the room.]

These two stanzas harp on the reported quality of the information: "Men seiden,"
"anothir seide," "seide the thridde," "somme seiden eke," "Another spake." The
narration is at pains to signal that Hoccleve does not know these facts about
himself directly. Instead, other people make the observations that he dutifully
recirculates through his subjective *I*: "Men seiden I loked as a wilde steer." The
bricolaged, hearsay character of these reports exaggerates the self-difference that
is characteristic of being a symptomatic subject, when one's body broadcasts
involuntary signs, which in turn call forth others' diagnostic interpretations. As
the previous chapters have explored, this symptomatic determination often catalyzes new articulations of the self to gloss and interpret one's own bodily signs.
But in Hoccleve's case, not only are his behaviors during his illness caused rather
than intended, he cannot even witness them—except through others' eyes,
belatedly. He is uniquely excluded from the authority to narrate and explain
them, even though he inhabits the *I* that they continue to constitute.

Hoccleve's failure of self-awareness is reiterated in the contents of the
descriptions. During his illness, he was beast-like: he had the gaze of a spooked

ox, a "bukkish" brain, and the erratic, darting foot-steps of a roe. The animal imagery echoes the language of wildness used to characterize his illness else-where: it is a "wilde infirmite," a "siiknesse savage," and a "wildenesse" (C40, 86, 107). In obeying the dictates of his misfiring material body, he seems less than human. The terms "brayn," "heed," and "brainseke" meanwhile draw attention to the physical substrate of his cognition, the organ where something has gone awry. Both animal and physiological vocabularies foreground the determining force of his material body. The reports also enumerate the social norms that Hoccleve has failed to uphold. He held his head too high, waved his feet "to and fro" when he should have been still, and during attempts at conversation, his eyes flickered away, seeking the corners of the room. These vignettes of failed sociability are made uncanny by the peculiarly mediated character of the *I* that inhabits them: "Chaunged had I m[y] pas, somme seiden." Hoccleve was physically present, as these testimonies insist, but the *I* that now tries to tell its story was also absent, not there to be cognizant, thanks to this illness "wiche me oute of mysilfe caste and threwe" (C42). Hoccleve's *I* in these stanzas is a cobbled-together affair, yoking his own powers of self-articulation to what lies outside of those powers, what "men seiden," which nonetheless forms a crucial passage of his biography. The most vertiginous thing about these reports is their necessarily third-person mode.

Personal action that outpaces self-awareness is a consistent theme of Hoc-cleve's poetry. Already in *La Male Regle* and in the long prologue to the *Regiment of Princes* Hoccleve has experimented with a poetic avatar similar to that in the *Series*—autobiographically grounded, comically anxious, a bit at odds with the discourses he invokes, and pathological. *La Male Regle* is an extended petition to the personification *Helthe*, with whom the speaker is out of favor, and in the *Regiment* the narrator suffers a morbid thoughtfulness that his interlocutor diagnoses as *malencolie*, or melancholia.[10] This habituated persona of Hoccleve is a variation on the figure of the hapless Chaucerian nar-rator, who embodies passivity and artlessness within an encompassing frame-work of knowing wit. In *La Male Regle* and the *Regiment*, Hoccleve raises Chaucerian irony to such a pitch that its focus shifts, moving away from the interplay between a narrator's earnestness and the world that outpaces him (as in Chaucer's *House of Fame* or the General Prologue) and settling instead on a self constantly differing from itself. Readers' ability to take stock of this persona that cannot see to its own edges gives Hoccleve's poems much of their dramatic tension: Can the literary work recoup the expressive authority that the poet-narrator seems to fumble? The game is one of risking poetic authority as far as he can, and what he wagers returns redoubled as bravura. Such play with humility and ambition, weakness and artistic clout was central to the fifteenth-century reception of Chaucerian poetics.[11] What makes Hoccleve's corpus unique in the literary milieu is his personalization of these dynamics. Lee Patterson calls Hoccleve "the most strenuously autobiographical poet of early English literature," who constantly dramatizes "both his particularity as this specific person and, more important, his own *sense* of his particularity," especially by means of "the urgent specificity, the dogged relentlessness, and the sheer ubiquity" of his self-descriptions.[12] Personalizing and pathologizing Chaucerian irony are Hoccleve's standard practice.

In the *Series*, Hoccleve does something new with his accustomed role by stretching it between two distinct versions of pathological self-difference. One, his madness, is unprecedented in the previous autobiographical poems, and it acts as a hard kernel of personal alterity that is handled and pondered over the course of the work. It is the primal scene of what will emerge as Hoccleve's central anxiety, the interpretive vulnerability of his own signifying. The other version of morbid self-difference, more familiar from Hoccleve's earlier work, is what he calls "the thoughtful maladie," which keeps him awake on the November night described in the *Series*' prologue (P21). There, Hoccleve carefully distinguishes between this thoughtfulness and (in the line immediately following) a "siknesse" that scourged him previously, presumably his madness (P22). As he remarks, "I sy [saw] wel, sithin [since] I with siknesse last / Was scourgid, cloudy hath bene the favour / That shoon on me ful bright in times past" (P22–24). Sickness has led to cloudy favor, which is fuel for insomniac ponderings. It is the interaction between these two pathologies, the ongoing "thoughtful maladie" and the discrete event of "siknesse," that generates Hoccleve's complaint.

When he recounts the creation of his complaint, he narrates it in quasi-symptomatic terms:

> The greef aboute myn herte so sore swal
> And bolned evere to and to so sore
> That nedis oute I muste therwithal.
> I thoughte I nolde kepe it cloos no more,
> Ne lete it in me for to eelde and hore,
> And for to preve I cam of a womman,
> I braste oute on the morwe and thus bigan. (P29–35)

[The grief around my heart swelled so severely and bloated ever more and more so painfully that I necessarily must burst out with it. I thought I would not keep it closed any more, nor keep it in me to age and grow gray, and to prove I came from a woman, I burst out on the morrow and thus began.]

On this account, the poet-narrator's mounting grief exerts such painful pressure that he cannot "kepe it cloos" and has to "braste oute" with what will be the "Compleinte" itself. The reference to his own birth ("to preve I cam of a womman") has the effect of associating his outpouring with his natural, corruptible body, but it also colors the next line with the suggestion of self-parturition. He bursts out from his physicalized grief to begin "on the morwe," to articulate himself anew. The verb ("braste oute") is only partly agential. It is more as a body, swollen with the night's grief and *maladie*, that he surges into lament. These symptomatic origins act as a compositional alibi, initially concealing the social agenda of Hoccleve's writing, or the simple fact that what he writes is intended for readers. Instead, the complaint is initially portrayed as both a flourish of self-creation and the gushing of embodied affect.

From its start, then, the *Series* emphasizes both the solipsistic enclosure and the fragmentation that Hoccleve's insanity has imposed on the self-narrating subject. But as soon as these are introduced, Hoccleve sets about trying to delimit their consequences. He initially does so by two means, normalizing his illness within a providential framework and sequestering it in the biographical past. His madness is cast both as something well-nigh universal and as something over and done. Thus the first stanza of "My Compleinte" remarks not only on the far-flung news of Hoccleve's madness ("as many a man wel knewe") but also the on common knowledge ("as men may se") that God visits adversity on people all the time:

Almyghty God, as liketh his goodnesse,
Vesiteth folke alday, as men may se,
With los of good and bodily sikenesse,
And amonge othir, he forgat not me. (C36–39)

[Almighty God, as pleases his goodness, visits people continually—as anyone can observe—with loss of property and bodily sickness, and among others, he did not forget me.]

Hoccleve is one "amonge othir," and "bodily sikenesse" forms a generic-sounding pair with "los of good," synecdoches for misfortune in all its variety. Against the idiosyncratic specificity of his "wilde infirmite" and its fallout, Hoccleve marshals the truisms of a Boethianism that would have been familiar to all his readers: Fortune is fickle, and it is part of God's goodness to teach us as much. Or, as Hoccleve remarks, "Whoso that taketh hede ofte may se / This worldis [world's] chaunge and mutabilite" (C116–17). Of course, Hoccleve's investment in these commonplaces of consolation can only be partial because they fail to capture the peculiarities of his identity, that constant fascination of his poetry. But Boethianism offers a starting point in his efforts to reclaim and renarrate this piece of his biography.

Hoccleve combines the imagery of Fortune's plunging wheel with a more hopeful plot of reconciliation and return. Although his "memorie" was absent for a while, it has been five years since God "Made it for to retourne into the place / Whens it cam" (C50, 54–55). "And evere sithin," he continues,

> thankid be God oure Lord
> Of his good and gracious reconsiliacioun,
> My wit and I have bene of suche acord
> As we were or the altercacioun
> Of it was. (C57–61)

> [And ever since—thanked be God our Lord for his good and gracious reconciliation—my wit and I have been of such accord as we were before it was changed.]

His wit is "hoom come agein," and God "hath made myn helthe home repeire [return]" (C64, 278). Drawing on the imagery of *Christus medicus*, Hoccleve notes that the "curteise [courteous] leche [physician] moost soverain" purged "the grevous venim [poison] / That had enfectid and wildid my brain" (C234–36). Despite the universal vicissitudes of fortune, then, Hoccleve insists on giving thanks for his recovery, as though to stabilize it and publicize it at once. Ethan Knapp rightly notes a tension between, on the one hand, the "fundamentally Augustinian language of procession and return," according to which Hoccleve's "true self vanishes into exile but is vouchsafed a return by God's grace," and, on the other hand, the pervasiveness of mutability, or the "unpredictable ebb and flow that patterns both fortune in the world and also, even more threateningly, the cohesion of a sane self."[13] What kind of self-assurance can be built on the foundation of "this worldis chaunge"?

Yet the tension between these two conventional sets of images is itself entirely conventional, and if this were the only conundrum, then the posture of penitential trust in God with which "My Compleinte" concludes would be sufficient to reconcile the counterpoised ethical standpoints. Hoccleve prays, in the final stanza of "My Compleinte,"

> Laude and honour and thanke unto thee be,
> Lorde God, that salve art to al hevinesse.
> Thanke of my welthe and myn adversitee.
> Thanke of myn elde and of my seeknesse.
> And thanke be to thin infinit goodnesse
> And thi giftis and benefices alle,
> And unto thi mercy and grace I calle. (C407–13)

> [Praise and honor and thanks be to you, Lord God, that are salve to all sadness. Thanks for my wealth and my adversity. Thanks for my age and my sickness. And thanks be for your infinite goodness and all your gifts and benefits, and I call upon your mercy and grace.]

This speech act is the present-tense establishment of an intimate reciprocity between *I* and *thou*. Hoccleve's call is sustained by God's "mercy and grace," and the ups and downs of life, *seeknesse* as much as *welthe*, are swallowed up in the category of God's *giftis*. And yet this prayer does not quite do the job. As the immediately ensuing debate in the "Dialoge" makes clear, God's surety is not enough. Social recognition is required. As James Simpson observes, "The very fact that Thomas intends to publish the *Complaint*, as part of his poetic and social rehabilitation, implies the insufficiency of solitary resignation."[14] Ethan Knapp makes a similar point about the jump between the "Compleinte" and "Dialoge": "as the abrupt stylistic transition from the high rhetoric of theological resignation to this raucous banter should make clear, the 'Dialoge' serves retroactively to question the adequacy of the previous pose."[15] The *Series*' fascination with the social reception of the protagonist's words and actions, his symptoms and his text, ultimately destabilizes the prayer's moment of apparent dyadic steadiness. Hoccleve's prayerful stanza, as much as the rest of the work, is *for readers*—and he is anxious to know, or at least to imagine, what his readers think about it.

Hoccleve admits as much in his grievances leading to the final prayer. He objects to the fact that his recovery has not been sufficiently recognized, or, as he says, "For though that my wit were hoom come agein, / Men wolde it not so undirstonde or take [accept]" (C64–65). "That I was hool [healthy]," he complains, "thei not ne deme kowde [they could not believe it]" (C289). He reports that "manie oone [many a one]" says of him that "'Although from him his siiknesse savage / Withdrawen and passed as for a time be, / Resorte [Return] it wole [will], namely in suche age / As he is of'" (C85–89). Under conditions of "passinge [extreme] hete," these skeptical commentators predict, "'Assail him wole [will] agein that maladie'" (C92–93). Contingent facts like his age or the warmth of the weather, the reasoning of these predictions runs, can bring his madness back, and health is more an accident of circumstance than a steady state. These rumors focus on Hoccleve's unique bodily condition and medical history, and no doubt register the growing prominence in medieval English society of humoral and physiological models. The claims here are not about the instabilities of fortune that govern all human life but about Hoccleve's unique physical susceptibilities. Public opinion insists on the continuity between Hoccleve's past self and his present one. This reinforces the *Series*' evident conviction that what matters for subjectivity is an external point of view, one focused on the apprehensible body and beholden to collectively distributed knowledge, not self-consciousness.

This outward, social perspective is the crux of Hoccleve's unhappiness in "My Compleinte." It is also what he really cares about. Rather histrionically, he compares the ambient skepticism about his health to a martyrdom: "Sith that time" of his cure, he remarks, "have I be sore sette on fire / And lyved in greet turment [torment] and martire [martyrdom]" (C62–63). "Greet turment" comes not from Hoccleve's original illness but from the diagnostic and prognostic rumors that swirl around him. While the friction between health's return and fortune's mutability can be resolved in a posture of obedience to God, Hoccleve finds no comparable way of resigning himself to the social field, or, as he says, "hou in my skyn to tourne" (C303). This is a tellingly somatic metaphor for the ways he comes to embody his misrecognition.

The Social Life of Symptoms

The circumstances in which these predictions of relapse reach Hoccleve's ears turn out to be central to what bothers him about them. They are third-person remarks, overheard rather than exchanged conversationally. Hoccleve has listened in on them, as he says, when "I in Westmynstir Halle, / And eke in Londoun, amonge the prees [crowd] went" (C72–73). In this crowd, the whole "worlde" presents "a straunge countinaunce," and those who were once accustomed to speak to Hoccleve now their "heed [heads] they caste awry [turned away], / Whanne I hem [them] mette, as [as if] they not me sy [saw]" (C70, 76–77). For his part, Hoccleve "leide [gave] an eere [ear] ay [always] to" these comments as he "by wente" (C134), but he does not pause in his urban transit. Instead, he remarks, "Kepte I me cloos, and trussid me my weie [took myself off], / Droupinge and hevy and al woo bistaad [woebegone]" (C145–46). He allows the speculations to stream around him, without stopping to answer them.

London's busy urban byways lend verisimilitude to what is a peculiar effect of these scenes; namely, they render Hoccleve nearly absent from the scene of his bodily presence. In a repetition of his madness—when he was a body without a reflective subjectivity in attendance—Hoccleve among these crowds is again physically there but apparently lacking powers of self-accounting. He acts as though "I had lost my tunges keie [tongue's key]" because "Whatso that evere I shulde answere or seie, / They wolden not han holde it worth a leke" (C144, 142–43). The oblique and anonymous character of the crowd's prognosis recalls the pieced-together, hearsay reports of his madness. The metropolitan scene's quotidian immediacy, focalized through Hoccleve, contrasts with the masses' abstraction. The whole milieu wears a stranger's averted countenance, and the imagery implies that there is no chance for face-to-face dialogue. The poem thus sets the *prees* at an angle where it cannot be addressed. It never resolves into an identifiable set of individuals, instead remaining an unappeasable *they*.

These street scenes are saturated with urban malaise and melancholic alienation, but there is, I think, yet another context for the overheard rumors and averted faces. The crowd also functions as a menacing analogue for readership. The absent but anticipated audience of literary writing always wears a "straunge countinaunce" for its author. Even if the direct addressees of a work are known, their reactions cannot be. Hoccleve's consistent and explicit attentiveness to his poetry's status within discursive exchange means that he is often performatively recalibrating his poetic voice for its projected readership. In his poetry, imagined addressees' actual and ineradicable autonomy saturates with anxiety their figuration in the text, and the ultimately unforeseeable nature of readers' responses returns to the poetic *I* as a flurry of demands, to which

Hoccleve portrays himself breathlessly responding. These anxious, tremulous modulations of Hoccleve's persona are one of the pleasures of his poetry, and in the *Series'* street scenes, the material form that this persona assumes shifts from text to body. The move may seem counterintuitive for all the reasons that writing is generally counterposed to bodily presence: surely the body is more immediate, more responsive, more real. But Hoccleve here deploys symptomatic subjectivity to show that, in fact, bodily and textual materializations of the self are bound in the same signifying condition. When a self takes on material form in the social gaze, whether in language or flesh—Hoccleve seems to say—that self does not know or control what it means. But being an inescapably social creature, no one can escape such exposure and heteronomy. The episode of Hoccleve's madness is the starkest realization of this condition, namely, the subject's absence to its own signifying in the social gaze. The anonymous "prees" is the threatening mask that this context of reception is made to wear.

The urban milieu of averted gazes, symptomatic speculation, and corporealized shame is the incitement to Hoccleve's celebrated mirror scene. In retreat from the crowded London streets, Hoccleve ushers his readers into "my chaumbre at home whanne that I was / Mysilfe aloone" (C155–56). In this domestic solitude, Hoccleve reports,

> I streite unto my mirrour and my glas,
> To loke howe that me of my chere thought,
> If any othir were it than it ought,
> For fain wolde I, if it not had bene right,
> Amendid it to my kunnynge and myght.
>
> Many a saute made I to this mirrour,
> Thinking, "If that I looke in this manere
> Amonge folke as I nowe do, noon errour
> Of suspecte look may in my face appere.
> This countinaunce, I am sure, and this chere,
> If I it forthe use, is nothing reprevable
> To hem that han conceitis resonable."
>
> And therwithal I thoughte thus anoon:
> "Men in her owne cas bene blinde alday,
> As I have herde seie manie a day agoon." (C157–71)

[I went immediately to my mirror to see what I thought of my
expression, if it were otherwise than it ought to be, because gladly
would I have amended it according to my knowledge and ability if
it had not been right. Many a leap I made to this mirror, thinking,
"If I appear in this manner among folks as I do now, then no
error of suspicious look may appear in my face. This appearance,
I am sure, and this expression, if I use it abroad, is not at all
objectionable to those who have reasonable understandings." And
thereupon I at once thought thus: "Men in their own cases are blind
perpetually," as I have heard said many times before this.]

Hoccleve here checks his appearance against the norms of what is *right* and
how he *ought* to look, with the aim of pliantly amending any deviations he
finds. The process is an iterative one, as he leaps in front of the mirror time
and again, finding nothing amiss. But as he glosses his performance, the gaps
in the logic of the exercise become apparent: *if* when he is "amonge folke" he
looks just like he does now, and *if* his observers have "conceitis resonable,"
then he will be found unobjectionable. The qualifying clauses of his inner
speech expose the limits of the bedroom mirror, which cannot account for the
opacity and heterogeneity of the streaming crowd. Far from embodying a set
of fixed norms to which Hoccleve can conform himself, the *prees* has shown
itself to be implacable and *straunge*. The burden of responsiveness has been
embodied entirely by Hoccleve, who trembles, blushes, sweats, and teeters
on the brink of "folie" (C140). When he overhears claims that his illness will
"resorte [return]," then his "visage / Bigan to glowe for the woo and fere"
(C88–90). When he imagines what it would mean to "Answere amys" in the
"prees," he worries that "To harme wole it me turne and to folie" (C138–40).

Folie can mean a laughingstock, but it also denotes madness.[16] The poem
thus plays with the idea that the crowd's refusal to acquiesce to Hoccleve's
recovery will undo its physical reality. His interpreters seem about to become
the *cause* of his bodily disturbance rather than its witnesses. This is an intensification of their hermeneutic authority, bringing it to a reality-constituting
power, as though viewers could transform physiology to match their interpretations. Hoccleve's physicalized anxiety, which is closely related to the "thoughtful maladie" that keeps him awake in the work's prologue, acts as the means
by which the crowd's interpretive superpowers might become diegetically real.
The menace is amplified by the medium of language, within which Hoccleve's
bodily state is only apprehensible to readers as a verbal effect. Words make

bodies in poetry. The mirror scene shows Hoccleve trying and failing to prop up the fantasy that his bodily form might entirely *precede* his being seen by others, rather than being constituted in relation to them. He dreams that the lineaments of his corporeality could somehow legislate once and for all how he is seen. Despite "many a saute," the fantasy proves impossible to sustain. Hoccleve's interior monologue catches up with the irony straightaway, when he recalls the adage that people are always blind to their own situations.

Hoccleve's mirror scene also functions as an embedded miniature of "My Compleinte" itself. Just as Hoccleve before his glass tries to reduce the social character of embodiment to a self-guaranteeing form, so the poem presents itself as an attempt to make self-articulation a closed circuit, whether in the form of the poet's self-curative "brast[ing] oute" in the prologue or his obedient reciprocity with God at the end. But Hoccleve's text, like his body, cannot escape its fundamental orientation toward other people. In his poetry, language and the human self share a fundamentally social ontology. Both respond ceaselessly to the reactions of others, but these reactions can be glimpsed only obliquely, in uncertain fragments. In "My Compleinte," this sociality does not reduce to intersubjectivity. It is something more impersonal and structural, all around the *I*, constituting it but not entirely comprehensible to it. When Hoccleve composes his expression in front of the mirror and anticipates "If that I looke in this manere / Amonge folke as I nowe do," his activities differ little from those of the literary writer who he also is, who in his chamber composes an autobiographical poem and anticipates what happens *if I am written in this manner.* In an abyssal mirroring that is appropriate to the episode's reflexive character, the mirror scene captures Hoccleve both written and writing, anticipating the scene of his apprehension by others, which he will always nonetheless miss. It is this misalignment that gives his body and his subjectivity its tremulous animation.

Alternatives

It is at the conclusion of the "Dialoge" that the *Series* arrives at an apparently satisfactory détente between poetic persona and projected audience, one that acts as the ground for the remainder of the composition. But before Hoccleve reaches this final orchestration of authority and address, he proposes several other models to replace his futile interchange with the implacable *prees* and his unsustainable fantasy of self-sufficient expressive enclosure.

One possibility is to reject the fleeting impersonality of the crowd in favor of sustained interpersonal exchange. "Man by hise dedis and not by his lookes / Shal knowen be," he assures himself (C202–3). Given the uselessness of his attempts "To peinte countenance, chere and look" for the urban crowd, Hoccleve turns to Matthew 7:16 (*a fructibus eorum cognoscetis*) to vaunt the sense of taste over sight: "Bi taaste of fruit men may wel wite and knowe / What that it is. Othir preef is ther noon" (C149, 204–5). The stanza then pulls the verb toward its more abstract meaning of "putting to the test," as Hoccleve urges those who doubt him to "Taaste and assay" if he is well (C210).[17] A few lines later he glosses "assay" as conversation: "By communynge [conversing] is the beste assay" (C217). The virtues of conversation will be played out in the "Dialoge" following "My Compleinte," where the banter between Hoccleve and his friend seems to instantiate an entirely different disposition of language, one that escapes the impersonal menace of both crowd and readership. This sudden vaunting of conversation is an about-face from Hoccleve's previous reports of his silence in the crowd, as though he had lost his "tunges keie," and his resolution to "peinte countenaunce" instead of speaking (C144, 149). In revising his earlier stance to praise dialogue, his point seems not to be that he was wrong before but that the social world is at fault for having demanded his wordless scuttling through the streets. "As it is writen in bookes," he scolds his interpreters, people are best known through talking to them (C203). Chatting about "thingis mene [ordinary]" is what stands to demonstrate the "homely resoun" shared by all those who (as he remarks in front of the mirror) "han [have] conceitis [understandings] resonable" (C218, 221, 168). I will have more to say about Hoccleve's conversation with his friend later in the chapter, and in anticipation of that I note in passing that the dyadic symmetries of conversation do not so easily escape the pressures of the wayward material signifier or the impersonal social field. What Hoccleve and his friend spend all their time talking about, as we will see, is the poet's bodily vulnerabilities and Hoccleve's readership.

The other attempt in the "Compleinte" to dismiss the unmasterable character of the social field is to replace Hoccleve's idiosyncratic voice with that of authorized literary tradition. While from the beginning of his narration Hoccleve draws on Boethian and penitential commonplaces, the Boethian tradition begins to operate differently when his diegetic avatar encounters it *as text*. The potentially transformative power of this literary discourse is announced by an abrupt turn in Hoccleve's self-characterization, when he veers from lamenting that his "troubly liif hath al to [too] longe endurid" to declaring that whatever other people say, "I not ne recche [care]" because "nowe mysilfe to mysilfe have ensurid" (C302, 307, 304). The apparent catalyst for this novel self-assurance is the "lamentacioun / Of a wooful man in a book," which Hoccleve has read "this othir day" (C309–10). The dialogue between the "wooful man" and Reason then is quoted for more than fifty lines before Hoccleve reveals that he could not finish reading the text because "He that it oughte [owned] agen [again] it to him took" (C374). The disruptive claim of the book's proprietor does not occur before Reason delivers a piece of crucial advice. In an especially intricate play of voices, Reason answers the woeful man by ventriloquizing him, speaking in the man's voice to tell him what he should and should not say. Reason advises him not to "grucche and seie, 'Whi susteine I this?'"—or, in other words, not to ask personalizing etiological questions. Instead,

> "thou shuldist thinke in thin herte,
> and seie, 'To thee, lorde God, I have agilte
> So sore I moot for myn offensis smerte,
> As I am worthi. O Lorde I am spilte
> But thou to me thi mercy graunte wilte.
> I am full sure thou maist it not denie.
> Lorde, I me repente, and I the mercy crie.'" (C365–71)

> ["You should think in your heart and say, 'To you, Lord God, I
> have done wrong so grievously that I must suffer for my offenses,
> as I deserve to. O Lord, I am destroyed unless you will grant mercy
> to me. I am very sure you will not deny it. Lord, I repent, and I cry
> mercy to you.'"]

A. G. Rigg has identified the source of Hoccleve's borrowed text as the *Synonyma* of Isidore of Seville, or, as John Burrow further clarifies, an epitome probably containing no more than the passages translated.[18] Whether readers know the source or not, Reason's advice is immediately recognizable as a consolation on the model of Boethius.

Within the sealed solitude of "My Compleinte," the inset text breathes new vocabulary and style into Hoccleve's interior monologue, more aureate than what has come before. An august literary and ethical tradition suddenly appears at the base of Hoccleve's doleful self-reflections. The same is true of the briefer evocation of Psalm 30 earlier in the poem: "As seide is in the sauter

[Psalter] might I sey, / 'They that me sy [saw], fledden awey fro me'" (C78–79). As David Lawton has argued, both the Psalms and Boethius's *Consolation* were among the most important sources for "public interiorities" in the English fifteenth century, and both were especially important to Hoccleve.[19] In each, God acts as a stabilizing force for the vicissitudes of doubt, despair, and alienation, and divine authority guarantees the genres' moral authority. The concluding prayer of "My Compleinte" (C407–13) is straightforwardly a reiteration of Reason's proposed script, shifted to the key of praise and thanksgiving. As recommended, Hoccleve thanks God for "My punischement" and the opportunity "my giltis to repente" (C395, 403). The prayer concludes similarly to Reason's model, crying for God's mercy. As discussed above, with this devotional utterance, Hoccleve appears temporarily to find his way from idiosyncrasy to collective tradition and from a self scattered in symptoms' gossipy report to a dialogic "I" stabilized against a divine other.

However, this "I" is a generic one. When Hoccleve repeats Reason's model script for the "wooful man" in his final prayer, utterances come unstuck from the specificities of person: the Boethian penitent should say what Reason says, which is what Hoccleve decides to say too. The frictionless movement of these phrases from speaker to speaker foregrounds their universality. Hoccleve's references to "my giltis" and "my sinful governaunce" lack any of the specificity used to characterize his personal history in the rest of the poem (C403, 406). Moreover, Hoccleve finds himself effortlessly everywhere in this textual tradition: he is its reader, as the detail of the borrowed book insists; he is its latest writer, as his concluding prayer ratifies; he identifies with the "wooful man" in need of consolation, but he is also like Reason because he has learned to speak in Reason's voice. As it is presented here, the Boethian literary tradition demands no grappling with the self's constitution through experiences of its own particularity and entails none of the *I*'s anxious accommodation of its outsides—the constant themes of Hoccleve's first-person poetry. Perhaps unsurprisingly the idiosyncrasy of Hoccleve's circumstances soon disrupts the Boethian paradigm. The book lender who takes his book hastily back again—a plot twist that Burrow judges to be a "convenient fiction"—functions like a bolt of pure contingency, breaking open the borrowed text's coherence.[20] And very soon, with similar happenstance, Hoccleve's friend will come knocking on his chamber door.

Intimate conversation and authoritative literary tradition, then, are two communicative paradigms that "My Compleinte" raises as alternatives to the symptomatic abjection Hoccleve suffers. Both return in the "Dialoge," the second act of the *Series'* frame narrative. There, the literary tradition that Hoccleve eventually settles on is not Boethian but Chaucerian. As Hoccleve tries out the model of his predecessor, Chaucer is made to signify a field of vernacular literary production that preserves authorial personality and that masters the ironic interplay between a limited self and its social field. Hoccleve's lofty praise for Chaucer in the *Regiment of Princes* is well-known, where he apostrophizes "O maistir deere and fadir reverent, / Mi maister Chaucer, flour of eloquence."[21] But Hoccleve's Chaucer in the *Series* is a cannier figure than the "Mirour of fructuous entendement" eulogized in the *Regiment*.[22] Hoccleve's Chaucer comes into fullest view at the end of the "Dialoge," but he also appears at the *Series'* outset. As numerous readers have observed, the start of the *Series'* prologue invites comparison to the opening of the *Canterbury Tales*:[23]

> Aftir that hervest inned had hise sheves,
> And that the broun sesoun of Mihelmesse
> Was come, and gan the trees robbe of her leves,
> That grene had ben in lusty freisshenesse,
> And hem into colour of yelownesse
> Had died and doun throwen undirfoote,
> That chaunge sanke into myn herte roote. (P1–7)

> [After the harvest had brought in its sheaves of grain and the brown season of Michaelmas had come and proceeded to rob the trees of their leaves, which had been green in lusty freshness, and had dyed them the color of yellow and thrown them down underfoot, that change sank into my heart's root.]

Chaucer's "Whan that Aprill . . ." depicts exactly the world of "lusty freisshenesse" that has passed out of Hoccleve's setting. Chaucer's poem came into existence on the strength of the engendering "vertu" of springtime flowers, while Hoccleve contrasts his own melancholic generation with the fallow landscape. If Chaucer's Zephyrus has breathed new life into the "tendre croppes" and springtime nature prods the birds in their "corages," then in Hoccleve's "broun sesoun of Mihelmesse" a change comes over him that will engender its own gloomy fruit: "chaunge sanke into myn herte roote."[24] The "freisshenesse" lost in line 4 returns in the speaker's own meditations, when this change "*freisshly* broughte it to my remembraunce / That stablenesse in this worlde is ther noon" (C8–9). The autumnal *chronographia* sets up a delicate play of correspondences and differentiations between narrator and scene, distinct from but evocative of the heady cosmic sweep of Chaucer's springtime.

Both Chaucer's and Hoccleve's openings delay the introduction of the first-person pronoun, but each to different effect. Compare the first appearance of *I* in each poem. As Chaucer writes,

> Bifel that in that seson on a day,
> In Southwerk at the Tabard as I lay
> Redy to wenden on my pilgrymage
> To Caunterbury with ful devout corage,
> At nyght was come into that hostelrye
> Wel nyne and twenty in a compaignye.[25]

> [It happened that in that season on a day, in Southwerk at the Tabard Inn as I lay ready to go on pilgrimage to Canterbury with fully devout spirit, at night there had come to that hostelry well twenty-nine people in a company.]

The comparable passage in Hoccleve reads:

> And in the ende of Novembre, uppon a night,
> Sighynge sore, as I in my bed lay,
> For this and othir thougtis wiche many a day,
> Byforne, I tooke, sleep cam noon in myn ye,
> So vexid me the thoughtful maladie. (P17–21)

> [And at the end of November one night, sighing deeply as I lay in my bed on account of this and other thoughts that for many days before I'd had, no sleep came to my eyes, so troubled me the thoughtful malady.]

Hoccleve has followed Chaucer in placing himself in bed. While Chaucer-the-pilgrim waits in anticipation of his journey's start the next morning, Hoccleve stews in the grief that will burst out of him "on the morwe" (P35). Chaucer's *I* is immediately followed by the introduction of the other pilgrims, "sondry folk, by aventure yfalle / In felaweshipe," in a transition that diverts readers' expectations of a dream vision in the direction of estates satire and, eventually, of the tale-telling game.[26] Hoccleve remains isolated, teeming with thoughts.

The *Series* likewise turns away from the genre of dream vision that the restless nighttime vigil seems to call for, but Hoccleve has nothing similar to Chaucer's twenty-nine pilgrims to fill out what comes next—just his "thoughtful maladie."

These inaugural evocations of the *Canterbury Tales* serve to mark the *Series* as an expansive and ambitious poem—though one that does not anticipate its totality in its origins. The General Prologue is a masterpiece of scale, zooming from the motions of the zodiac to a cozy bed in Southwerk, and then out again to the sundry company, whose possibilities turn out to be too rich to realize fully in the existing versions of the *Tales*. One could never guess from Hoccleve's prologue—or at least could not guess correctly—what the entirety of the *Series* will be. The narrator-poet's anguish and his fragmentation into component faculties ("my remembraunce," "myn ye," "my spirite," "myn herte," P8, 20, 27, 29) suggest that this troubled self will be the topic, but in fact, by the end of the "Dialoge" Hoccleve's persona no longer preoccupies the *Series*. Similar to the *Canterbury Tales*, the *Series* as a whole proves itself concerned with the collocation of heterogeneous discourses and with the interface between orality and textuality. Moreover, Hoccleve follows Chaucer in using "links," or contextual frames, for inset parts of his work, to represent a dynamic milieu of discursive production and first-order interpretation. But such work-wide homologies receive only the barest hint in the prologue. Hoccleve's initial evocations of the Chaucerian tradition serve instead to pose the question of whether he will make his way to something like the many voices of the *Canterbury Tales*, or remain mired in his intricately divisible subjectivity. How, this opening asks, will the *Series* handle the sociality of language?

Etiological Dialogue

The juxtaposition between the conclusion of "My Compleinte" and the start of the "Dialoge" is the most abrupt and surprising textual joint in the *Series*. After Hoccleve's prayer and following a textual rubric ("Here endith my compleinte and begynneth a dialogue"), he recounts that just when he "endid my compleinte in this manere," someone then comes knocking "at my chaumbre dore sore / And criede alowde, 'Howe, Hoccleve, art thu here?'" (D1–3). With this voice, the poem receives a transformative jolt. The sketchily delineated November "morwe" on which Hoccleve began his complaint becomes a socially permeable scene, subject to quotidian vagaries. The standoffishness of the *prees* and the universality of the prayer are punctured when someone calls Hoccleve's name.

Hoccleve invites this "good frende of fern agoon [long standing]" to come inside, and "right anoon I redde hym my compleinte" (D8, 17). The nature of "my compleinte" is abruptly clarified. Though Hoccleve seems to end the first poem in the dialogic voice of prayer, with his performative call to God ("And unto thi mercy and grace I calle," C413), the "Dialoge" straightaway marks this preceding section as a written artifact.[27] The textual rubric hundreds of lines earlier that marks the beginning of Hoccleve's complaint ("Here endith my prolog and folwith my compleinte," between lines 35 and 36) on an initial reading seems to dwell outside of the diegesis, explicable as a retrospective addition during compilation. As with the Latin textual divisions in Chaucer's "Knight's Tale," for example, readers might readily classify it as a bit of para-text distinct from narratorial enunciation. But the opening of the "Dialoge" discloses the relevance of the earlier rubric and announces that the medium of Hoccleve's lament is not "direct and impassioned utterance" but poetic composition.[28] What "braste oute" with all the immediacy of a bodily purge was actually a literary work in elegant rhyme-royal stanzas.

In this way, the poet-narrator's grasp of his situation, which has often appeared so limited in "My Compleinte," here leaps out in front of readers' expectations. Hoccleve catches us in the textual illusion of his voice. There is a winking glibness in how he then folds the sustained duration of reading "My Compleinte" into barely a line: "I redde hym my compleinte, / And, that done" (D17–18). Yet the friend's response seems to take the advantage back from Hoccleve just as suddenly. "'Hast thou maad this compleint forth to goo / Among the peple?'" his friend asks and then urges, "'Nay, Thomas, war [beware], do not so. / . . . Kepe al that cloos for thin honours sake'" (D23–25, 28). The friend's phrase "among the peple" suggests that Hoccleve's poem is just as unprepared to circulate to readers as his embodied self was to circulate in the streets of London. In what superficially looks like a comforting gesture, the friend characterizes Hoccleve's urban acquaintances in much friendlier terms than Hoccleve himself has done, assuring him that "'In as good a kinde / As thou hast stonde amonge men or [before] this day / Stondist thou nowe'" (D33–35). Yet the friend's reassurance implies deep skepticism about Hoccleve's point of view. He may be trying to dissuade the poet from paranoia, but even more vertiginous is the notion that Hoccleve's social perceptions have been all wrong. The friend's comments make the connection between the mirror scene and "My Compleinte" quite neat: both illustrate, perhaps, the impossibility of comprehending one's social milieu or oneself in it.

Part of the friend's argumentative arsenal deals in etiology. "'Thy bisy studie,'" he claims, "'Hath causid thee to stirte into the plyt [enter into the trouble] / That thow wer in'" (D302–4). Responding to Hoccleve's plans to return to writing, he worries, "'Thy brayn, par cas, therto nat wole assente'" (D297). The friend presents it as a settled fact that "'of studie was engendred thy seeknesse,'" and so, he demands incredulously, "'Woldest [Would you] now agayn / Entre into that laborious bisynesse / Syn it thy mynde and eek thy wit had slayn?'" (D379–82). The friend explains that he would give himself the very same advice to stop writing "'if so [thus] causid seeknesse on me fil [fell]'" (D388). The friend's etiological worries gain plausibility by continuing the imagery of heat that has been used before to characterize the causes of Hoccleve's illness. The friend remarks,

> "Thogh a strong fyr that was in an herth late,
> Withdrawen be and swept away ful cleene,
> Yit aftirward, bothe the herth and plate
> Been of the fyr warm, thogh no fyr be seene
> There as that it was, and right so I meene.
> Althogh past be the grete of thy seeknesse
> Yit lurke in thee may sum of hir warmnesse." (D309–15)

["Though a strong fire that was recently in the hearth has been withdrawn and swept away entirely, yet afterward both the hearth and plate are warm from the fire, though no fire can be seen there where it was, and just so is what I mean. Although the greater part of your sickness is past, yet some of its warmth may yet lurk within you."]

The extended metaphor of the hearth is undergirded by the "warmnesse" that belongs, materially, both to "seeknesse" and to fire. The body, like the hearth, is subject to the influence of physical properties. The terms of the friend's conceit echo the prognostic rumors that circulated in the crowd: "'Whanne passinge hete is,' quod thei, 'trustith this. / Assaile him wole agein that maladie'" (C92–93). The "thoughtful hete" that vexes Hoccleve on his walks home "fro Westminstir" pulls him toward the "folie" that he fears (C183–84, 140).

It is a striking feature of Hoccleve's self-characterization in the "Compleinte" and "Dialoge" that he puts forward no coherent counteretiology. He tells no clear story of why he went mad or how his "wilde infirmite" came to be. Instead, he draws intermittently on a variety of explanations, usually to combat what he takes to be mischaracterization, and he shows no apparent interest in these explanations' internal consistency. Are his past madness and his current melancholy intertwined or distinct? It depends. Sometimes he treats them as unrelated, sometimes as uneasily proximate. The prologue names them differently—"siknesse" versus "thoughtful maladie" (P21–22)—but the terminological distinction is not maintained, as rumors circulate that Hoccleve's "maladie," meaning his insanity, will return (C93). As we have seen, Hoccleve sometimes treats his madness as an all-purpose misfortune, sometimes as a purgative penance, and sometimes as a physiologically explicable illness caused by "the grevous venim / That had enfectid and wildid my brain" (C234–35). The point where Hoccleve most directly attaches his insanity to sin is just after reading the dialogue of Reason and the "wooful man," and so it seems less like a personal admission than the poet's provisional adoption of a ready-made discourse. It is easy then to disagree with Penelope Doob's claim that Hoccleve's topic in the *Series* "is the sinful madness of mankind" and that the work implies that "sin is the worst madness, the only madness that really matters."[29] If the autobiographical portion of the *Series* had ended with the "Compleinte," then Doob's interpretation would be plausible—but the "Dialoge" overturns that penitential finale and restores a plurality of causes and meanings to his insanity.

Hoccleve actually draws an elaborate distinction between his illness and sinful behavior. He tells his friend that the identities of "homicide," "extorcioner or a robbour," "coin clipper," and "werriour / Agein the feith" all proceed from moral weakness—what he calls the "freelte [frailty] / Of man hymsilfe"—because "God to man yove hath [has given] liberte" to choose "to do wel or no" (D64–74). Hoccleve's situation is entirely different, he explains, because sickness is removed from the sphere of agency: "this is al another caas, sothly. / This was the strook of God; he yaf me this" (D78–79). Declaring that his insanity was the stroke of God seems intended to stop further etiological speculation on his friend's part, especially his warnings about the physiological effects of writing. Nonetheless, the *Series'* continues to confound understanding of Hoccleve's madness all the way through the poet's final etiological claims, when he tells his friend, "'Trustith right wel, that nevere studie in book / Was cause why my mynde me forsook, / But i[t] was causid of my long seeknesse, / And othirwyse nat in soothfastnesse'" (D424–27). The explanation raises more questions than it answers. What is this "long seeknesse"? Does it connect his insanity to the "thoughtful maladie" after all (P21)? Or metaphorically to his "sinful governaunce" (C406)? What kind of explanation is it to source one sickness to another? As Matthew Boyd Goldie points out, "To admit he still has a long-standing, even recurring sickness, contradicts his arguments for recovery."[30]

Rather than answering any such questions, Hoccleve follows his mystifying etiology with a call to cease all causal speculation. "'That men kneew I had seeknesse is ynow [enough],'" he says, "'Thogh they make of the cause no serchynge, / Ther cometh but smal fruyt of swich deemynge. / To yow told have I treewely the cause'" (D430–33). Causation is dismissed rather than clarified. As they continue talking, Hoccleve insists, "'he lyveth nat that can / Knowe how it standith with another wight [person] / So wel as himself'" (D477–79). This assurance in self-knowledge is a stark reversal of Hoccleve's previous dependence on other people for any account of his madness. Without quite resolving the problem of his bodily and epistemological limits, he here shoulders past them, continuing to claim his authority to write. And it is shortly after this that the friend changes his tune. First he admits, "'Had I nat taastid [tested] thee, as that I now / Doon have, it had been hard, maad me to trowe [to make me believe] / The good plyt [condition] which I feele wel that thow / Art in'" (D485–88). Though still expressing caution, he concedes that now "'I am seur [sure] that thy disposicioun / Is swich that thow maist more take on hoonde / Than I first wende in myn oppinioun'" (D519–21). It seems, then, that here are the fruits of face-to-face conversation that Hoccleve looked forward to in the "Compleinte": "By communynge [conversing] is the beste assay [test]" (C217). His rhetoric and arguments have apparently convinced his friend of his "good plyt" and strengthened "disposicioun."

And yet this act of dialogic persuasion is not entirely convincing. Hoccleve's many contradictory accounts of his insanity do not add up to a valid rebuttal of his friend's concerns. His final, seemingly decisive etiological explanation—that his madness came from his "long seeknesse"—seems to bind his illness even more firmly to his present condition. As Ethan Knapp notes, these are signs that "despite the Friend's apparent acquiescence we are not meant to take Hoccleve's malady as something yet done away with."[31] The question remains, however, what interpretive significance these lingering suspicions and unanswered queries might have. My sense is that the artificial, illogical quality of the friend's capitulation points to the fact that he is not, in fact, a good avatar for the social exteriority of audience. As I have argued earlier in the chapter, the "prees" functions as a figure for textual readership, an entity that is necessarily impersonal and abstract to some degree. In the "Dialoge," Hoccleve's friend steps in as a substitute for the crowd. His role as literary audience is made clear by the fact that Hoccleve "redde hym my compleinte," and the ensuing debate can be taken to be one of interpreting both Hoccleve's corporeality and his text (D17). What was previously figured as the London crowd, with its fragmentary whispers and "straunge countinaunce," here gets an affable makeover. But Hoccleve's dissatisfaction with this solution is apparent almost as soon as it is in place. What is at stake throughout the debate between Hoccleve and his friend is whether Hoccleve should circulate his work "Amonge the peple" and continue writing (D24). The alterity of audience is still out there, beyond the "chaumbre dore," preoccupying those inside (D2). The friend's ultimately facile agreement with Hoccleve's account of himself is a sign of the poet growing bored with the dialogic conceit. The abrupt folding of the friend's resistance can be taken as a minor Brechtian estrangement effect, which recalls that the scene is staged and it is the author who is pulling the strings. As the "Dialoge" moves toward its conclusion, Hoccleve begins playing with such effects more and more openly. Without having resolved the constitutive vulnerabilities of the signifying condition, the poem gradually withdraws its attention from Hoccleve's riven and symptomatic self and turns instead to the task of staging the author's metatextual power.

The Comforts of Convention

From the point that the friend concedes and admits that Hoccleve should write his composition as he planned to do, things start moving very fast. The poem shifts into a stagily literary register, completing the *Series'* turn away from symptomatic corporeality. Not only does Hoccleve's body no longer interrupt his rhetorical agenda (as it did in "My Compleinte"), but he henceforth declines to make it the topic of his remarks. This represents another step in the poet-narrator's ascent from what has been portrayed as the expressive abjection of his insanity.

   Now, having convinced his friend of his health, he talks with him about his noble patron, Humphrey, Duke of Gloucester, to whom he owes a commission. The two praise the Duke's military prowess and virtue, and Hoccleve worries over how to write a work worthy of him (D534–616). He announces his previous plan of translating Vegetius's *De re militari* but dismisses the idea since Humphrey's chivalric valor is already so great (D561–65). These verses here are on eminently conventional footing: according to a familiar dynamic, the praise heaped on the patron redounds on the accomplishment and author-ity of the poet. Gloucester is yet another figure for Hoccleve's audience, one whose glory gilds the poet-narrator but also backs him into a rather narrow range of attitudes, the scant spectrum from cautious reverence to respectful humility. John Burrow has made the case that Hoccleve's most important autobiographical role is that of "dependent or petitioner," but in this case the position seems not to have captured the poet's imagination.[32]

It is in the midst of the encomium to Duke Humphrey that Hoccleve's friend gives voice to what is perhaps the most winklingly erudite and self-reflexive stanza of the *Series*. He advises Hoccleve that for a "prince so famous" he needs to write "good mateer and vertuous" and continues:

"Thow woost wel, who shal an hous edifie
Gooth nat therto withoute avisament
If he be wys, for with his mental ye
First is it seen, purposid, cast and ment,
How it shal wroght been, elles al is shent.
Certes, for the deffaute of good forsighte,
Mistyden thynges that wel tyde mighte." (D638–44)

["You know well, whoever will build a house goes to it not without
deliberation if he is wise, for it is seen first with his mental eye,
proposed, forecast, and planned, how it shall be made, or else all
is ruined. Certainly, for the lack of good foresight, things happen
poorly that might have happened well."]

The metaphor insists that a literary work, like a house, requires a plan, which is seen first with one's "mental ye" and then executed. The lines derive from a passage in the *Poetria Nova* of Geoffrey of Vinsauf, quoted in Latin alongside the stanza in the manuscripts. As Ellis observes in his editorial notes, "Within the terms of the fiction, it is Friend who acts as translator of the proverb, and Hoccleve, acting as scribe of his own work, who supplies the marginal gloss."[33] However, even as the friend delivers this writerly advice, it is he who begins to seem anticipated—"purposid, cast and ment." The meaning of the analogy, delivered here with metatextual virtuosity, slyly suggests that the poet has been in control all along. Hoccleve alienates the learned advice from his own persona, but the effect is to point out wittily the disjunction between his diegetic avatar and the real agency that has planned and emplotted the avatar's movements throughout.

This clever insistence on literary totality is a real departure for the *Series*, which seems to rebuke the poem's previous efforts to stage contingency—for instance, in the taking back of the borrowed book, in the knock at Hoccleve's door, and in the "wilde infirmite" itself. The analogy seems instead aligned with the failed reasoning of the mirror scene, where the way that Hoccleve's face was "seen, purposid, cast and ment" was imagined to determine his status in the crowd. In any case, despite the flourishing introduction of the Galfrid-ian metaphor here, the *Series* continues to pursue its contingency effects. For example, the fifth and final textual component of the *Series*, a misogynistic story from the *Gesta Romanorum*, is said to be added at the whim of Hoccleve's friend, against the poet-narrator's wishes. As David Watt remarks, "The *Series* is not the book that Thomas initially planned to make."[34] The prominent anal-ogy of the house "seen, purposid, cast and ment," then, seems more like a turn in the poem's rhetoric than a reliable emblem of the *Series'* poetics. The friend's advice to Hoccleve might be taken instead as nudging advice to readers: the totalizing force of the maker's "forsighte," he implies, demands interpreters' retrospective vantage on the completed design. Hoccleve's audience, in other words, is here being asked to bear the burden of literature's ontological dou-bleness, its division into textual artifact and narrative illusion, total design and time-bound action. If in "My Compleinte" Hoccleve's poetic persona was fragmented by the signifying condition—between subjective responsiveness and his materialization beyond himself, between the moment of writing and that of reading—now that work of adjustment is assigned to readers.

The reference to Geoffrey of Vinsauf is also a Chaucerian allusion, echo-ing the characterization of Pandarus's scheming in the first book of *Troilus and Criseyde*, where the go-between's plotting gives another turn to the Galfridian metaphor of writing and house building:

> For everi wight that hath an hous to founde
> Ne renneth naught the werk for to bygynne
> With rakel hond, but he wol bide a stounde,
> And sende his hertes line out fro withinne
> Aldirfirst his purpos for to wynne.
> Al this Pandare in his herte thoughte,
> And caste his werk ful wisely or he wroughte.[35]

[For every person who has a house to build runs not to begin the work with hasty hand, but will wait a while and send out his heart's line to measure how to attain his purpose. All this thought Pandarus in his heart, and laid out his work prudently before he began it.]

Although the Latin gloss indicates that Hoccleve was not dependent on Chaucer's version, the passage nonetheless assumes Chaucerian resonance in the increasingly dense web of allusions to the English poet in the final two hundred lines of the "Dialoge."[36] The dominant conceit of this final part of the poem is that Hoccleve finds himself in the same position as the poet-narrator in the *Legend of Good Women.* Just as in the *Legend* Chaucer is rebuked for slandering women in his *Troilus and Criseyde,* Hoccleve stands accused by his earlier poem, the "Letter of Cupid." As the friend tells him, "'Thow woost wel, on wommen greet wyt and lak [blame and reproach] / Ofte haast thow put'" (D667–68). As Chaucer undertakes the *Legend* in recompense, so Hoccleve is urged, "'Sumwhat now wryte in honour and preysynge / Of hem [them]. So maist thow do correccioun / Sumdel of thyn offense and misberynge'" (D673–75).

"'The Wyf of Bathe take I for auctrice,'" the friend declares as he rounds out his warnings about the hostility Hoccleve has excited among his women readers, "'That wommen han no ioie ne deyntee [pleasure] / That men sholde upon hem putte any vice. / I woot wel so, or lyk to that, seith shee'" (D694–97). The lines echo a passage in the Wife of Bath's Prologue where she, furious about Jankyn's misogynist proverbs, declares, "I hate hym that my vices telleth me, / And so doo mo [more], God woot, of us than I."[37] Like the friend's Galfridian advice on "good forsighte," this allusion to the Wife of Bath is double-edged. Invoked as a supposedly chastening "auctrice," the Wife also brings the model of the *Canterbury Tales* even closer to the *Series.* She is Chaucer's creation, and the friend's reference to her playfully alludes to the ontological status of the friend as well, who, like the Wife, is a fictionalized figure of both speech and reception. The friend interacts with the poet-narrator even as his naturalistic chitchat, falling neatly into prosodic form, registers the author's skill in colloquial versifying.

That Hoccleve is showily assuming the Chaucerian mantle is made even more obvious when he responds to his friend's warning about women's anger by reiterating Chaucer's elaborately reflexive disclaimers in the General Prologue. There Chaucer warns that "thogh that I pleynly speke in this mateere" and even though he reports the pilgrims' unvarnished words, his language should not be counted "vileynye" because "Whoso shal telle a tale after a man, / He moot reherce as ny as evere he kan / Everich a word"—and to do otherwise would be to "telle his tale untrewe."[38] Hoccleve gives a likewise wide-eyed self-defense. In the case of "th'epistle of Cupyde," he says, "was I noon auctour" (D760). Rather, "I nas in that cas but [I was in that case nothing but] a reportour / Of folkes tales. As they seide, I wroot" (D761–62). He follows this with a winking statement of poetic principles:

> "Whoso that shal reherce a mannes sawe,
> As that he seith moot he seyn and nat varie,
> For, and he do, he dooth ageyn the lawe
> Of trouthe. He may tho wordes nat contrarie." (D764–67)

> ["Whoever will report a man's speech, as that man says must he say and not vary it, for if he does, he acts against the law of truth. He may not alter those words."]

These echoes of the Chaucerian humility topos are of course also claims to Chaucerian poetic invention. It is within this playful discourse of modesty and masculine beleaguerment that Hoccleve's poetic persona comes newly alive. An air of insouciant bravado pervades, for instance, his very slanted retelling of the Adam and Eve story (D722–28). "'What world is this? How undirstande am I?'" he demands histrionically (D774), in a bathetic echo of Arcite's deathbed queries in the "Knight's Tale."[39] He is suddenly in the midst of a broadly comic performance while his friend, the earnest straight man, urges him to take on what sounds like a very secular penitential assignment, to redeem himself in ladies' eyes.

Hoccleve's women critics, as they are depicted in the "Dialogue," are a parody and triumphant diminution of the fearsome power of the interpreters whom Hoccleve has faced over the *Series'* frame. In the frame narrative's concluding section, the implacability of the London crowd becomes feminine waspishness and bad reading. When Hoccleve shifts his address to "My ladyes all," his words sound like those he might have wished to speak to the "prees" when he was quaking and blushing instead: "I am al othir to yow than yee weene. / By my wrytynge hath it and shal be seene" (D806, 811–12). Similarly, the tone of Hoccleve's final submission to his lady readers—"I lowly me submitte" (D813)—sets up a striking contrast to the obedient thanksgiving with which "My Compleinte" concludes. There, God is invoked as a principle of

self-stabilization against the jointly corporeal and social wildness of the symptomatic self. That Boethian voice is parodied by the penitential imagery at the
end of the "Dialogue." Instead of "Laude and honour and thanke" to God, it is
"honur and plesance / Of yow, my ladyes" with which Hoccleve will now be
concerned (C407, D821–22). In place of the purifying power of "myn elde and
of my seeknesse," his new project of literary translation "shal pourge, I hope, /
My gilt as cleene as keverchiefs dooth sope" (C410, D825–26).

Declaring that his friend as well as his women readers have failed to notice
that the offending book concludes "vertuously," Hoccleve remarks, "'For had
yee red it fully to the ende, / Yee wolde seyn it is nat as yee wende'" (D780,
783–84). This is an oblique return to Geoffrey of Vinsauf's well-planned house:
to appreciate the writer's foresight and intent, readers must read to the end. In
the case of the "Letter of Cupid," this supposedly means reading to the proof
that Hoccleve is blameless; in the case of the *Series'* frame narrative, it means
following the poet-narrator into his confident embodiment of the Chaucerian
tradition and thus his fitness to write. As a solution to the vulnerabilities of
the signifying condition—or, more accurately, as a feint and dodge away from
them—Hoccleve winds up trivializing the radical exteriority of audience in
the figure of his lady critics, who are made to embody the peevishness of bad
reading. In this sense, the *Series* indeed seems to be an "antifeminist contin-
uation of the *Letter of Cupid*," as Karen Winstead has argued.[40] With all of
Hoccleve's faux submission and comic penitence at the close of the "Dialogue,"
his audience is invited into the presumptively masculine space of *good* readers, who can appreciate the jibes at women's expense. Hoccleve's own persona
continues to be gently mocked as well, for instance, as he frets over his wife's
"hokir [scorn] and greet desdeyn" (D741)—but this is all within the familiar
conventions of antifeminism, where men's downtroddenness stabilizes gender
solidarity, a solidarity that here buoys up Hoccleve's newly achieved Chaucerian persona. At the end of the *Series'* frame, "My ladyes all" make it possible
for Hoccleve to appear in a body that is primarily masculine rather than symptomatic, constituted more by his authorial corpus than by the pathological
quaverings of his flesh.

Over the "Compleinte" and "Dialogue," then, Hoccleve has comported
himself toward a spectrum of addressees—first and most captivatingly the
prees of London, followed by God, his friend, an aristocratic patron, and a
hostile female readership. These figures function as avatars for the *Series'* context of reception, which is necessarily permeated by contingency and uncertainty. Each of the *Series'* versions of audience calls forth a different iteration

of the poet-narrator, and in retrospect his persona's transformations seem to constitute a plot of semiotic ascent, from symptom to art. Hoccleve begins the "Compleinte" with neither body nor social identity under his control. The murmuring urban *prees* affixes his insanity—that episode of pure, non-subjective bodiliness—to his person, and the crowd's gaze ongoingly incites ungovernable bodily responsiveness. Such flailing contingency is precisely the opposite of the foresight implied in the later allusion to Geoffrey of Vinsauf, where the poet slyly assures his readers that all apparent wildness has been "seen, purposid, cast and ment" (D641). To trust in that metaphor is to affirm the quasi-Chaucerian, masculine persona with which the "Dialoge" closes. And yet the Galfridian analogy will not do for the *Series* as a whole, which goes on after its frame narrative to stage the happenstance of literary making again and again.[41] Instead of functioning as a metapoetic key, "who shal an hous edifie" represents one pole of a profound ambiguity that Hoccleve locates in authorship. "Thomas Hoccleve" is both the artful agent of his poems and their contingent outcome. As their origin and cause, he is responsible for the unforeseen meanings they will assume independently of him—a fact to which he cannot stop responding. The metapoetic image that the *Series* offers for the signifier's ineradicable contingency is Hoccleve's symptomatic body. It is between the "mental ye" and madness, between "forsighte" and symptom, that Hoccleve's literary persona and his poetry unfold.

Chapter 8

From Noise to Narration
in the *Book of Margery Kempe*

The category of voice has been indispensable for scholars interpreting the *Book of Margery Kempe*. "Margery's voice rings clearly from the text," remarks one reader; another comments, "In her *Book* we hear recorded, however tidied, much of the accent of an authentic voice, the voice of a medieval English woman"; a third writes, "The *Book*'s overwhelming effect is one of immediacy, 'as if' a voice is talking, rather than a pen writing"; and "At issue in the text of Margery Kempe is authorial voice."[1] Yet *voice* remains an elusive concept in literary scholarship, in part because of the numerousness of its meanings.[2] Voice alternately signifies speech-sound, likeness to oral delivery, individual style, personal authenticity, and narration as such. In literary criticism, it functions as a catachresis, or a metaphor that cannot be defiguralized. Like the legs of a table or the face of a clock, a text's *voice* names something with no proper or literal name—since sonic voice is precisely what written script does without. This vocal catachresis works by referring to a scene of bodily presence, an occasion of speech that lies outside and prior to the written work. The image of the embodied, speaking author then rises up alongside the written work as the text's ostensible cause but also as its figural emission. In practice, this figural voice functions to gather up the multiple idioms that compose the text into a speaking persona, even as this persona's coherence wavers among the multitudinous vantages and speech acts constituting the written work.

It is difficult to think of a work more concerned with the traffic between authorial body and narrating voice than the *Book of Margery Kempe*. In the opening proem, it describes the text's genesis from Margery's oral self-narration; the work is packed with quotations of Margery's direct speech, whether in meditative dialogues or in contentious scenes of contemporary life; and the most distinctive signs of Margery's sanctity are her "krying and roryng [crying and roaring]," which time and again are described breaking through her resistances and ringing out.[3] The *Book*'s unstinting insistence on its protagonist's utterances is no doubt what has led scholars to their interest in Margery's voice, and the present chapter shares that interest, though it declines to accept voice as something given or integral, something to be simply found in the text. Instead, the following pages focus on the ceaseless production and dispersal of voice within the apparatus of symptomatic subjectivity. Margery's crying is a symptom, a kind of zero-degree voice that signifies by claiming a causal origin outside of systems of conventional meaning and intentional expression. But to lay claim to such a symptomatic origin always requires more speaking. An interlocking chain of enunciations takes shape, stretching from unverbalized *roryng* through Margery's many speech acts, whether in vignettes of fifteenth-century England or in mystical dialogues with Christ, and ultimately to the narrating voice of the *Book* itself. What finally counts as Margery's voice is a figural effect achieved by her enunciations' ceaseless routing through circuits of symptom and explanation, noise and narration.

The *Book of Margery Kempe* is a work of Middle English prose recounting the exceptional spiritual career of a middle-class laywoman. It chronicles her meditations, mystical dialogues, feats of holiness, and tribulations in England and abroad over a period of roughly twenty-five years. The text does not adhere to a single generic scheme, instead mixing elements of hagiography, spiritual handbook, devotional meditation, confession, and the visionary writings associated with medieval women like Mary of Oignies (d. 1213), Bridget of Sweden (d. 1373), and Catherine of Siena (d. 1380). Its narration is in the third person, and Margery is generally referred to as "this creatur," though it records a multitude of experiences that would have been exclusive to Margery's first-person point of view. By its own account, the *Book* records its central figure's self-narration as taken down by a pair of scribes.[4] The first section ("Book I") seems to have been committed to writing in 1421 as a stand-alone work, perhaps in a garbled shorthand script. After some mishaps, the text was eventually recopied by a second scribe in 1436, with an addition ("Book II") focused on Margery's travels when she was in her sixties. The entirety of the *Book* was complete in 1438 and survives in one copy, now British Library, Additional MS 61823, which was owned and annotated by Carthusians at Mount Grace Priory during the later fifteenth and the sixteenth centuries.

The constitution of voice is a constant concern for the *Book of Margery Kempe* in part because laywomen's spiritual authority was no easy matter in fifteenth-century England. One path to religious power and sanctity was through visionary experience, which depended on the visionary's being overmastered by forces outside herself, by divine presence and the gifts of the spirit. It is to this paradoxical authority of subjection that Michel de Certeau refers in his suggestive essay "Mystic Speech," where he remarks that "what is renewed" in mystical and visionary literature "is the relation between the signifier and the constitution of the subject: do we exist to speak to the other, or be spoken by him?"[5] Karma Lochrie, commenting on Certeau's essay in light of the *Book of Margery Kempe*, remarks that the "mystical text sets up a void" that then "inhabits" the visionary subject, where the "divine will" can speak.[6] The logic of (as Certeau has it) "being spoken" and of a void-ridden self where alien significations unfold connects the figure of the visionary to that of the symptomatic subject. Each one acts as a medium for forces exterior to the self. And when the visionary's divine overpowering becomes evidenced on the body, such bodily signs constitute (in the idiom of the present study) symptoms. Margery's periodic fits of shouting literalize—and *corporealize*—the logic of the visionary condition. Her vocalizations occur at the tangent point where symptoms touch speech and compulsion joins articulation. When Margery cries, God speaks through her, as he explains: "I geve the [you] gret cryis and roryngys for to makyn the pepil aferd [afraid] wyth the grace that I putte in the."[7] This noisy, concussive overthrow makes room for God inside Margery's voice, and her cries crystallize what in the pages that follow I explore as Margery's *first heteronomy of voice*, her coercion by a divine imperative that is both violent and authorizing.

However, her utterances are also under the sway of a second heteronomy. Her cries make her radically vulnerable to others' interpretations. Amid the institutions and social contexts of late medieval England, it was not enough for visionary experience to come from God. That origin had to be demonstrated and recognized, in part by distinguishing it from other possible causes: physiological, psychological, demonic, and deliberate. Establishing the proper etiology of holy phenomena was anything but straightforward, and in the milieu of late medieval etiological imagination, elaborate protocols were being developed to test the signs of sanctity. The early fifteenth century, when Margery Kempe was producing her *Book*, witnessed the growing importance of the discourse of *discretio spirituum*, or the discernment of spirits. This etiological scrutiny of sanctity gave a new twist to symptomatic subjectivity. As we have seen, a symptom is what appears on the medium of a living person but originates from other powers. The symptomatic subject has no special claim to understand her bodily signs because these signs' causation—and therefore their meaning—lies outside the bounds of first-person knowledge. In the normative framework of medieval medicine, patients relied on the expertise of practitioners who could link bodily phenomena to physiology, environment, and regimen. In situations of spiritual discernment, expert opinion was also deemed necessary, and this was particularly true in the case of holy women, who, in the gendered hierarchies of late medieval Christendom, were thought less discriminating and more vulnerable than their male counterparts, in part because of their physiological constitution.[8] Yet visionaries also *gained* interpretive authority from the signs they bore, and the experiential nature of many sanctifying signs maintained the importance of visionaries' first-person perspective, even under the scrutiny of clerical experts. Mysticism thus constituted a site of etiological contestation.

What is striking about the *Book of Margery Kempe* is how concerned it is to stage the *twofold* heteronomy that both symptoms and visionary experience entail—namely, their external causes and their subsequent construal (and misconstrual) by other people. While the divine etiology of "mystic speech" is an important concern throughout the tradition of visionary literature, the *Book*'s degree of explicit attention to the second heteronomy, the vulnerability of symptoms once they enter the social field of interpretation, is unprecedented. The *Book*'s unflagging inclusion of others' resistance, hostility, and misinterpretation contributes to the irreducibly public character of Margery's sanctity, or what Sarah Beckwith calls "the social dimension which makes her mysticism distinctive."[9]

In the pages that follow, I show how Margery's crying crystallizes around itself a consistent narrative pattern, one that sutures the narration's first- and third-person perspectives into their tightest and most polarized relation. This reiterated microdrama of embodiment, agency, and causation is made a leitmotif of Margery's spirituality. The text repeatedly stages the production and reception of Margery's cries, I argue, as a means of incorporating her voice's dependencies and alterities into the *Book*'s own narrating voice. In this repeated *fort-da* game of discursive authority, Margery's command over voice is lost and regained, lost and regained. If, in Freud's account, rendering an object "gone" (*fort*) and "there" (*da*) again, over and over, is what helps the child master loss, in the *Book* the crucial form of losing and finding happens in the prose, where Margery's authority is constantly obscured and rediscovered.[10] The narration draws voices that lie outside of Margery—beyond her person, exterior to her perspective, and out of her control—into its own ken. In turn, the *Book*'s textual narration is tethered by a series of metonymic links to Margery's embodied voice. By yoking "roryn [roaring]" to explanation and "noyse" to meaning, the repeated narration of Margery's cries makes these vocalizations into the irritating grain of sand around which the *Book* forms its pearl, the text itself.

Perspectives on a Symptom

One day in 1414, on the hillside where Jesus was crucified, Margery Kempe is overcome with bodily convulsions that she has never experienced before. This moment, her visit to Mount Calvary, is the climax of an eventful pilgrimage to Jerusalem and the culmination of a series of somatized emotions that have shaken her throughout the holy city. Here, at the site of Christ's suffering on the cross, something new overtakes her:

> And whan thei cam up onto the Mownt of Calvarye sche fel down
> that sche mygth not stondyn ne knelyn but walwyd and wrestyd
> wyth hir body, spredyng hlr armys abrode, and cryed wyth a lowde
> voys as thow hir hert schulde a brostyn asundyr, for in the cité of
> hir sowle sche saw veryly and freschly how owyr Lord was crucifyed.
> Beforn hir face sche herd and saw in hir gostly sygth the mornyng
> of owyr Lady, of Sen John and Mary Mawdelyn, and of many other
> that lovyd owyr Lord. And sche had so gret compassyon and so
> gret peyn to se owyr Lordys peyn that sche myt not kepe hirself fro
> krying and roryng thow sche schuld a be ded therfor. And this was
> the fyrst cry that evyr sche cryed in any contemplacyon. (I.28)

> [And when they came up on to the Mount of Calvary, she fell down
> because she could not stand or kneel, but writhed and wrestled with
> her body, spreading her arms out wide, and cried with a loud voice
> as though her heart would have burst apart, for in the city of her
> soul she saw truly and freshly how our Lord was crucified. Before
> her face she heard and saw in her spiritual sight the mourning of
> our Lady, of Saint John and Mary Magdalene, and of many others
> that loved our Lord. And she had such great compassion and such
> great pain to see our Lord's pain, that she could not keep herself

from crying and roaring though she should have died for it. And
this was the first crying that ever she cried in any contemplation.][11]

Margery's perceptible actions in this scene are all actions of incapacity: she
falls, she struggles against "hir body," she flails her arms in a gestural echo
of Christ on the cross, and she cries because she cannot keep herself from
doing so, even on pain of death. Her body and voice register the overthrow
of everyday capacities, and on this busy pilgrimage site her bellowing would
necessarily have incited etiological questions from onlookers: *What is happening to that woman? Why is she shouting?* Yet at the moment these queries arise
from the populated scene, they are already answered for readers. Margery cries
on account of what she sees in the "cité of hir sowle" and because she feels
"so gret compassyon and so gret peyn." The narration stitches together two
different points of view, spectatorial observations of Margery (how she looks
and sounds) and what she alone experiences. The final sentence shifts to yet
another vantage, that of retrospection, which looks back on this "krying and
roryng" to place it as the "fyrst" in a series that will go on to be characterized
for "many yerys aftyr this tyme" (I.28).

In this inaugural scene of Margery's crying, a fluidity of narrative focalization is established that recurs in subsequent portrayals. Focalization is a
narratological term for investigating standpoint ("Who sees?"), as distinct
from voice ("Who speaks?"). It directs attention to how what is presented
in narrative ongoingly entails a locus of perception, which may shift independently of changes in speaker.[12] The shifts in focalization in the scene on
Mount Calvary are subtle (more dramatic ones are discussed below), but they
are discernible in the distinction between two sets of images—the crucifixion
perceived within Margery's "gostly sygth" and her thrashing body on the hillside. Readers both look *with* Margery, "in the cité of hir sowle," and look *at*
her. As Sarah Salih observes, the *Book* tends to give "both exterior and interior
perspective on her bodily manifestations of saintliness."[13]

This flexibility of narrative vantage, its focal restiveness, is among the
Book's most important and distinctive techniques of etiological persuasion.
In scenes like this one, the *Book*'s prose takes care to portray Margery's bodily
signs both as phenomena in need of causal explanation, as they appear to
those standing nearby, and as effects proceeding inexorably and unmistak-
ably from God's grace, as they are experienced by Margery. Effect and cause
compose a single narrative unit that unfolds across a split in point of view.
Margery's vantage testifies to what I above called her first heteronomy of voice,

or the irresistible divine influence over her expressions. She feels this power of God in her body via her own loss of physical control. Onlookers' perspectives manifest the second type of heteronomy: the opacity of this cause-and-effect relationship to other people, which makes the meaning of her cries dependent on contingent processes of interpretation. Margery's body is crucial to representing both modes of heteronomy, but it operates differently in each case. To register God's power, her body acts a medium of sensation and felt compulsion; it is a locus of experience, focalized through Margery. For other people, her body is a source of sense data and social information demanding interpretation—sound, tears, motion, gesture, and spectacle. Throughout the *Book*, the gap between one vantage and the other, between first- and third-person focalization, constitutes a space of interpretive waywardness. This is where misunderstanding and skepticism arise but also where there is room for Margery's explanations and self-narration. "Not only could [Margery] howl," Nicholas Watson observes, but "she could analyze the causes, effects, history, and significance" of her cries.[14]

In the *Book of Margery Kempe*, then, what symptoms are good for is drawing three realms—divine, personal, and social—into tense interaction. Of course, this is just one of the concerns of the *Book*'s narration. At other moments, the anxious awareness that other people are watching recedes into the background. In Margery's visions, for instance, scenes of private conversation with Christ overwrite the quotidian world of fifteenth-century England. These episodes attain what feels like a degree of narrative autonomy as they unfold without interruption over many pages and accrue diegetic vividness and reality. In them, only minimal traces of textual mediation recall the ongoing pressures of social perception—like the third-person narration that continues to refer to Margery as "this creatur." Another type of scene functions more like a play, adopting a dramatic standpoint in which readers, like onlookers, follow Margery's actions and words from the outside, as when she delivers her withering rebuttals to the Archbishop of York and his retinue (I.52). In contrast to both the meditative and dramatic styles of narration, scenes focused on Margery's paramystical symptoms tend to emphasize and even exaggerate the difference between Margery's experience and other people's, rendering that disjunction a crucial element of her cries' significance.

Margery's crying is closely related to other physical symptoms of her sanctity. The accompanying gestures of falling and flailing on Mount Calvary suggest as much, as does her cries' frequent occurrence together with uncontrollable weeping ("sche wept, sche sobbyd, sche cryed so lowde"; "sche wept wyth gret sobbyng and lowde crying," etc. [I.29, 30]). Crying and weeping, however, remain distinguishable, the former being essentially auditory, while the latter is defined by tears.[15] The *Book* itself distinguishes between them by giving them different narrative trajectories: Margery's weeping occurs through the entirety of the action, but her crying begins abruptly on Mount Calvary and is withdrawn ten years later, when God tells her, "'I schal takyn awey fro the thy criyng that thu schalt no mor cryin so lowde ne on that maner wyse as thu hast don befor thei thu woldist [I shall take away from you your crying, so that you will no longer cry so loudly, nor in the way you have before, even if you should want to]'" (I.63; 194). "Holy tears" have a strong legacy in Christian tradition,[16] while disruptive vocalizations have fewer precedents in hagiographical literature.[17] As Nicholas Watson remarks, "Despite all medieval and modern efforts to find parallels, her crying aligns her with nobody."[18] If medieval grammarians were to classify her cries, they would likely place them in the category of *vox confusa*, or *vox inarticulata illiterata*, because the *Book* tends to portray them as *inrationalis* and *inscriptilis*—spoken without reasoned intention and incapable of being written out in letters. They are instances of *sonus simplici vocis*, the sounding of bare voice.[19]

At the end of the passage from Mount Calvary quoted above, the narration switches its focalization once more, this time to a more comprehensive temporal vantage. Turning away from the particulars of the scene, the narrating voice assumes a posture of retrospection by deeming Margery's hillside cries the "fyrst" in a pattern that extends "many yerys aftyr this tyme" (I.28). This broadening-out of the point of view effects a shift from what Gérard Genette calls singulative narration—"narrating once what happened once," in this case, the events on Mount Calvary—to iterative, or frequentative, narration—"relating one time what happened numerous times."[20] Thus, the text continues:

And this maner of crying enduryd many yerys aftyr this tyme for owt that any man myt do, and therfor sufferyd sche mych despyte and mech reprefe. The cryeng was so lowde and so wondyrful that it made the pepyl astoynd les than thei had herd it beforn and er ellys that thei knew the cawse of the crying. (I.28)

[And this kind of crying lasted for many years after this time, despite anything that anyone might do, and she suffered much contempt and much reproof for it. The crying was so loud and so amazing that it astounded people, unless they had heard it before, or else knew the reason for the crying.] (104)

These lines both explain something about Margery's crying and embody a further narrative mode, that of retrospection. On this account, people's knowledge of the "cawse of the crying" is what makes the difference between their contemptuous befuddlement and their proper recognition of her sanctity. Such etiological understanding is what the prose of the *Book* labors to produce in its attention to both the public shock of her vocalizations and Margery's experience of how they are produced. The narrative voice's peeling away from the time and place of the Jerusalem pilgrimage also has the effect of showing its flexibility and range, as it speaks from a position of encompassing hindsight.

The *Book*'s habit of shifting among focal positions answers to a variety of rhetorical needs. Singulative narration of Margery's cries, like the vivid recounting of the events on Mount Calvary, has an evidentiary function, sketching the circumstantial details of what happened, almost as though for a canonization dossier. Iterative narration plays a more explanatory role, fitting particular instances into larger patterns and perhaps connecting them to received models of sanctity. The shifts in focalization play a crucial aesthetic function, as they rapidly circulate the reading audience through different perceptual experiences: the painful overwhelming of self-possession, as Margery feels her heart ready to "brostyn asundyr [burst asunder]"; the perceptions of onlookers, who encounter her flailing, shrieking form; and the reflections of a retrospective vantage, which gathers up particular instances in its encompassing backward regard. Thus are readers made to feel and understand the logic of paramystical signs.

The *Book*'s constant effort to satisfy a variety of expectations bespeaks its unsettled genre commitments—to visionary revelation, devotional guide, and hagiographical vita.[21] Sarah Salih argues that where the *Book* "is original is in its combination of apparently incompatible [textual] models," for it "draws on a number of disparate traditions, often reworking them in the process, to produce a probably unique performance of visible, visionary, preaching, remade virgin in the world."[22] Amy Hollywood provides another genealogy for the *Book*'s perspectival shifting in her account of thirteenth-century women mystics, where she shows "the tendency of the [male, clerical] hagiographer to translate mystical into paramystical phenomena, or internally apprehended into externally perceptible experiences."[23] Over the course of the fourteenth century, Hollywood argues, demands for the physical authorization of female sanctity were internalized in women's visionary writings and became constitutive of the genre. Women needed to manifest bodily signs of their sanctity, which were then available to observation and evaluation in a way that private experience was not.

These complex signifying imperatives and generic expectations reflect the fact that women's holiness was among the most contested categories of spiritual authority in the later Middle Ages.[24] The new models of female sanctity that gained prominence starting in the later twelfth century incited corresponding growth in the discourses *regulating* pious women. Women's visionary authority demanded demonstrations that God was the direct cause of their exceptional insights and behaviors.[25] From the reign of Pope Innocent III (1198–1216), the standards of proof for miracles were growing more arduous, and the papacy claimed new oversight of the cults of the saints. As Dyan Elliott has argued, the Fourth Lateran Council's attention to the regulation of sanctity and the threat of heresy culminated, by the end of the fourteenth century, in a situation where "women's faith and religious practices [would] be increasingly scrutinized from a skeptical standpoint, and the women themselves [would] ultimately be required to prove their orthodoxy."[26] Such changes are part of not only the history of the Church and adjacent religious practices but also the broader unfolding of late medieval etiological thought. The many different causes that might be at the root of something—of a cure at a shrine, a visionary experience, or a fit of crying—became the occasion for the Church's etiological adjudication.

The developing discourse of the "discernment of spirits" is particularly relevant in this regard. Spiritual discernment had its scriptural basis in 1 John 4:1: "Dearly beloved, believe not every spirit, but try the spirits if they be of God [*probate spiritus si ex Deo sint*]: because many false prophets are gone out into the world." The medieval revival of John's injunction was a deeply ambivalent response to the proliferation of devotional styles that began in the late twelfth century; Nancy Caciola calls the resulting discourse a "practice of institutionalized mistrust regarding individual claims to visionary or prophetic authority."[27] The "spirits" to be tested were the causal forces behind apparent miracles, revelations, prophecies, and other tokens of sanctity. Before a revelation or sign could be authenticated, other causes had to be ruled out— demonic ruse, a pseudo-mystic's calculating imposture, worshippers' unwitting self-deception, or a simple physiological origin. Interest in the discernment of spirits was high during Margery Kempe's lifetime. One of Margery's spiritual models, Saint Bridget of Sweden, was the topic of intense, ongoing clerical controversy about the authenticity of her revelations. These controversies catalyzed efforts to establish criteria for evaluating visionary phenomena. Bridget's spiritual advisor Alfonso de Jaén wrote an influential work on the topic, the *Epistola solitarii ad reges*, which in turn became an important source for one of Bridget's most powerful detractors, the prominent theologian and chancellor of the University of Paris Jean Gerson (1363–1429), who was Margery Kempe's contemporary.[28] In England, the discourse of discernment was less exclusively an outward-looking mode of clerical investigation, and it assumed more introspective forms in vernacular devotional treatises like the "Pistle of Discrecioun of Stirings" and "Tretis of Discrecyon of Spirites" (often found together in manuscripts), as well as in the *Chastising of God's Children* and Walter Hilton's *Scale of Perfection*.[29] However, England's ongoing conflicts over Lollardy and the contested line between reform and heresy meant that inquisitional procedures were never far off.

What both inquisitional and self-reflective versions of *discretio* shared was an interest in the conditioning *causes* of experience, or what stood at the root of perceptions, feelings, and behaviors as their incitement and thus as an indicator of their true significance. The *Book of Margery Kempe* responds to the etiological fascinations of *discretio*. As Sarah Beckwith remarks, "The clerics in the book of Margery Kempe are obsessed with the *sources* of her knowledge,"[30] and the *Book* is full of occasions in which Margery must explain the origins and circumstances of her insights. The *Book*'s generic hybridity and its shifting focalization—as Sarah Salih writes, its combination of "the first-person perspective of women's mystical writings with the third-person perspective of male-authored hagiography"[31]—are tactics to answer the crossed demands on her sanctity, of laying hold of saintly power directly, as a visionary, and of its explanatory validation in institutional and social frameworks. Her story documents the support of prominent clerics and fellow Christians, even as she claims a paramystical authority that eschews subordination to the institutional church, in a text that "embraces disobedience more frequently and openly than any other female revelations."[32] Through its orchestration of focalization, imagery, and voice, the narration of the *Book* performs an awareness that Margery's holiness depends on the divine origins of her devotional and mystical experiences but also on the human recognition of those origins, a recognition that is at stake in the *Book*'s efforts at etiological representation and persuasion.

The Crying Plot

Between Margery's "fyrst cry" on Mount Calvary and the end of the *Book*'s long first part ("Book I"), Margery's paramystical shouting occurs or is discussed substantially in thirty-four of fifty-nine chapters, sometimes multiple times per chapter. This reiteration makes her crying one of the *Book*'s most insistent manifestations of her visionary status. In many of its depictions, Margery's crying follows a habituated narrative pattern, a sort of underlying plot. As I have argued elsewhere, this plot tends to entail a sequence of three phases—*interiorization*, *vocalization*, and *reception*—each linked with distinctive events, subjective states, syntactical structures, and positions of focalization.[33] While the entirety of the plot is certainly not played out every time Margery's cries are mentioned, its outlines are often discernible in even brief discussions. The plot's structure helps give consistency to the *Book*'s portrayal of Margery's paramystical sanctity and to the rhetorical demands that these bodily signs place on the narrative. The significance of Margery's cries, then, lies not just in their divine origin and their contested reception but in how the *Book* consistently regulates literary form in response to them.

One Palm Sunday in Margery's hometown of King's Lynn, a "worshepful doctowr of divinté" preaches a sermon on Christ's love. The preacher dwells on Christ's suffering for mankind and often repeats "thes wordys, 'Owr Lord Jhesu langurith [languishes] for lofe'" (I.78). As Margery listens, she begins to undergo a transformation:

> Tho wordys wrowt so in hir mende whan sche herd spekyn of the
> parfyte lof that owr Lord Jhesu Crist had to mankynde and how der
> he bowt us wyth hys bittyr Passyon, schedyng hys hert blood for owr
> redempcyon, and suffyrd so schamful a deth for owr salvacyon, than
> sche myth no lengar kepyn the fir of lofe clos wythinne hir brest,
> but, whethyr sche wolde er not, it wolde aperyn wythowteforth
> swech as was closyd wythinneforth. And so sche cryed ful lowde and
> wept and sobbyd ful sor as thow sche schulde a brostyn for pité and
> compassyon that sche had of owr Lordys passyon. And sumtyme
> sche was al on a watyr wyth the labowr of the crying, it was so lowde

and so boistows, and mech pepil wondryd on hir and bannyd hir ful fast, supposyng that sche had feynyd hirself for to cryin. (I.78)

[Those words so worked in her mind, when she heard speak of the perfect love that our Lord Jesus Christ had for mankind, and how dearly he bought us with his bitter passion, shedding his heart's blood for our redemption, and suffered so shameful a death for our salvation, that she could no longer keep the fire of love within her breast, but, whether she would or no, what was enclosed within would insist on appearing outwardly. And so she cried very loudly and wept and sobbed very bitterly, as though she would have burst for pity and compassion that she had for our Lord's Passion. And sometimes she was all of a sweat with the effort of the crying, it was so loud and violent, and many people wondered at her and cursed her roundly, supposing that she had pretended to cry.] (225)

As this example suggests, the "crying plot" tends to be set in motion by something objectively present—here, a sermon; elsewhere a pious image (I.46) a liturgical spectacle (I.57), a holy man's grave (I.60), or a quotidian scene, like an animal being struck (I.28). As Margery watches and listens, the narration's focalization tends to move inward, to become more exclusively first person. This initial phase of the plot, then, is one of *interiorization*. On this Palm Sunday, the standpoint sets out from a relatively neutral or "dramatic" stance, describing and quoting the sermon's theme as any onlooker might have done. It then begins to shift into the ambit of Margery's perceptions, as she "herd spekyn" the sermon's contents. The mediating effects of her consciousness come increasingly to the fore and seem to transform the contents of the sermon. The familiar events of the Passion are imbued with new urgency. The movement of interiorization happens similarly on Mount Calvary, where Margery comes to see not only the pilgrimage site around her but "veryly and freschly how owyr Lord was crucifyed." In that episode, it is "beforn hir face" that she sees Mary and John mourning—but this somatic reference points not to the common physical space she shares with other people but to the domain of "hir gostly [spiritual] sygth." In a manner that becomes familiar over the course of the *Book*, readers follow the narration as it is pulled centripetally into Margery's private devotional sensorium.

Meanwhile, not only is Margery's consciousness allowed to alter what readers perceive in the scene, but her perceptions are described *working on her*, or in the words of the Palm Sunday scene, they "wrowt" on "hir mende." Her internal state lurches into metamorphosis. The prose builds suspense with its open "so" clause (the preacher's words "wrowt *so* in hir mende"): in what manner, to what effect, do these words work on Margery's mental state? Readers await resolution across the paraphrased details of the sermon, and this stretching of syntax is characteristic of the crying plot. For instance, another passage (which is in fact a renarration of Margery's crying on Mount Calvary) opens with a long, hypotactic *when* clause, that crescendos—*then*—with her outburst:

> And, whan thorw dispensacyon of the hy mercy of owyr sovereyn savyowr Crist Jhesu it was grawntd this creatur to beholdyn so verily hys precyows tendyr body, alto rent and toryn wyth scorgys, mor ful of wowndys than evyr was duffehows of holys, hangyng upon the cros wyth the corown of thorn upon hys hevyd, hys blysful handys, hys tendyr fete nayled to the hard tre, the reverys of blood flowyng owt plenteuowsly of every membr, the gresly and grevous wownde in hys precyows syde schedyng owt blood and watyr for hir lofe and hir salvacyon, than sche fel down and cryed wyth lowde voys, wondyrfully turnyng and wrestyng hir body on every syde, spredyng hir armys abrode as yyf sche schulde a deyd. (I.28)

> [And when through dispensation of the high mercy of our sovereign savior, Christ Jesus, it was granted to this creature to behold so truly his precious tender body, all rent and torn with scourges, more full of wounds than a dove-cote ever was with holes, hanging upon the cross with the crown of thorns upon his head, his blessed hands, his tender feet nailed to the hard wood, the rivers of blood flowing out plenteously from every limb, the grisly and grievous wound in his precious side shedding out blood and water for her love and her salvation, then she fell down and cried with a loud voice, twisting and turning her body amazingly on every side, spreading her arms out wide as if she would have died.] (105–6)

The syntactic suspense built up across a sentence like this one mimics the pressure and intensity gathering within Margery, demanding its outlet in vocalization. The subordinate *when* clause is here filled out with imagery drawn from Richard Rolle's *Meditations on the Passion*. The borrowed and conventional nature of these contents is instructive. It is not necessarily *what* Margery perceives but *how* she perceives it that makes the difference. This is why the emplotment of focalization, or the carefully signaled process of interiorization, is central to the narrative form of the crying plot.

In the Palm Sunday passage, it is with the resolution of the open "so" clause that the plot shifts to its next phase, vocalization. Here, Margery's body comes abruptly to the fore, where it is described in polarized terms of interiority and exteriority and agency and compulsion. She "myth no lengar kepyn the fir of lofe" inside of herself, and her efforts at self-enclosure give way under the imperative that what was "closyd wythinneforth" must appear "wythowteforth." The double use of "wolde" emphasizes Margery's loss of agency: "whethyr sche *wolde* [intended, consented] er not," the fire of love "*wolde* [would]" appear. Margery's body becomes a container for the fiery, pressurized contents within, strained to the point of bursting—"as thow sche schulde a brostyn for pité and compassyon." This grammar of oppositions set into wrenching and conflicted motion is among the *Book*'s most powerful aesthetic means to depict God within Margery, or the divine overpowering of her own agential powers, which I have termed the first heteronomy of her voice. Medieval studies has in recent years grown adept at recognizing the porous and fluid models of subjectivity circulating in premodern cultures, and visionary women have served as exemplars of such permeability.[34] Yet in these moments, when Margery is undergoing her paramystical overthrow, it is important to notice that the narration actually hardens the binary oppositions that define the boundaries of Margery's person. The force field separating "wythinneforth" from "wythowteforth" becomes highly charged, and its puncturing is what gives the crying plot its cathartic release.

By this point in the plot, focalization has been on the move. It has traveled from an unmarked observer's stance inward, "wythinneforth," while the interior pressure builds against Margery's self-enclosure. There is then something paradoxical about the climactic moment of crying. It is enormously intimate, transpiring "in hir mende" and "wythinne hir brest," but it is also the point at which experiential content is evacuated. At the instant of vocalization, the "fir of lofe" functions like a simple physical force. Margery becomes all causal entailment, all physical action and reaction, through what is almost a hydraulics of affect and sound.

A similar transformation is evident in another scene of Margery's crying, when her vocalizations erupt during a mass on Good Friday. The vision of the Passion that Margery perceives "wyth hir gostly eye"

wrowt be grace so fervently in hir mende, wowndyng hir wyth pité
and compassyon, that sche sobbyd, roryd, and cryed, and, spredyng
hir armys abrood, seyd wyth lowde voys, "I dey, I dey," that many
man on hir wonderyd and merveyled what hir eyled. (I.57)

[worked by grace so fervently in her mind, wounding her with
pity and compassion, so that she sobbed, roared, and cryed, and,
spreading her arms out wide, said with a loud voice, "I die, I die,"
so that many people were astonished at her, and wondered what was
the matter with her.] (179)

Here Margery's devotional contemplation becomes physicalized as it works
fervently on her mind, an adverb that connotes heat and fever, while the images
wownd her. Such concretizing diction helps to shift from mental to somatic
phenomena. The devotional content of Margery's thoughts—"hys precyows
body betyn, scorgyd, and crucifyed" (I.57)—falls away as the narration turns
instead to the representation of her observable symptoms. While it is somewhat unusual for Margery to speak articulately in the midst of her crying, it
is not unprecedented in the *Book*. Her repeated phrase "I die! I die!" places
her first-person pronoun under a double negation. She pronounces her own
death, in a hyperbolic metaphor of the self-loss she undergoes. To pronounce
one's own death is always a paradoxical speech act, and here it announces
self-extinction at the same time that, amid the gathered congregation of worshippers, it extravagantly enacts Margery's speaking presence. But the *I* is also,
simultaneously, not Margery's. It is Jesus who dies on the cross on Good Friday, and at the moment when Margery cries out, the liturgical tableau in front
of her includes the eucharistic host enclosed in the chancel wall to commem-
orate Christ's entombment. It may well be Christ who speaks in Margery's
person, replacing her *I* with his own to announce, "I die! I die!" The phrase,
like Margery's crying, thus poses anew Certeau's query about whether mystic
speech stands "to speak to the other, or be spoken by him."[35] It functions as a
crystallization of the overdetermined and mercurial significance of Margery's
symptomatic voice.

In the Good Friday scene, the flailing of Margery's arms and the loudness
of her voice are not recounted as actions reflectively considered and carried
out, nor are they described as something Margery herself experiences. Instead,
they seem to be seen and heard by someone else, a perspective that is swiftly
attached to the "many man" who "merveyled what hir eyled." This brings us

to the final movement of the crying plot, when focalization bursts out along the same trajectory as Margery's voice and lands among the "pepil." Suddenly readers do not perceive through Margery's experiential lens but rather witness the "creatur" from the point of view of others, as spectacle. This new perspective allows readers to apprehend events as though for a second time, now with onlookers' puzzlement and skepticism, as when (in the Palm Sunday passage) they "wondryd on hir and bannyd [cursed] hir ful fast, supposyng that sche had feynyd hirself for to cryin."

This accusation of hypocritical feigning is especially notable. Suspicions of deception depend upon the separation of first-person and third-person knowledge; the accusation entails witnesses' exteriority to Margery's private experience. In the case of her Palm Sunday crying, the narration has just recounted Margery's experience so intimately that it would seem to eliminate, for the reader, all possibility of hypocrisy and pretending. And yet the final turn to the befuddled, skeptical reception of her cries has destabilizing effects. If over the course of Thomas Hoccleve's "Compleinte" and "Dialoge" (as the previous chapter argued) the corporeal and social heteronomies of the symptomatic body are eventually subsumed into the achievement of a commanding narrative voice, the *Book of Margery Kempe* does something rather different. It never overcomes the disjunctions between God, mystic, and other people, and it also never ceases to include them within the breadth of its narrative voice.

It is the achievement of the crying plot to link in one vector of narration Margery's felt experience, her paramystical symptoms, and these symptoms' reception by other people. When devotional affect becomes physical force and overpowers Margery's self-control, it bursts into a peopled soundscape, a social field of interpretation. At the point of vocalization, the narration leaps from its intimacy with Margery to a suddenly external standpoint, and in the process it generates the shock of encountering wildly unexpected utterance. The obscure indexicality of these cries, the fact that they testify to divine power without naming it, means that they demand explanation. Margery's voice, then, becomes a special locus of etiological contestation.

Etiologies of Voice

Many readers attest to how unsettling the final act of the crying plot can be, when the *pepil* around Margery hear her cries but do not recognize their

divine origins. In addition to the *Book*'s constant reiteration of onlookers' baf-
flement and mistrust, even many of Margery's clerical supporters, like her
confessor in Rome, are said to "mystrosten [mistrust]" her cries (I.33), and in
one vision, the twelve Apostles actually "comawndyd hir to cesyn and be stille"
(I.73). Allowing so much airtime to oppositional opinions was unconventional
in medieval women's visionary literature, in part because women's claims to
authority were so tenuous. In spite of this, the "*Book* devotes much attention
to the reactions to the cryings, exaggerating rather than trying to obscure how
controversial they were," as Sarah Salih observes.[36] Nicholas Watson understands the *Book*'s inclusion of such controversy as a means of implicating its
audience, by "continually tempt[ing] readers into refusing [Margery], should
their faith and trust not be supple enough." "The *Book* demands that readers
believe in Kempe," Watson continues, "but it also gives them every opportunity to number themselves among her doubters or opponents."[37] Rosalynn
Voaden identifies archetypes for Margery's revilement in the Gospels, but she
finds that the *Book*'s overreliance on the topos undermines her authority and
ultimately disrupts the *Book*'s project: her "successful construction as a visionary is fatally compromised by her simultaneous construction as an object of
abuse."[38] What Watson and Voaden notice, I think, is a crucial effect of the
Book's narrative style. It never ceases to reproduce the divergence between the
divine origins of Margery's vocalizations and their hostile reception. It continuously dramatizes the fractious misalignment of her voice's divine and social
heteronomies.

One of the ways this friction is staged is through the *Book*'s rehearsal of
other people's etiological explanations. For instance,

> summe seyd it was a wikkyd spiryt vexid hir; sum seyd it was a
> sekenes; sum seyd sche had dronkyn to mech wyn; sum bannyd hir;
> sum wisshed sche had ben in the havyn; sum wolde sche had ben in
> the se in a bottumles boyt; and so ich man as hym thowte. (I.28)

> [some said it was a wicked spirit that tormented her; some said it was
> an illness; some said she had drunk too much wine; some cursed her;
> some wished she was in the harbor; some wished she was on the sea
> in a bottomless boat; and so each man as he thought.] (105)

As the laity here practice their own form of *discretio spirituum*, Margery's crying becomes the incitement to etiological imagination and disputation. On

this account, what it means to have one's visionary voice enter public circulation is to find it construed according to a jostling host of causal models, which are particularized in their explanations but united in their hostility to Margery's sanctity. The causes proffered (demon, sickness, drunkenness) verge into the sneering wish that she were dead, "in the se in a bottumles boyt." A similar passage occurs when Margery is struck with her crying in Norwich:

> And many seyd ther was nevyr seynt in hevyn that cryed so as
> sche dede, wherfor thei woldyn concludyn that sche had a devyl
> wythinne hir whech cawsyd that crying. And so thei seyden pleynly
> and meche mor evyl. . . . Sum seyde that sche had the fallyng evyl,
> for sche wyth the crying wrestyd hir body turnyng fro the o syde
> into the other and wex al blew and al blo as it had ben colowr of
> leed. And than folke spitted at hir for horrowr of the sekenes, and
> sum scornyd hir and seyd that sche howlyd as it had ben a dogge
> and bannyd hir and cursyd hir and seyd that sche dede meche harm
> among the pepyl. (I.44)

> [And many said there was never a saint in heaven that cried as
> she did, and from that concluded that she had a devil within her
> which caused that crying. And this they said openly, and more evil
> talk. . . . Some said she had epilepsy, for while she cried she wrested
> her body about, turning from one side to the other, and turned
> all blue and gray, like the color of lead. Then people spat at her in
> horror at the illness, and some scorned her and said that she howled
> like a dog, and cursed her.] (142–43)

As in the previous passage, both demonological and pathological explanations are offered, but they amount to the same thing: a discrediting hostility, which the *Book* does not hesitate to fold into its narration.

These etiological outbursts from Margery's fellow Christians illustrate her cries' vulnerability on their wayward path to recognition, a vulnerability that arises in part from the kind of signifier that a natural sign is. Her crying, like any symptom, is not mimetic, nor does it originate within the shared conventions of a language. Instead, it depends for its meaning on interpreters' knowledge of the causal relations out of which the sign emerged. Those who hear Margery crying lack access to the first-person experience of God within her, triggering her voice. As a result, the inarticulacy of Margery's cries licenses

onlookers' own causal attributions, and in the *Book*'s struggles over their interpretation, this incomprehensibility acquires a reflexive and almost allegorical
status. Her voice's wordless, boisterous noise seems to distill the unfinished
quality of all enunciation, which in each case awaits an apparatus sufficient
to guarantee its meaning. No matter what the source of a sign, once it enters
discursive circulation, it loses touch with its origins and demands the labor of
buttressing explanation.

It is this very dynamic that makes room for Margery's voice to unfurl itself.
"The language of the body always requires glossing," Sarah Salih observes of
the *Book*.[39] If, as Diana Uhlman writes, Margery's "cries have probably been
the purest, unmediated oral expression and proof of Kempe's contact with
the divinity," they are also in many cases what licenses her entry into more
rational and explanatory discourses, as she tries to provide the information
necessary for interpreting them.[40] Margery carries out this contextualization
when she confesses, when she defends herself, when she submits to empirical
tests, and when she recounts the feelings and visions that have accompanied
the tokens of her sanctity.[41] She also searches out authorities for the verifica-
tion of her visions and thus to help close the gap between her own first-person
experience and its recognized causes. Authentication has a backward-forward,
metonymic logic: etiological explanation secures recognition of the divine origin of her original cry, which in turn licenses her continuously speaking, to
explain herself.

The *Book*'s most extended episode of etiological disagreement takes place
when a friar famous for his preaching arrives in King's Lynn.[42] If the friar's reputation for powerful oration precedes him, Margery's vocal repute circulates
as well. Before he delivers his first sermon in town, a parish priest approaches
him to warn him about a woman who "oftyn tymes, whan sche herith of the
Passyon of owr Lord er [or] of any hy devocyon, sche wepith, sobbith, and
cryeth," and so, the priest advises, "therfor, good ser, yyf sche make any noyse
at yowr sermown, suffyr it paciently" (I.61). In a familiar sequence of events,
Margery finds herself unable to listen without breaking out into shouts and
weeping: "Sche kept hir fro crying as long as sche myth, and than at the last
sche brast owte [burst out] wyth a gret cry and cryid wondyr sor [with amazing severity]." On this first occasion, the "good frere suffyrd it paciently and
seyd no word therto [about it] at that tyme."

The next time the friar is set to preach, Margery watches "how fast the
pepyl cam rennyng." She prays to Jesus, first by imagining the joy of "the
pepyl" if "thu [you] wer here to prechyn thin owyn persone." She then asks

that God "make thi holy word to sattelyn in her sowlys [settle in the people's souls] as I wolde that it schulde don [do] in myn." That way, "as many mict [might] be turnyd be hys [the friar's] voys as schulde ben be thy voys yyf thu [if you] prechedist thyselfe" (I.61). Though Margery's prayer is for the spiritual success of the friar's preaching, it also signals the latent competition over God's voice that is brewing. Though Margery casts herself in the role of model listener, an ideal for how "the pepyl" should receive the "holy word," her passive reception has already been belied by her crying during the friar's first sermon. At each occasion of his preaching she attends, her voice as well as his will be in play, and she has a very different, paramystical claim to speak with the power of Christ's "owyn persone."

Through a series of escalatingly antagonistic encounters, the friar bans Margery from his sermons "les than [unless] sche wolde levyn [cease] hir sobbyng and hir crying" (I.61). Various authorities intercede on Margery's behalf, explaining to the friar that Margery cannot control her crying because it is a "gyft of God," as she knows "be [by] revelacyon" (I.61). The chapter spends quite a lot of effort enumerating her defenders, who include the parish priest, another priest who "knew the cawse of hir crying," a Carmelite friar who "had knowyn the sayd creatur many yerys of hir lyfe and belevyd the grace that God wrowt in hir," a bachelor of law who had acted as her confessor, and a "worschepful burgeys [most worthy burgess]" who would soon become mayor of Lynn (I.61). Presenting this dossier of elite endorsements is clearly one of the chapter's purposes, and they are not narrated from Margery's point of view (she is absent from their scenes of appeal) but are reported neutrally, as befits their evidentiary character. However, the friar refuses to give "credens [credence] to the doctowrys wordys ne the bachelerys," and he rejects Margery's cries' divine etiology. Instead, he trusts "mech in the favowr of the pepil" and makes common cause with "summe men" who have grown "mor bolde, for hem thowt that her opinyon was wel strenghthyd er ellys fortifyed be this good frer [bolder, for they thought that their opinion was much strengthened by this good friar]" (I.61; 188).

In refusing to believe her cries come from God, the friar offers Margery his own diagnosis:

> he seyd, yyf sche myth not wythstond it whan it cam, he levyd it
> was a cardiakyl er sum other sekenesse, and, yyf sche wolde be so
> aknowyn, he seyd, he wold have compassyon of hir and steryn the
> pepil to prey for hir, and undyr this condicion he wolde han paciens

in hir and suffyr hir to cryen anow, that sche schulde sey that it was
a kendly seknes. (I.61)

[he said, if she could not withstand it when it came, he believed
it was a heart condition, or some other sickness, and if she would
acknowledge this to be so, he said, he would have compassion on
her and urge people to pray for her. And, on this condition, he
would have patience with her and allow her to cry enough, if she
would say it was a natural illness.] (190)

What began as a clash of voices has become an impasse over symptomatic causation. If Margery concedes a physiological origin for her crying in
"kendly," or natural, illness, she can rejoin the congregation of devotional
listeners. But such an admission would strip her cries of their spiritual authority, and their symptomatic structure would point back only to the physical
body. The stalemate between Margery and the preaching friar arises from a
clash of perspectives as well as from competing claims to godly voice. As the
various town authorities have already rehearsed, Margery knows "be [by] revelacyon" that God causes her crying—"and that was unknowyn to the frer." It
is unknown to him because he would have to rely on Margery's own account
to know it, and he prefers instead his naturalistic, and humiliatingly deflating,
explanatory logic. His physiological account participates in a strand of *discretio spirituum* that was gaining ground in the fifteenth century, what Dyan
Elliott has deemed the "gradual pathologization of women's spirituality."[43] Of
course Margery rejects his explanatory bargain: "And hirself [she herself] knew
wel be revelacyon and be experiens of werkyng it was no sekenes, and therfor
sche wolde not for al this world sey otherwyse than sche felt. And therfor thei
myth not acordyn [agree]" (I.61). Her private revelations and her *experiens* of
her cries make her certain of their divine etiology. Indeed, these revelations
and experiences are precisely what the *Book* itself is occupied with portraying.
Through reiterated episodes, readers come to know what "was unknowyn to
the frer."

Maintaining the divine etiology of her cries means that Margery cannot
enter the church when the friar is preaching, an exclusion that causes her "so
mech sorwe that sche wist not [did not know] what sche myth do" (I.61). But
the chapter is designed to show the expendability of listening's consolations
when matched against the license to speak for and with God. When Margery's
confessor charges her not to disobey the friar's request and to stay away from

his sermons, she settles on a peculiar substitution: "whan he prechyd in o [one] chirche sche schulde gon into another." This becomes her routine: "Whan sche was alone be hirself in on [one] cherch and he prechyng the pepil in an other, sche had as lowde and as mervelyows cryis as whan sche was amongys the pepil" (I.61). Two churches and two voices: the friar continues to preach to the "pepil," and Margery continues to cry. Her vocalizations in the empty church make an apt illustration of Certeau's description of mystic speech as what "is at the same time *beside* the authorized institution, but outside it and *in* what authorizes that institution, i.e., the Word of God."[44] Margery is outside, next-door, to institutional authority, but within the authorizing presence of God. The two churches might appear like two distinct options. The preacher's venue of communal instruction is contrasted with Margery's perfectionist solitude, and his homiletic address is inverted in her cries that only index, but do not articulate, the divine relation that causes them. Yet Margery's unpeopled church is also an image for the *Book* itself. It is a structure to hold and frame Margery's voice, an institutional form that has here gone feral, turned over to Margery's reinvention of it. Though no one else is present in the scene, the reverberations of her cries are not lost; they make their way into the narrative record and reach us. The church's solitude is haunted by the wish to be speaking for and with God "amongys the pepil" and by the spectral promise of absent listeners—another name for which is readers.

I, Thou, and They

Margery's bold speech acts, the narrative makes clear, are made against enormous pressures. Not least of these is the injunction that she should "forsake this lyfe . . . and go spynne and carde as other women don" (I.53), and the threat that she might be burned as a "fals lollare [Lollard]" (I.13). Voice does not pass from this laywoman's subjective interiority to public expression without friction. Importantly, the *Book* actually embeds this social disapprobation into the structure of the crying plot. This is made clear in a passage just after Margery's "fyrst cry" on Mount Calvary. When the narration shifts to its iterative mode, it reports as a general fact of Margery's crying that "as sone as sche parceyvyd that sche schulde crye, sche wolde kepyn it in as mech as sche myth [might] that [so that] the pepyl schulde not an herd [have heard] it for noyng of hem [and grown annoyed]." It is *so that* people will not be irritated that she struggles to contain the impulse to cry. This crucial hypotaxis helps explain the shape of subjectivity at the center of the crying plot and the *Book* at large. A bit later in the same chapter, the point is made again. After elaborating on the hostility of the "pepil" and also the "gret clerkys" who refuse to believe that Margery cannot keep from crying, the narration continues: "And therfor, whan sche knew that sche schulde cryen, sche kept it in as long as sche mygth and dede al that sche cowde to withstond it er ellys [or else] to put it awey til sche wex as blo as any leed [became as blue as lead]" (I.28). It is *because* of the hostility and counterexplanations enumerated in the previous sentences, "therfor," that Margery struggles to contain the impulse to cry. If we think that it is Margery's *self*-control being battened down in her crying—when "sche myt not kepe hirself fro krying and roryng thow sche schuld a be ded therfor"—these passages insist that we recognize her would-be silence as the product of social pressure. The line between *wythinneforth* and *wythowteforth*, which corresponds to the physical outline of Margery's body enclosing the "fir of lofe clos wythinne hir brest," turns out to be a social boundary, policed by the annoyance of the *pepyl*. Paramystical embodiment, which is also symptomatic embodiment, becomes an occasion for feeling the social constitution of subjectivity.

What is remarkable about the crying plot, then, is how it deploys a set of binary oppositions—"wythinneforth" and "wythowteforth," agency and passivity, self and other, silence and voice, first-person and third-person perspectives—to effect the kaleidoscopic remapping of *three* realms into one body and one voice: the divine, the personal, and the public. God, self, and the social world are shown to be endlessly reflecting and distorting one another, with Margery's body as their shared medium and master figure. These realms interpenetrate. For instance, the social world is manifest not just in onlookers' perceptions and reactions but in the pressurized boundaries of Margery's body, generated from the normative injunction to keep quiet. Yet the social is present also in the divinely outbursting pressure to vocalize, to somehow bring forth what she experiences so it can be apprehended by others. The overlapping positions are operated by the *Book's* "topography of personal pronouns," which effect a "distribution of positions" that make its distinctive *modus loquedi* possible. These phrases comes from Certeau's "Mystic Speech," where Certeau claims that mystic texts "always define themselves as being entirely the product of inspiration," and in every case, "divine utterance is both what founds the text, and what it must make manifest."[45] But what this account of the paradoxical congress of *I* and *thou* does not capture about Margery's mysticism is the degree that it is always posited for others. The *Book* constantly defines itself not only as a product of inspiration but also of a foundational need to communicate with fellow Christians. When Christ assures Margery of their mystical mutuality ("I am in the, and thow in me"), this shared identity is triangulated through a third position, another locus in the "topography of personal pronouns," the *they*: "thei that worshep the [you] thei worshep me; thei that despysen the thei despysen me, and I schal chastysen hem therfor. I am in the, and thow in me. And thei that heryn the thei heryn the voys of God" (I.10). *They*—they who praise, they who despise, they who hear Margery—turn out to be essential to the *Book*'s grammar of speaking and listening, experience and interpretation. And in a sense, this triangulation should not surprise us. Breaking open mysticism's dyadic colloquy and making it communicable are the very functions of narration and textualization. Turning what Margery has "in felyng and werkyng" toward its social dissemination is the ongoing project of the *Book*.

The *Book*'s portrayal of its own textual etiology offers a further gloss on the structure of its mystic speech. By its own account, the text is the result of a collaborative process of composition undertaken by Margery, who could neither read nor write, and two scribes. The proem, or introductory section of the *Book*, details the convoluted process that ultimately produces the written version of Margery's story. Weird orthography, failing eyesight, tricks of memory, public opinion, death, and inscrutable divine will all contribute to the slowness and difficulty of transforming Margery's oral recounting into the form of a book. As David Lawton quips, "There is simply no account of textual mediation as complex and circumstantial, almost wantonly obscure, as that provided by *The Book of Margery Kempe*."[46] But this emphasis on the dense materiality of the text is counterbalanced, as Lawton acknowledges, by the proem's underscoring "the dependence of the writing on Kempe's dictation and memory—literally, on her voice."[47] Though she relies on two amanuenses, she is said to be present and in control at both scenes of inscription. Reinforcing Margery's role as author, the conclusion of Book I remarks that "this lityl boke" was made thanks to "the help of God and of hirselfe that had al thi tretys in felyng and werkyng" (I.89). The phrase implies that Margery possessed the *tretys*, the text of the *Book*, first as a matter of what she felt and did, "in felyng and werkyng."

If personal experience is presented as the *Book*'s first medium, from which it travels its twisting path into written script, the proem nonetheless declines to affirm Margery's authorship in the conventional way, by metonymic identification of text and individual. Instead, much like the portrayals of Margery's crying, it sets up a *circuit* of expressive power, here shared out among God, Margery, the two scribes, and the social milieu to which the *Book* is addressed.[48] In medieval texts, prefatory materials tend to act as privileged sites for defining interactions of audience and text. Here the proem does not so much discount Margery's authorship as give an account of its heteronomous etiology, where she is nonetheless at the center. Again, this is like Margery's "roryng," that species of vocalization that the *Book* seeks spectacularly to divorce from Margery's agency and intentions, even as it grounds it viscerally in her body. My reading is similar to that of Sarah Salih, who contends that "the writing of the *Book* can be seen, not as a further layer of alienation from the self, but as the reclamation of the authority to tell of the self."[49] I would add that such authority is constituted over the course of the *Book* paradoxically, by Margery finding her powers of expression again and again limited, coerced, overridden, muzzled, or misconstrued. Each of these occasions, incorporated into the narrative, becomes an opportunity for more speaking, for explanation and response, and for enfolding the voices of dissent, resistance, enmity, and alterity into the capacious and encompassing medium of the *Book*'s narration. This is what I have called the *Book*'s *fort-da* game of discursive authority.

The upshot of the proem's account of textual production is that readers are asked to recognize Margery's personal voice as a constantly present component of the third-person narration that recounts the diegetic events of the *Book*. To say that this narrating voice is *her* voice is to embrace the catachrestic logic that the *Book* invites; it refers what is written to a scene of bodily presence, an occasion of speech that lies outside and prior to the written work. Margery's utterance is conjured alongside the text as its ostensible cause but also as its figural emission. Her body and voice function to gather up the multiple idioms that compose the text, even as their coherence necessarily dissolves in the multitudinous vantages and speech acts constituting the *Book*'s line of narration. As Ruth Evans argues, the *Book*'s voice "emerges indirectly, through a mixture of third-person past tense narration and direct speech. The reader must actively construct a meaning for this voice rather than passively hear it."[50]

Modern readers have disagreed about the significance of the narration's oscillation in and out of Margery's own perspective. For instance, John Erskine takes the fact that the narration "relate[s] events to which she [Margery] was plainly not a party" to mean that the *Book* "operates in a fictional or creative mode."[51] Lynn Staley Johnson claims that "Kempe's experience is described by an omniscient, third-person narrator, presumably the scribe, whose ability to recount both God's intimate speech to her as well as the experience of Kempe herself renders him a powerful 'witness' to her life."[52] Felicity Riddy thinks that the "perspective is autobiographical, except there is the formal oddity that the narration is in the third person and not the first."[53] Since the first sentence of the 1940 scholarly edition, uncertainties about the *Book*'s narration have been funneled into questions of authorship, with Sanford Meech announcing the impossibility of studying the *Book* "until one has given the best answer one can to the question, 'Whose language it is?'"[54] Scholars weighing in on the evidence can be grouped roughly into three camps: those attributing the *Book*'s language primarily to Margery Kempe,[55] those giving the second scribe a dominant role in the *Book*'s composition,[56] and those who elect to jettison authorship in order to analyze the *Book* as "the product of the occasion of its creation" and as a "relational" artifact "in the sense that it arose out of and was embedded in social interaction."[57]

The forensic work of recovering who is responsible for the words and ideas of the *Book* remains an important ongoing project, though one that cannot rely too heavily on the evidence of the *Book*'s narrating voice. After all, we are accustomed to attributing to individual authors the interplay of free indirect discourse, dramatic reportage, bird's-eye views, and characters' dialogue that constitutes the "omniscient" narration of nineteenth-century novels; writers accomplish such effects by making use of the transpersonal affordances of language. Of course, the *Book* differs from the genre of the novel by asking readers to recognize the actual contributions of the narrative figure Margery to the creation of the narratorial voice that describes her. The *Book*'s claim to truthfulness, entailed in its genre commitments, continuously directs readers to the implied scene of a real "literacy event" that has brought together Margery's subjective experience with what frames it, examines it, and exceeds it.[58] As Rory Critten observes, "The *Book* manifests a clear desire to create the impression of Kempe's closeness to her work at the moment of its reinscription."[59] But these injunctions to reality and bodily proximity do not escape the figural logic of literary voice that I described at the outset of this chapter. Margery's voice—ascending from her cries through ever wider rings of responsiveness and ultimately to the vast sprawl of the text's narration—is always pictured originating from her body, that fleshly switchpoint for God's desires, her own, and other people's. The fantasy of the *Book*'s narration ceaselessly departing from and returning to Margery's body is one of the text's great fascinations.

The final chapter of the *Book of Margery Kempe* begins by returning to her paramystical symptoms. Although by this point in her life Margery is no longer visited by fits of uncontrollable vocalization, she is still prone to violent weeping, and on this occasion she does so until "thei that seyn [saw] hir wepyn and herdyn hir so boistowsly sobbyn wer takyn wyth gret merveyl and wondyr what was the ocupasyon of hir sowle [wondered what was preoccupying her soul]" (II.10). A young man approaches her and expresses a "fervent desir to have undirstondyng what myth be the cawse of hir wepyng," because, as he remarks, "'I have not seyn a persone so plenteuows in teerys as ye ben, and specialy I have not herd beforn any persone so boistows in sobbyng as ye ben'" (II.10). It is the noisy excess of her weeping that makes the youth seek explication, and in reply, in a translation of her symptoms, she explains her shame for offenses against God and her wonder at the miracle of salvation. The two converse at length and become friends. Here, then, is the final and rather upbeat iteration of Margery's etiological drama: her puzzling, "boistows" noise creates an occasion for self-narration, teaching, and friendship that is eventually folded into the *Book*. The episode concludes with the young man's delight: he "was ful glad to ben in hir cumpany."

It is shortly after this last repetition of the crying plot that the *Book* pivots toward its conclusion. It ends with a long prayer, cosmic in its scope, which Margery was accustomed for "many yerys" to pray (II.10). Perhaps surprisingly, then, the *Book* will not draw to its close in the third-person narration that largely constitutes it and through which it has been modulating Margery's point of view and many others' over its dozens of chapters. Instead, the *Book* concludes in the first-person voice of Margery's prayer.

Near the start of her prayer, Margery speaks to God about her paramystical symptoms—"my crying, my sobbyng, and my wepyng"—and "what scornys, what schamys, what despitys, and what reprevys [reproofs]" she suffers on account of them (II.10). She prays that all the world may be made "to knowyn and to trowyn [believe]" that her cries are "thi werke" and "the gyft of the Holy Gost," over which she herself has no power (II.10). This wish for etiological transparency, for the causal and semantic clarity of her paramystical voice, is also a wish to realize its evangelical power. She prays "that as many men mote be turnyd be my crying and my wepyng as me han scornyd therfor er schal scornyn into the werdys ende [that as many men may be turned by my crying and weeping as have scorned me for it or shall scorn unto the world's end]" (II.10; 293). The preceding events of Book II (which take place when Margery is in her sixties) have shown that scorn is not something that Margery's biography ever leaves behind, and her noisy devotions are apparently revilement's surest catalysts. But here in her prayer that scorn is linked to her cries' obverse possibility of "turnyng," or conversion. The vignette at the start of the chapter, when her cries' draw the young man into conversation and spiritual friendship, functions as a concrete realization of this idea. Whatever interpretive exposure and heteronomy her symptomatic voice brings with it, it is also, on this account, a means of opening out from within herself the disruptive presence of God and drawing all those who hear her into the possibility of their *turnyng*, their transformation.

As the prayer goes on, Margery calls for divine mercy for an astounding array of people—for the pope and the cardinals, for all the archbishops and bishops, for the whole order of the priesthood, for all the men and women religious, for the king of England and all Christian kings, all lords and ladies, for Jews, Saracens, "and alle hethen pepil," for heretics, misbelievers, false tithe-payers, thieves, adulterers, "alle myschevows levarys [wicked livers]," for all who are tempted, for her confessors, for "al the pepil in this world," friends and enemies, the sick, all those in prison, "alle creaturys that in this world han spokyn of me eythyr good er ylle [or ill]," all the souls in purgatory, and many more (II.10). The maximalist, even universalist, reach of Margery's prayer is anticipated in the ambitions of the *Book*'s narrative voice, which has encompassed exterior vantages, skepticism, incomprehension, and ridicule. Its narration too can hold within its ample bounds whoever speaks "eythyr good er ylle"; it can give a place to the sinful as well as the virtuous, to the saved as well as the unsaved. The *Book* achieves this not so much by dissolving other voices into its own but by introjecting them, where they continue to speak *in propria persona*. The *Book* seems to trust that their clamorous, dissenting cacophony belongs in its narration and should be kept. The unfurling line of textual discourse corresponds, then, to a potentially infinite medium of inclusion, which swallows every circuit of misunderstanding and misinterpretation into its expansive energies and manages still to be Margery's voice, as the culminating first-person prayer argues, as she asks for grace for anyone who trusts her prayers or will trust them unto the world's end: "I pray the, Lord, grawnt hem for the multitude of thi mercy. Amen."

Coda

Symptomatic bodies, as the preceding chapters have shown, give form to medieval selves. The Summoner's *saucefleem* face bespeaks his scabrous disposition in the *Canterbury Tales*. The characters of exempla embody their past actions in the cipher of disease. Physiognomy reads personality in, say, the forehead's breadth and the ears' hairiness, and the Galenic theory of complexion testifies to innate temperament as well as the contingencies of daily environment. Yet alongside these expressive functions, symptoms are also means of recognizing what is *not* the self. The medical description of Arcite in the "Knight's Tale" shows the Theban knight constituted by subpersonal forces at war within him. Jonathas's hand hangs alone onstage in the *Croxton Play of the Sacrament*, alienated from the rest of his fallen body. Medieval leprosy acts not only as a moralistic signifier but as a destroyer of embodiment's legible forms. And Thomas Hoccleve finds himself tethered to an episode of insanity that is beyond his conscious recall. Symptomatic bodies are the strange material things that we also are—but that we exceed and that exceed us. Symptomatic subjectivity is the performance of self inflected by just these conditions.

The present study has been about the etiological labor that transpires between bodies and selves, or the work of piecing together cause-and-effect chains to make physiology and person mutually comprehensible, at least in part. In the later Middle Ages, such etiological work was often medical in tenor. England in the fourteenth and fifteenth centuries witnessed unprecedented growth in the textuality of *phisik*, largely for non-university audiences. Attending to *phisik*'s conceptual language, we discover medieval readers and writers experimenting with how to understand, and how to influence, persons' material constitutions. Yet the tasks of explaining and narrating bodies did not need to be medical. What I have characterized as the etiological imagination of the later Middle Ages addressed itself to a welter of forces, articulated in various discourses, which together constituted the period's discontinuous logic of causal implication. What *phisik*'s growing importance did mean for poetry and narrative was that medicine's naturalistic system became available alongside other explanatory idioms, to be set in concert with them or deployed against them. In the *Testament of Cresseid*, for instance, the hypercoherence shared between the poem's medical and punitive logics is disrupted by the affective tradition of leprosy. In the *Book of Margery Kempe*, Margery's paramystical cries stage the heteronomy of symptoms to disarm naturalistic explanation and construct a more capacious voice for personal spiritual authority. Whatever its other effects, England's remarkable growth in the accessibility of medical writings roiled the causal entailments of the self and made them ripe for reimagining.

Symptomatic Subjects, then, explores what in late medieval England came to be written at the fraught interface between physical causation and embodied agency. In doing so, it returns to some of the central concerns of the "history of the body," the interdisciplinary subfield that flourished in the 1980s and 1990s, often with scholars of the Middle Ages at its center.[1] The original force of the "history of the body" lay in the phrase's torque of denaturalization: what seems natural and given—the body in its fleshly palpability—turns out to be the result of historically contingent processes. *Symptomatic Subjects* comes back to that crucial insight, to the social construction of the body, to investigate the operations of that construction in all their phenomenological density and variegation. Generally speaking, scholarship on the body's history has excelled at reconstructing the somatic templates and disciplinary scripts of particular discourses—of chivalry, laywomen's piety, and medieval antisemitism, for instance. Yet *phisik* calls for a way of reading that is sensitive to the discourse's relative weakness or nonhegemony in the fourteenth and fifteenth centuries, when it asserted less control than appeal. I have sought to understand medicine's simultaneous prevalence and provisionality by attending to medieval writers' habits of setting "termes of phisik" among competing idioms, to create volatile economies of forces. The churn of unreconciled discourses in these texts and the symptomatic subjects portrayed in the eye of the storm give some sense of what accounting for material bodies was like in the era of etiological imagination. By following the history of the body as well as cutting new paths, *Symptomatic Subjects* traces one approach to a phenomenology of medieval selfhood, an approach that passes through the articulations (medical and otherwise) of a certain gap in embodiment—between somatic materiality and felt experience, or between having and being a body.

The Wound Man in Wellcome Library MS 290, I suggested at the outset of Chapter 1, makes a supple emblem for the body's in-betweenness. The
Wound Man's gaze reaches viewers from a point suspended between a diagram's abstraction and the urgency of individual suffering. He not only bears
his injuries with placid calm but seems actively to present them to view, in a
polarized interplay of determination and agency. Jack Hartnell has recently
argued that the illuminations in Wellcome Library MS 290 show the influence of one of the earliest printed works of medical learning, the *Fasciculus
medicinae*, first published in Venice in 1491.[2] While the Wound Man's iconography is attested from the start of the fifteenth century, it seems likely (on the
basis of Hartnell's reasoning) that this English iteration was painted under the
influence of print. Does this reperiodization set the Wellcome Wound Man
beyond the bounds of my arguments, concerned as they are with late medieval
England? I hope rather that it opens them to the porous and uncertain periodization of embodiment. The etiological ferment of causal systems unrationalized in terms of one another continued into the early modern period, together
with the promiscuous textual cultures of *phisik* that went with it.[3] Of course,
there are other stories to tell about this ensuing era, about the rise of medical
humanism in figures like Thomas Linacre (d. 1524) and John Caius (d. 1573),
about the founding of the Royal College of Physicians in 1518 and subsequent
developments in medicine's centralization and regulation, about printing's
impact on the circulation of scientific knowledge, about human dissection
and Renaissance anatomy, and about the eventual rise of empiricist natural
philosophy and experimental medicine. These new developments, each and
all, can be seen to move in the direction of systemization, regularity, and the
dawning of what would come to be solidified, more boundedly, as modern
medicine. But the arguments of *Symptomatic Subjects* suggest the possibility,
and the potential usefulness, of other narrative trajectories for *phisik*, even
beyond the later Middle Ages. For the play of determination and counter-
determination, of symptoms in excess of their stabilized codification—all the
disruptive energy entailed in the simultaneity of being and having a body—
hardly ceases with the rise of a new medical rationality. Today, as in the Middle
Ages, medicine is one idiom among others for speaking about embodiment.
This book has explored the complex and contentious narration of material
selves during one age of etiological imagination, but that project—of conceiving our lives in the full rush of the world's causes, where we suffer, seek care,
and tell our stories—continues into the present.

Notes

INTRODUCTION

1. *Troilus and Criseyde* II.1037–9, in *Riverside Chaucer.*

2. *Troilus and Criseyde* II.1042, in *Riverside Chaucer.*

3. *Troilus and Criseyde* II.1043, in *Riverside Chaucer.*

4. See, for instance, *Troilus and Criseyde* I.419–20, I.484–91, and II.1527–33, in *Riverside Chaucer.*

5. For an overview, see Voigts, "Scientific and Medical Books" and "Multitudes of Middle English Medical Manuscripts"; Getz, "Charity, Translation, and the Language of Medical Learning in Medieval England"; Jones, "Information and Science" and "Medicine and Science"; Keiser, "Scientific, Medical, and Utilitarian Prose"; and Taavitsainen and Pahta, "Vernacularisation and Medical Writing." For an important early study, see Robbins, "Medical Manuscripts in Middle English."

6. These are the "natural things" that constitute and regulate living bodies: *elementa, commixtiones, compositiones, membra, virtutes, operationes, spiritus.* See Joannitius and Constantine the African, "Johannicius," 151.

CHAPTER 1

1. It appears on fol. 53v. For a description of the manuscript, see Romero-Barranco, *The Late Middle English Version of Constantinus Africanus' Venerabilis anatomia* and Moorat, *Catalogue of Western Manuscripts on Medicine and Science in the Wellcome Historical Medical Library*, 1:185–86. On the illuminations, see Scott, *Later Gothic Manuscripts*, 2:275–77 and especially Hartnell, "Wording the Wound Man," which details the iconography's medieval and early modern history.

2. These are Middle English versions, respectively, of a pseudo-Galenic anatomical treatise on the internal structures of the body (fols. 1–41) and of Copho's *Anathomia Porci* (41v–53).

3. See Hartnell, "Wording the Wound Man," on the original linking of text and image.

4. Examples survive in churches in Poundstock and Breage (Cornwall) and West Chiltington (Sussex). For more on the "Sunday Christ," see Astell, "Memorial Technai" and Reiss, *The Sunday Christ.*

5. For the point that earlier examples of the Wound Man are cued to greater textual information, see Hartnell, "Wording the Wound Man."

6. *Canterbury Tales* I.673, 650, and 664, in *Riverside Chaucer*; hereafter cited in text by line number.

7. *MED*, s.v. "saucefleume" (n.) and (adj.).

8. For references to medieval medical writings on saucefleme and related pathologies, see Curry, *Chaucer and the Mediaeval Sciences*, 37–53, which includes discussion of *gutta rosacea*, morphew, and leprosy; Aiken, "The Summoner's Malady," on scabies; Garbáty, "The Summoner's Occupational Disease," on syphilis; and Grigsby, *Pestilence in Medieval and Early Modern English Literature*, 82–87, on leprosy. I remain unconvinced by these several attempts to diagnose the Summoner beyond *saucefleem*. Though the Summoner's symptoms call out for readers' conjecture about his condition, in body and soul, it seems to me that just this restless diagnostic incitement, rather than any nosological certainty, is the intended effect—an effect that matches the suggestive and allusive mode of the portraits generally. The dictional choice of *saucefleem* is significant: the word is relatively technical and the condition, relatively unserious; Chaucer might have chosen *lepre*, a much more common term, had he sought its dire connotations. Nonetheless, for a thoughtful reconsideration of leprosy and the Summoner, see Whearty, "The Leper on the Road to Canterbury."

9. Siraisi, *Medieval and Early Renaissance Medicine*, 102.

10. Bartholomaeus Anglicus and Trevisa, *On the Properties of Things*, 1:639.

11. See Robertson, *Nature Speaks*, esp. chap. 3.

12. See Patterson, *Chaucer and the Subject of History*, 26–32.

13. Both medieval Latin and modern English translations of Galen's *Tegni* cited from Kaye, *A History of Balance*, 158. The *Tegni* was "the most widely read and studied of the Galenic texts in the thirteenth and fourteenth centuries" (165).

14. Du Cange, s.v. "symptoma" and "sinthoma"; *DMLBS*, s.v. "symptoma"; and *MED*, s.v. "sinthome."

15. Holmes, *The Symptom and the Subject*, 11–12.

16. See *Trotula*, ed. Green, 65.

17. Augustine, *De doctrina christiana* book II, chap. 1 (*PL* vol. 34, p. 36).

18. Augustine, *De doctrina christiana* book II, chap. 1 (*PL* vol. 34, p. 36).

19. Augustine, *De doctrina christiana* book II, chap. 1 (*PL* vol. 34, p. 36).

20. Bacon, *De signis*, 83.

21. Bacon, *De signis*, 83.

22. For English, Joannitius and Constantine the African, *Isagoge*, 154; for Latin, Joannitius and Constantine the African, "Johannicius," 171.

23. Several twentieth-century phenomenological writers offer powerful conceptual tools for thinking about experiences of sickness and pain. See especially Merleau-Ponty, *Phenomenology of Perception*; Ricoeur, *Freedom and Nature*; Scarry, *The Body in Pain*; and Leder, *The Absent Body*.

24. Scarry observes that the experience of pain "contains not only the feeling 'my body hurts' but the feeling 'my body hurts me,'" which is to say, "the person in great pain experiences his own body as the agent of his agony." See *The Body in Pain*, 47.

25. Augustine, Sermon 277, 5. I thank Timothy M. Harrsion for bringing this sermon to my attention.

26. Augustine, Sermon 277, 6.

27. Augustine, Sermon 277, 8. The translator notes: "The Latin has *stomachus*. But would any English speaker not know what the stomach is? The admirable Messrs Lewis and Short inform us that the primary reference of *stomachus* is to the esophagus or alimentary canal—and which of us knows what that is?"

28. Caroline Bynum's scholarship on this is paradigmatic; see especially *The Resurrection of the Body in Western Christianity*, *Fragmentation and Redemption*, and *Holy Feast and Holy Fast*.

29. Getz, "Medical Education," 86.

30. For instance, see Kibre, "The Faculty of Medicine at Paris."

31. On Florence, see Park, *Doctors and Medicine*, 15–46. For England's lack of salaried physicians, see Rawcliffe, *Urban Bodies*, 291–92.

32. In fact England had already been the scene of precocious medical vernacularity. While in most of western Christendom, vernacular medical writing can be traced from the eleventh century, in England it began in the late ninth century with the Alfredian reforms; see Cameron, *Anglo-Saxon Medicine* and Bonser, *The Medical Background of Anglo-Saxon England*. After the Conquest, vernacular medical writing was not resumed until the Anglo-Norman texts of the thirteenth century; see Kealey, *Medieval Medicus* and *Anglo-Norman Medicine*, ed. Hunt. However, the new wave of vernacular medical writing in the fourteenth and fifteenth centuries was on a considerably larger scale than the Anglo-Saxon developments.

33. Getz, "Charity, Translation, and the Language of Medical Learning in Medieval England," 3.

34. Jones, "Medicine and Science," 434. For an important early account of the production of medical texts in England, which also considers Singer's hand-list, see Robbins, "Medical Manuscripts in Middle English."

35. Jones, "Information and Science," 101.

36. Voigts, "Multitudes of Middle English Medical Manuscripts," 188.

37. The database is available as a CD-ROM (Voigts and Kurtz, *Scientific and Medical Writings*) and in an expanded version online, Voigts and Kurtz, *Voigts-Kurtz Search Program*. The total number of codices (1,200+) is cited from the introduction to the CD-ROM. Also see Voigts, "Multitudes of Middle English Medical Manuscripts."

38. Search conducted January 14, 2018. The total number of texts is somewhat inflated by prologues (when they are found) being counted separately from the works themselves.

39. The standard scholarly reference work on the manuscript witnesses of medieval Latin medical and scientific writings is Thorndike and Kibre, *Catalogue of Incipits*. The catalogue can be searched electronically via Voigts and Kurtz, *Voigts-Kurtz Search Program*.

40. Voigts, "Scientific and Medical Books," 380.

41. See Bylebyl, "The Medical Meaning of *Physica*" and Wallis, *Medieval Medicine*, xxii–xxiii.

42. For an introduction to these developments, see Siraisi, *Medieval and Early Renaissance Medicine*, chaps. 1, 3.

43. Burnett, "Gerard of Cremona," 191.

44. Beullens, "Burgundio of Pisa," 104.

45. McVaugh, "Nature and Limits of Medical Certitude," 63–64.

46. McVaugh, "Nature and Limits of Medical Certitude," 62.

47. *MED*, s.v. "phisik" (n.) 1(a)–(f)—a set of meanings not unlike modern English's "medicine."

48. Chauliac cited from *MED*, s.v. "lẹche-craft" (n.) 1(a), and Paston cited from "phisĭk(e" (n.) 1(e).

49. Cited from Voigts, "Fifteenth-Century English Banns," 264; orthography modernized and some punctuation added. For more on the banns, see Chapter 2.

50. Pseudo-Bacon, "On Tarrying the Accidents of Age," 207.

51. For these conditions, see Park, "Medicine and Society."

52. Slack, *The Impact of Plague in Tudor and Stuart England*, 176.

53. For English, Joannitius and Constantine the African, *Isagoge*, 140; for Latin, Joannitius and Constantine the African, "Johannicius," 151.

54. Joannitius and Constantine the African, *Isagoge*, 150.

55. See Carey, "What Is the Folded Almanac?" and, for a sensitive reading of one example, Silva, "Opening the Medieval Folded Almanac."

56. Rawcliffe, *Medicine and Society*, 3.

57. It should be emphasized that the plague did not result in any large-scale discrediting of medieval medical science or its practitioners. On the continuities between plague medicine and traditional medical theory, see Arrizabalaga, "Facing the Black Death." The bibliography on medieval medical responses to the Black Death is immense; for an astute introduction to the issues, see Carmichael, "Universal and Particular," 21.

58. Horrox, *Black Death*, 167–72 (original in Latin).

59. Modern English translation cited from Horrox, *Black Death*, 159; Latin from Hoeniger, *Der schwarze Tod*, 153.

60. Horrox, *Black Death*, 158; Hoeniger, *Der schwarze Tod*, 153.

61. Horrox, *Black Death*, 158; Hoeniger, *Der schwarze Tod*, 152.

62. Siraisi, *Medieval and Early Renaissance Medicine*, 128.

63. On the extreme rarity of medieval plague treatises in England invoking sin and divine wrath, see Keiser, "Two Medieval Plague Treatises," esp. 300–01. An adaptation of the plague tract of John of Burgundy by the Dominican Thomas Multon is the *only* known work of Middle English medicine to offer an extended statement about plague as divine retribution for sin.

64. John of Burgundy, "Treatises on Plague," 571.

65. This number was obtained using the manuscript information and dates in Keiser, *Works of Science and Information*, 3662–64, 3856–58.

66. John of Burgundy, "Treatises on Plague," 578–79.

67. John of Burgundy, "Treatises on Plague," 579.

68. John of Burgundy, "Treatises on Plague," 578.

69. John of Burgundy, "Treatises on Plague," 580.

70. John of Burgundy, "Treatises on Plague," 580.

71. John of Burgundy, "Treatises on Plague," 586.

72. Horrox, *Black Death*, 163; Hoeniger, *Der schwarze Tod*, 156.

73. The text survives in eight complete manuscripts and four fragments; see *Dives and Pauper*, ed. Barnum, xi.

74. *Dives and Pauper*, ed. Barnum, 117.

75. *Dives and Pauper*, ed. Barnum, 118.

76. *Dives and Pauper*, ed. Barnum, 146.

77. *Dives and Pauper*, ed. Barnum, 152.

78. *Dives and Pauper*, ed. Barnum, 141.

79. *Dives and Pauper*, ed. Barnum, 143.

80. *Decrees of the Ecumenical Councils*, ed. Tanner, 1:245.

81. *Decrees of the Ecumenical Councils*, ed. Tanner, 1:245–46.

82. *Decrees of the Ecumenical Councils*, ed. Tanner, 1:246.

83. Amundsen, "Medieval Catholic Tradition," provides representative examples at 89–90.

84. Amundsen, "Medieval Catholic Tradition," 89.

85. *Canterbury Tales* I.421–26, in *Riverside Chaucer*.

86. *Canterbury Tales* I.17–18, in *Riverside Chaucer*.

87. To be sure, late medieval medicine did develop largely naturalistic structures of explanation, but the scope and authority of those structures were acknowledged to be limited. For an important account of learned medicine's eschewing moralism and supernatural explanations, see Demaitre, "The Description and Diagnosis of Leprosy."

88. For a negative evaluation, see Curry, *Chaucer and the Mediaeval Sciences*, 3–36. For more positive accounts, see Ussery, *Chaucer's Physician*, 91–139 and Rawcliffe, "Doctor of Physic." Jill Mann argues for an ambivalent portrayal in *Chaucer and Medieval Estates Satire*, 91–99.

89. I borrow the phrase "specific rationality" from Kieckhefer, "The Specific Rationality of Medieval Magic."

90. For English, Joannitius and Constantine the African, *Isagoge*, 140; for Latin, Joannitius and Constantine the African, "Johannicius," 151.

91. Avicenna, excerpt from the *Canon*, 716.

92. For the Aristotelian definitions of *scientia* most important in the Middle Ages, see the *Nicomachean Ethics* 6.3–8 (1139b–1142a) and the *Metaphysics* 1.1–2 (981b–982b). For discussion and further bibliography, see Livesey, "*Scientia*."

93. O'Boyle, "Medicine, God, and Aristotle," 188. For a history of the *accessus* form, see Quain, "The Medieval *Accessus ad Auctores*."

94. O'Boyle, "Medicine, God, and Aristotle," 189–90.

95. Middle English renderings of Henri's writings can be found in Cambridge, Peterhouse MS 118, I, fols. 1–169v and II, fols. 1–65v and London, Wellcome Library MS 564, fols. 146–70v.

96. Henri de Mondeville, *Chirurgie des Heinrich von Mondeville*, 69.

97. Henri de Mondeville, *Chirurgie des Heinrich von Mondeville*, 85.

98. Aristotle, *Metaphysics* I.1 (981a), emphasis added. English adjusted from Aristotle, *Aristotle's Metaphysics*; Latin is that of William of Moerbeke—Aristotle, *Metaphysica*, liber 1, cap. 1.

99. Aristotle, *Metaphysics* I.1 (981a). English adjusted from Aristotle, *Aristotle's Metaphysics*; Latin from Aristotle, *Metaphysica*, liber 1, cap. 1.

100. Kaye, *A History of Balance*, 6, emphasis original.

101. Kaye, *A History of Balance*, 473.

102. Kaye, *A History of Balance*, 16.

103. Kaye, *A History of Balance*, 472.

104. Kaye, *A History of Balance*, 476.

105. As Danielle Jacquart notes, learned medical debates at the start of the fourteenth century show "a more acute awareness of the difficulty of applying authoritative general rules to individual cases." Jacquart, "Theory, Everyday Practice," 140.

106. As Marion Turner writes, "Late medieval writers not only had an understanding of the impulse to fit illness into narrative structures but also understood the inherent limitation that emplotment and narrativization entails" ("Illness Narratives in the Later Middle Ages," 62). On this topic, also see Jones, "The Surgeon as Story-Teller." Narrative's epistemological efficacy has been theorized by modern philosophers of history; see especially Mink, "Narrative Form as Cognitive Instrument."

107. For further discussion, see Chapter 4.

108. English modified slightly from Henry, *Book of Holy Medicines*, 149–50; French from Henry, *Livre de Seyntz Medicines*, 85–86.

CHAPTER 2

1. *Canterbury Tales* I.424, 421, in *Riverside Chaucer*.

2. Bartholomaeus Anglicus and John Trevisa, *On the Properties of Things*, 1:435, orthography modernized.

3. Avicenna, excerpt from the *Canon*, 716.

4. My translation. Aristotle, *Analytica posteriora* I.ii (71b), p. 286.

5. Cited from McVaugh, *Rational Surgery of the Middle Ages*, 40.

6. On this tradition of "rational surgery," see McVaugh, *Rational Surgery of the Middle Ages*, 9–11 and passim.

7. Grothé, "Le Ms. Wellcome 564," 380, 271; discussed in McVaugh, *Rational Surgery of the Middle Ages*, 254.

8. Lanfranc of Milan, *Lanfrank's "Science of Cirurgie,"* 20, orthography modernized.

9. Nutton, "The Seeds of Disease," 4. Also, see van 't Land, "Internal Yet Extrinsic."

10. Guy de Chauliac, *Cyrurgie*, 12.

11. Cited from Kaye, *A History of Balance*, 155; the citation is from Galen's *Tegni*.

12. See McVaugh, "'Experience-Based' Medicine," 113–17.

13. Middle English renderings of Henri's writings can be found in Cambridge, Peterhouse MS 118, I, fols. 1–169v and II, fols. 1–65v and London, Wellcome Library MS 564, fols. 146–70v.

14. Henri de Mondeville, *Chirurgie des Heinrich von Mondeville*, 67–68.

15. Translation cited from McVaugh, *Rational Surgery of the Middle Ages*, 46; for Latin, see Henri de Mondeville, *Chirurgie des Heinrich von Mondeville*, 60.

16. McVaugh, *Rational Surgery of the Middle Ages*, 48; for Latin, see Henri de Mondeville, *Chirurgie des Heinrich von Mondeville*, 330–31.

17. Apparently, the list of contingencies is Mondeville's late addition to his composition and is thus not included in the French translation of 1314. See McVaugh, *Rational Surgery of the Middle Ages*, 48 and Jacquart, *La Médecine médiévale dans le cadre parisien*, 62–69.

18. Henri de Mondeville, *Chirurgie des Heinrich von Mondeville*, 81: si nihil de contingentibus omittatur, hoc est, si sciat cyrurgicus in praedictis, scilicet patiente, membro laeso etc. omnia particularia vel contingentia intueri et unicuique ipsorum medicinam congruam adaptare.

19. Henri de Mondeville, *Chirurgie des Heinrich von Mondeville*, 81.

20. McVaugh, *Rational Surgery of the Middle Ages*, 48.

21. Another version in circulation: "Vita brevis, ars vero longa; occasio praeceps, experimentum periculosum, iudicium difficile." On the medieval history of the *Aphorisms*, see O'Boyle, *The Art of Medicine*, 86.

22. *Parliament of Fowls*, lines 1–2, in *Riverside Chaucer*. The Middle English translation of Guy de Chauliac's *Chirurgia magna* has the pithy rendering, "The lyf is schort, the craft forsothe is long, experiment is deceyvable, dome [judgment] is hard" (*Cyrurgie*, 11, orthography modernized).

23. Translation cited from McVaugh and Salmón, introduction to Arnau of Vilanova, *Repetitio super aphorismo Hippocratus*, 294.

24. Cited from McVaugh, "'Experience-Based' Medicine," 113.

25. Renzi, *Collectio Salernitana*, 4:325, 515–16.

26. Arnau's exposition is conventionally known as the "Repetitio super Vita brevis," although its recent commentators hypothesize that it is more likely to have been a *reportatio*, or a student transcript of a master's oral commentary. See McVaugh and Salmón, introduction to Arnau of Vilanova, *Repetitio super aphorismo Hippocratus*, 269.

27. For Latin, see Arnau of Vilanova, *Repetitio super aphorismo Hippocratus*, 198; for English, see McVaugh and Salmón, introduction to Arnau of Vilanova, *Repetitio super aphorismo Hippocratus*, 271.

28. Cited from McVaugh and Ballester, "Therapeutic Method," 81.

29. Cited from McVaugh and Ballester, "Therapeutic Method," 84.

30. English cited from McVaugh and Ballester, "Therapeutic Method," 83–84. Original Latin can be found at Arnau of Vilanova, *Repetitio super aphorismo Hippocratus*, 257–58.

31. Cited from McVaugh and Ballester, "Therapeutic Method," 86.

32. McVaugh and Salmón, introduction to Arnau of Vilanova, *Repetitio super aphorismo Hippocratus*, 326.

33. Cited from McVaugh and Ballester, "Therapeutic Method," 76. Original Latin can be found at Arnau of Vilanova, *Repetitio super aphorismo Hippocratus*, 247–48.

34. See Tavormina, "The Middle English 'Letter of Ipocras.'"

35. See Keiser, "'More Light on the Life and Milieu of Robert Thornton."

36. Steiner, "Authority," 142.

37. Park, *Doctors and Medicine*, 15–46.

38. Rawcliffe, *Urban Bodies*, 291–92.

39. Getz, "Medical Education," 86.

40. Getz, "The Faculty of Medicine," 388.

41. Getz, "The Faculty of Medicine," 396.

42. For instance, see Jones, "Vernacular Literacy in Late Medieval England," 61–62, 355–59, and for the description of an especially salient manuscript (London, British Library, Harley MS 2374), see 123–26.

43. Jones, "Arderne, John." Apart from the sources on Arderne cited below, see also Citrome, *The Surgeon in Medieval English Literature*, 113–38.

44. Arderne, *Treatises of Fistula in Ano*, 1, orthography modernized.

45. Arderne, *Treatises of Fistula in Ano*, 2, orthography modernized.

46. Jones, "Four Middle English Translations," 68, 69.

47. Jones, "Four Middle English Translations," 65.

48. Voigts, "Multitudes of Middle English Medical Manuscripts," 189. Arderne's popularity is exceeded by alchemical authorities George Ripley and Raymond Lull as well as by Geoffrey Chaucer and John of Burgundy.

49. On Arderne's special relation to narrative, see Turner, "Illness Narratives in the Later Middle Ages."

50. Both Arderne's original Latin and its Middle English translation are cited from the editions in Jones, "Surgical Narrative in Middle English," 6 and 4, respectively, orthography modernized.

51. Jones, "Surgical Narrative in Middle English," 7 and 5, orthography modernized.

52. Jones, "Harley MS 2558," 50, 48.

53. *Paston Letters and Papers*, ed. Davis, 628. The letter was written between 1487 and 1495, orthography modernized.

54. On medieval medicine and women's literacy, see Green, "The Possibilities of Literacy."

55. *Paston Letters and Papers*, ed. Davis, 291, orthography modernized.

56. The manuscript is Cambridge, Countway Medical Library MS 19. For the link to the Paston family, see Jones, "Discourse Communities and Medical Texts," 33. For more on the manuscript, see Harley, "The Middle English Contents of a Fifteenth-Century Medical Book."

57. Finucane, *Miracles and Pilgrims*, esp. 59–71.

58. *Rotuli parliamentorum*, 158: *Petitiones in Parliamento* 9 Henry V.

59. Antonius of Florence, excerpt from *Summa Theologica*, 443.

60. Beck, *Cutting Edge*, 63, orthography modernized here and in subsequent citations.

61. Beck, *Cutting Edge*, 63.

62. Beck, *Cutting Edge*, 63–64.

63. Beck, *Cutting Edge*, 64.

64. I cite from the Modern English translation in the *Calendar of Plea and Memoranda Rolls*, 4:174–75. I have been unable to locate the ruling in its original Latin.

65. For English, Joannitius and Constantine the African, 154; for Latin, see Joannitius and Constantine the African, "Johannicius," 171. See discussion in Chapter 1.

66. Getz, "The Faculty of Medicine," 402.

67. On race as the tendency to "demarcate human beings through differences among humans that are selectively essentialized as absolute and fundamental," see Heng, "Invention of Race II," 332. On sex, see Cadden, *Meanings of Sex Difference in the Middle Ages*. On innate complexion, see Siraisi, *Medieval and Early Renaissance Medicine*, 102. For an overview of bodily difference in the Middle Ages more generally, see Green, "Bodily Essences" and "Diversity of Human Kind."

68. Demaitre, *Medieval Medicine*, 31.

69. Siraisi, *Medieval and Early Renaissance Medicine*, 123–27; Demaitre, *Medieval Medicine*, 44–50.

70. Fredborg, Nielsen, and Pinborg, "'De signis,'" 83. See discussion in Chapter 1.

71. For overviews of scholarship on leprosy, see Brenner, "Recent Perspectives on Leprosy" and Tabuteau, "Historical Research Developments on Leprosy." For accounts of the various roles persons with leprosy played, see Rawcliffe, *Leprosy in Medieval England*.

72. Demaitre, "The Description and Diagnosis of Leprosy."

73. Cited from Rawcliffe, *Leprosy in Medieval England*, 155.

74. Rawcliffe, *Leprosy in Medieval England*, 156.

75. Rawcliffe, *Leprosy in Medieval England*, 157, emphasis added.

76. Guy de Chauliac, *Cyrurgie*, 381, orthography modernized.

77. Jordanus de Turre, "The Symptoms of Lepers," 754.

78. Demaitre, "The Description and Diagnosis of Leprosy," 343.

79. This passage (*Lilium medicinae* I.2) is cited from Demaitre, *Leprosy in Premodern Medicine*, 20–22.

80. I explore this dynamic at greater length in Orlemanski, "How to Kiss a Leper."

81. English translation slightly altered from Richards, *The Medieval Leper*, 145–46. Latin from *Rymer's Foedera Volume 11*, 635–37.

82. Richards, *The Medieval Leper*, 145; *Rymer's Foedera Volume 11*, 635–37.

83. Richards, *The Medieval Leper*, 146; *Rymer's Foedera Volume 11*, 635–37.

84. Richards, *The Medieval Leper*, 146; *Rymer's Foedera Volume 11*, 635–37.

85. Richards, *The Medieval Leper*, 146; *Rymer's Foedera Volume 11*, 635–37.

86. Contagion assumed something like its modern meaning only after the advent of the plague in the mid-fourteenth century. See Touati, "Contagion and Leprosy."

87. Richards, *The Medieval Leper*, 145; *Rymer's Foedera Volume 11*, 635–37.

88. Krochalis and Peters, *The World of Piers Plowman*, 219.

89. Bacon, *Opera hactenus inedita*, 5:165.

90. *Three Prose Versions of the Secreta Secretorum*, ed. Steele, 216.

91. London, British Library, Royal MS 12 G IV. Other medical manuscripts containing physiognomic texts include London, British Library, Sloane MSS 213, 282, and 1313 and Egerton MS 2852, as well as Oxford, Bodleian Library, Ashmole MS 396 and Lyell MS 36.

92. See Voigts, "The 'Sloane Group.'" The "Sloane Group" manuscript with a physiognomy is London, British Library, Sloane MS 1313; the closely related manuscripts containing physiognomies are Cambridge, Gonville and Caius MS 336/725; New Haven, Beineke Library, Takamiya MS 33; and London, British Library, Additional MS 5467.

93. For alchemical texts accompanying physiognomies, see, for example, London, British Library, Sloane MSS 1128 and 2476, and Manzalaoui's description of the manuscript of Johannes de Caritate's *The Priuyté of Priuyteis* (*Secretum Secretorum*, ed. Manzalaoui, xxx). For works of divination accompanying physiognomies, see London, British Library, Sloane MSS 213 and 2030, Additional MS 15236, and Egerton MS 847.

94. See Mapstone, "The Scots *Buik of Phisnomy* and Sir Gilbert Hay."

95. London, British Library, Royal MS 12 C VI.

96. Williams, *The Secret of Secrets*, 1–2.

97. *Secretum Secretorum*, ed. Manzalaoui, 10 and 12, orthography modernized here and in subsequent citations.

98. *Secretum Secretorum*, ed. Manzalaoui, 12, 11.

99. *Secretum Secretorum*, ed. Manzalaoui, 10.

100. *Secretum Secretorum*, ed. Manzalaoui, 14.

101. *Secretum Secretorum*, ed. Manzalaoui, 10.

102. *Secretum Secretorum*, ed. Manzalaoui, 10.

103. *Secretum Secretorum*, ed. Manzalaoui, 10–11.

104. *Secretum Secretorum*, ed. Manzalaoui, 11.

105. *Secretum Secretorum*, ed. Manzalaoui, 14.

106. *Secretum Secretorum*, ed. Manzalaoui, 14.

107. Williams, *The Secret of Secrets*, 246–47.

108. *Secretum Secretorum*, ed. Manzalaoui, 11.

109. The dating is Manzalaoui's; see *Secretum Secretorum*, ed. Manzalaoui, xxvi.

110. I would like to thank M. Teresa Tavormina for sharing her unpublished notes on this manuscript.

111. Voigts, "Scientific and Medical Books," 348.

112. Voigts, "Scientific and Medical Books," 351.

113. Voigts, "The 'Sloane Group,'" 37, emphasis original.

114. See *Latin Technical Phlebotomy*, ed. Voigts and McVaugh, 24–25, 15.

115. Voigts, "Scientific and Medical Books," 383. This is Cambridge, Gonville and Caius MS 84/166.

116. Jones, "Argentine, John."

117. Jones, "Information and Science," 107.

118. Middle English cited from Voigts, "Fifteenth-Century English Banns," 264; orthography modernized and some punctuation added in this and subsequent citations.

119. Translation modified from Voigts, "Fifteenth-Century English Banns," 246–47.

120. Voigts, "Fifteenth-Century English Banns," 266.

121. Voigts, "Fifteenth-Century English Banns," 266–67.

122. I discuss Thornton's manuscript at length in Orlemanski, "Thornton's Remedies."

123. Scott, "Newly Discovered Booklets."

124. Scott, "Newly Discovered Booklets," 123.

125. Keiser, "Two Medieval Plague Treatises," 297–98; Scott, "Newly Discovered Booklets," 115.

126. Keiser, "Two Medieval Plague Treatises," 301.

127. Cant, "Thesaurus Pauperum," 159.

128. Cant, "Thesaurus Pauperum," 159–60.

129. Max Förster provides an edition of Lydgate's poem alongside the corresponding Latin stanzas in his "Kleinere mittelenglische Texte."

130. Edwards, "Lydgate Manuscripts." The manuscript count comes from Morrissey's thorough study, "'To al indifferent,'" 258. On versification, see Tavormina, "Three Middle English Verse Uroscopies," and bibliography therein.

131. See Orlemanski, "Thornton's Remedies," 249–53.

132. Lydgate, "Dietary," lines 1–4. The longer variant printed in Lydgate, *Minor Poems*, 702–7 is attested in only two of the fifty-nine manuscripts; see Morrissey, "'To al indifferent,'" 260.

133. Lydgate, "Dietary," lines 9–16.

134. See Olson, *Literature as Recreation in the Later Middle Ages*, esp. 39–89 and Stadolnik, "Gower's Bedside Manner," 164–68.

135. Arderne, *Treatises of Fistula in Ano*, 8.

136. Cooper, "Poetics of Practicality."

CHAPTER 3

1. "Sum Practysis of Medecyne," line 1, in Henryson, *Poems of Robert Henryson*, ed. Fox, 179–82, with notes at 475–87.

2. *DOST*, s.v. "guk" (n.), and "gowk" (n.). Elizabeth Leach, in *Sung Birds*, observes that in Marchetto of Padua's discussion of *vox* in the influential *Lucidarium*, "cu cu" (along with "cra cra") serves as an example of "nonarticulate" yet "literate" voices, "which cannot be understood and yet can be written down" (36).

3. See Godefroy, s.v. "jargon"; *OED*, s.v. "jargon" (n. 1) and "jargle" (v.); *DOST*, s.v. "jargoun" (n.) and "jargolyne" (vbl. n.); *MED*, s.v. "jargoun" (n.).

4. Henryson, *Poems of Robert Henryson*, ed. Kindrick, 147.

5. Goldstein, "Writing in Scotland," 239.

6. On medicine in late medieval Scotland, including the increasing numbers of learned practitioners and of Scottish medical manuscripts, see Comrie, *History of Scottish Medicine*, 1:55–104.

7. For an ingenious exploration of the poetic and speculative properties of Middle English medical writing, see Bower, "Similes We Cure By."

8. Yunck, "Satire," 135.

9. For the characterization here, see Gillespie, "The Study of Classical Authors," 223–29.

10. Tiffany, *Infidel Poetics*, 7, 16.

11. Tiffany, *Infidel Poetics*, 6.

12. Voigts, "Multitudes of Middle English Medical Manuscripts," 183.

13. Keiser, "Robert Thornton's *Liber de Diversis Medicinis*," 35, 33. For more on Thornton's medical writing, also see Orlemanski, "Thornton's Remedies."

14. All examples discussed in Chapter 2.

15. Bacon, "Errors of the Doctors According to Friar Roger Bacon," 30. For the original Latin, see Bacon, *Fratris Rogeri Bacon*, 153–54.

16. Monica Green calls the linguistic matrix of Anglo-Norman remedy collections "dizzyingly macaronic" and notes that "the English tolerance for willy-nilly mixtures of languages in recipe collections" is something she has "encountered to this degree in no other vernacular tradition"; see Green, "Salerno on the Thames," 231. Both systematic and "willy-nilly" language mixing continued into the fifteenth century. Linda Ehrsam Voigts has argued for the essentially bilingual character of late medieval medical textuality in England; see Voigts, "What's the Word?"

17. Cant, "Thesaurus Pauperum," 159. Also see Bishop, *Words, Stones, and Herbs*.

18. Hunt, *Plant Names of Medieval England*, xix–xxxvi.

19. Pliny, *Natural History*, Book XXIX, 198–99. On the humanist tradition of medical satire, see Carlino, "Petrarch and the Early Modern Critics of Medicine."

20. Cited from Fox, "Henryson's 'Sum Practysis of Medecyne,'" 454–55.

21. Nancy Pope provides an introduction, diplomatic edition, and translation of the text in "A Middle English Satirical Letter in Brogyntyn MS II.1." I have modernized orthography and silently altered Pope's translation at several points.

22. Edmond Faral describes the *herberie* as a minor genre that "figurait au répertoire des jongleurs, qui la débitaient comme une charge, comme une parodie des boniments de charlatans." See *Mimes français du XIIIe siècle*, ed. Faral, 59.

23. Translation modified from Ham, "Rutebeuf Guide," 22; French text drawn from *Mimes français du XIIIe siècle*, ed. Faral, 61–68, lines 48–51. Hereafter cited in text by line number.

24. Ham, "Rutebeuf Guide," 29.

25. Walsh, "Rubin and Mercator," 187.

26. Abrahams, "The Mercator-Scenes in the Mediaeval French Passion-Plays," 114.

27. *Mystères inédits du quinzième siècle*, ed. Jubinal, 2:299–300. The play is titled *La Passion de Notre Seigneur*.

28. Mann, *Chaucer and Medieval Estates Satire*, 91–99.

29. The remark about the cynical trade of physicians is from the description of the Physician in the General Prologue of the *Canterbury Tales* (I.442, in *Riverside Chaucer*). The best reference on the medical doctor in medieval satire remains Mann, *Chaucer and Medieval Estates Satire*, 91–99.

30. Pliny, *Natural History*, Book XXIX, 194–95.

31. Petrarca, *Invectives*, 34–36.

32. French drawn from Chrétien de Troyes, *Cligès*, ed. Méla and Collet, lines 5737–38; English from Chrétien de Troyes, *Cligès*, trans. Raffel, lines 5798–99.

33. See van D'Elden, "The Salerno Effect."

34. Chrétien de Troyes, *Cligès*, ed. Méla and Collet, line 5808; trans. Raffel, line 5869.

35. Chrétien de Troyes, *Cligès*, ed. Méla and Collet, lines 5882–83; trans. Raffel, lines 5942–43.

36. Chrétien de Troyes, *Cligès*, ed. Méla and Collet, lines 5932–33; trans. Raffel, lines 5992–94.

37. Cant, "Thesaurus Pauperum," 210, orthography modernized.

38. *Medieval Woman's Guide to Health*, ed. Rowland, 58, orthography modernized. For an important analysis of this treatise in light of five other English versions, see Green, "Women's Medical Practice and Health Care in Medieval Europe," 68–74.

39. Lochrie, *Covert Operations*, 118–31.

40. Lydgate, "Dietary," lines 9–10, 16.

41. Lydgate, "Dietary," lines 78–80.

42. Morrissey, "'To al indifferent,'" 264–69.

43. Getz, *Medicine in the English Middle Ages*, 45–53.

44. For discussion, see Chapter 2.

45. *Secular Lyrics of the XIV and XV Centuries*, ed. Robbins, 102.

46. *Secular Lyrics of the XIV and XV Centuries*, ed. Robbins, 102, lines 4–8, orthography modernized.

47. *Canterbury Tales* VII.2923–31, in *Riverside Chaucer*; hereafter cited in text by line number.

48. See Voigts, "Herbs and Herbal Healing," 227, for glosses on this passage.

49. On the danger of the recipe, see Kauffman, "Dame Pertelote's Parlous Parle."

50. The sole surviving manuscript witness is the Bannatyne Manuscript, Edinburgh, National Library of Scotland, Advocates' MS 1.1.6, fols. 141v–142v. For an earlier version of the reading advanced in this section, see Orlemanski, "Jargon and the Matter of Medicine in Middle English."

51. Goldstein, "Writing in Scotland," 252.

52. *OED*, s.v. "dia-, prefix2."

53. "Sum Practysis of Medecyne," lines 38–39, 51–52, in Henryson, *The Poems of Robert Henryson*, ed. Fox. Further citations are given parenthetically in the text by line number, with orthography modernized throughout. Translations are my own, based on Fox's notes as well as those in Henryson, *Robert Henryson*, ed. Parkinson. Many of Fox's and Parkinson's glosses remain tentative, as do my translations. At numerous points the meaning is obscure, likely due not only to the eclecticism of the poem's language but also to scribal corruption.

54. London, British Library, Royal MS 17 D I, fol. 4v. I have modernized orthography.

55. Mirfield, *Johannes de Mirfeld*, 48–49.

56. See Fox, "Henryson's 'Sum Practysis of Medecyne,'" 458.

57. Parkinson notes that the stanza form "had an association with flyting and grotesquery" in another fifteenth-century Scottish comic poem, Sir Richard Holland's *Buke of the Howlat*; see Henryson, *Robert Henryson*, ed. Parkinson, 227.

58. See Tavormina, "Three Middle English Verse Uroscopies"; Keiser, "Verse Introductions to Middle English Medical Treatises"; Hunt, "The Poetic Vein"; and Garrett, "Middle English Rimed Medical Treatise."

59. Cited from Tavormina, "Three Middle English Verse Uroscopies," 591.

60. Sigerist, "Bedside Manners," 139.

61. Henryson, *The Poems of Robert Henryson*, ed. Fox, 486.

62. See Jones, "Four Middle English Translations."

63. Jones, "Staying with the Programme," 207.

64. "*Here . . . must . . . an image appere owt, with woundys bleeding*": stage directions following line 712 in *Croxton Play of the Sacrament*, ed. Sebastian. The play is subsequently cited in the text by line number.

65. Lawton, "Sacrilege and Theatricality," 286.

66. Wright, "What's So 'English' About Medieval English Drama?" 87.

67. On which see Beckwith, "Ritual, Church and Theatre."

68. In particular Easter plays from fifteenth-century Germany offer a close analogue, in which a clownish servant "Rubin" appears alongside his master the *mercator*; see Walsh, "Rubin and Mercator." Some have suggested a connection to the "mock death and cure" in mummers' plays, though the records of such plays postdate the *Croxton Play*; see Chambers, *English Folk-Play*, 160–70.

69. John Sebastian judges that "the [metrical] alteration is appropriate to the change in tone and consistent with the habits of contemporary playwrights"; see *Croxton Play of the Sacrament*, ed. Sebastian, 81.

70. Lawton, "Sacrilege and Theatricality," 292.

71. Lanfranc of Milan, *Lanfrank's "Science of Cirurgie,"* 7, orthography modernized.

CHAPTER 4

1. A Middle English translation of Bernard's *Lilium* survives in Oxford, Bodleian Library, Ashmole 1505, though it has not been edited. Bernard's *Lilium* appears to have been well known in England; for instance, John Arderne's *Liber medicinalium* draws more extracts from the *Lilium* than from any other work; see Jones, "Arderne, John."

2. Bernard of Gordon, *Practica seu lilium medicinae*, 54–55. Incunabula pages not numbered; quotation drawn from what are pages 54–55 of the complete pdf of the digitized microfilm.

3. Mosher, *Exemplum in the Early Religious and Didactic Literature of England*, 1.

4. On the background and medieval history of exempla, I have relied particularly on von Moos, "The Use of Exempla in the *Policraticus* of John of Salisbury"; Mitchell, *Ethics and Exemplary Narrative in Chaucer and Gower*; and Roberts, "*Ars Praedicandi* and the Medieval Sermon."

5. See *De Inventione* 1.19.27–1.20.30 and *Rhetorica ad Herennium* 4.49.62.

6. Roberts, "*Ars Praedicandi* and the Medieval Sermon," 53–54.

7. Murphy, *Rhetoric in the Middle Ages*, 342.

8. Roberts, "*Ars Praedicandi* and the Medieval Sermon," 54.

9. Scanlon, *Narrative, Authority, and Power*, 81–134.

10. Scanlon, *Narrative, Authority, and Power*, 3.

11. Forster, *Aspects of the Novel*, 86, emphasis added. For further general reflections on the role of causality in narrative, see Currie, "Narrative Representation of Causes."

12. Scanlon, *Narrative, Authority, and Power*, 33.

13. Mitchell, *Ethics and Exemplary Narrative in Chaucer and Gower*, 17.

14. Mink, "Narrative Form as Cognitive Instrument," 132.

15. Mitchell, *Ethics and Exemplary Narrative in Chaucer and Gower*, 24.

16. Tubach, "Exempla in the Decline," 412, emphasis added.

17. Tubach, "Exempla in the Decline," 414.

18. Tubach, "Exempla in the Decline," 415.

19. Tubach, "Exempla in the Decline," 416.

20. Tubach, *Index Exemplorum*.

21. Tubach, "Exempla in the Decline," 411, 413.

22. For an overview, see Lindberg, *The Beginnings of Western Science*, 183–244.

23. See discussion in Chapter 8.

24. For further details, see McNiven, "The Problem of Henry IV's Health."

25. See Maidstone, "Miscellanea Relating to the Martyrdom of Archbishop Scrope."

26. Gascoigne, *Loci e Libro veritatum*, 228.

27. Gascoigne, *Loci e Libro veritatum*, 228.

28. *Canterbury Tales* II.669–70, in *Riverside Chaucer*.

29. von Nolcken, "Gascoigne [Gascoygne], Thomas."

30. See discussion in Chapters 1 and 2.

31. Henri de Mondeville, *Chirurgie des Heinrich von Mondeville*, 81.

32. McVaugh and Ballester, "Therapeutic Method," 76. For Latin, see Arnau of Vilanova, *Repetitio super aphorismo Hippocratus*, 247–48.

33. Jacquart, "Medical Scholasticism," 229–30.

34. Jacquart, "Theory, Everyday Practice," 140.

35. Siraisi, *Medieval and Early Renaissance Medicine*, 152. See also Jones, "Surgical Narrative in Middle English."

36. Jacquart, "Medical Scholasticism," 231.

37. The word *experimentum* could mean numerous things in medieval medicine, including an experience, a cure discovered empirically, or a specific narrative or case history. For further discussion, see Agrimi and Crisciani, "Per una ricerca su *experimentum-experimenta*."

38. Jacquart, "Medical Scholasticism," 232.

39. Jacquart, "Medical Scholasticism," 232.

40. See Siraisi, "How to Write a Latin Book of Surgery," esp. 100.

41. Jones, "The Surgeon as Story-Teller," 79: "by comparison with the Latin authors of surgery, the Arabic authorities had made very little use of narratives of individual cases of treatment."

42. See McVaugh, *Rational Surgery of the Middle Ages*, 230–41.

43. Jones, "Surgical Narrative in Middle English," 3.

44. Jones, "Surgical Narrative in Middle English," 6.

45. Getz, "The Faculty of Medicine."

46. Getz, *Medicine in the English Middle Ages*, 119n130.

47. Lanfranc of Milan, *Lanfrank's "Science of Cirurgie,"* 69–70, orthography modernized here and in subsequent citations.

48. Lanfranc of Milan, *Lanfrank's "Science of Cirurgie,"* 88.

49. See, for instance, Lanfranc of Milan, *Lanfrank's "Science of Cirurgie,"* 266.

50. Lanfranc of Milan, *Lanfrank's "Science of Cirurgie,"* 232.

51. Siraisi, "How to Write a Latin Book of Surgery," 101.

52. On the relation between saints and physicians, see Finucane, *Miracles and Pilgrims*, 60–71.

53. Mark 5:25–34; Luke 8:43–48.

54. Finucane, *Miracles and Pilgrims*, 59.

55. Guy de Chauliac, *Cyrurgie*, 10. Regarding similar attitudes expressed by Henri de Mondeville, see Macdougall, "The Surgeon and the Saints."

56. Lanfranc of Milan, *Lanfrank's "Science of Cirurgie,"* 9.

57. Arderne, *Treatises of Fistula in Ano*, 6, orthography modernized.

58. Arderne, *Treatises of Fistula in Ano*, 6, orthography modernized. For a compelling discussion of this passage from Arderne, see Turner, "Illness Narratives in the Later Middle Ages," 66–67.

59. Latin cited from Ziegler, *Medicine and Religion*, 208n101. Ziegler points out that Bersuire's story "is indeed taken from Arnau's *De parte operativa*, though it has acquired some dramatic elements which are absent in Arnau's original text" (208).

60. Macaronic Latin and Modern English translation both drawn from *A Macaronic Sermon Collection*, ed. and trans. Horner, 144–45.

61. *A Macaronic Sermon Collection*, ed. and trans. Horner, 144–45.

62. *A Macaronic Sermon Collection*, ed. and trans. Horner, 144–45.

63. *A Macaronic Sermon Collection*, ed. and trans. Horner, 146–47.

64. *A Macaronic Sermon Collection*, ed. and trans. Horner, 146–47.

65. Ziegler, *Medicine and Religion*, 180.

66. Ziegler, *Medicine and Religion*, 181–82.

67. *Decrees of the Ecumenical Councils*, ed. Tanner, 245–46. See discussion in Chapter 1.

68. *Decrees of the Ecumenical Councils*, ed. Tanner, 245.

69. For a compelling recent study of how physical and spiritual levels inform one another in the portrayal of the Seven Deadly Sins, see Langum, *Medicine and the Seven Deadly Sins in Late Medieval Literature and Culture*.

70. Bremond, Le Goff, and Schmitt, *L'"Exemplum,"* 31.

71. Isidore of Seville, *Etymologies* I.xxxvii.31, p.63.

72. *A Macaronic Sermon Collection*, ed. and trans. Horner, 34–35, 276–77, 440–41.

73. *A Macaronic Sermon Collection*, ed. and trans. Horner, 446–47.

74. *A Macaronic Sermon Collection*, ed. and trans. Horner, 446–47.

75. *A Macaronic Sermon Collection*, ed. and trans. Horner, 96–97.

76. *A Macaronic Sermon Collection*, ed. and trans. Horner, 98–99.

77. *A Macaronic Sermon Collection*, ed. and trans. Horner, 426–27.

78. *A Macaronic Sermon Collection*, ed. and trans. Horner, 426–27.

79. O'Mara and Paul, *A Repertorium of Middle English Prose Sermons*, 354.

80. Mirk, *Mirk's Festial*, 43.

81. *Ancrene Wisse*, ed. Millett, 69, including text in note 2; orthography modernized.

82. For overviews of medieval disability studies, see Godden and Hsy, "Analytical Survey: Encountering Disability in the Middle Ages" and Hsy, "Disability."

83. Metzler, *Disability in Medieval Europe*, 46.

84. For an overview, see Brenner, "Recent Perspectives on Leprosy" and Tabuteau, "Historical Research Developments on Leprosy." Important studies include Touati, *Maladie et société au moyen âge* and "Contagion and Leprosy"; Rawcliffe, *Leprosy in Medieval England*; and Demaitre, "The Description and Diagnosis of Leprosy" and *Leprosy in Premodern Medicine*. These scholars complicate and partly refute the perspectives in older studies like Brody, *Disease of the Soul* and Moore, *Formation of a Persecuting Society*.

85. On the role of medicine in *Piers Plowman*, see Gasse, "The Practice of Medicine in *Piers Plowman*," and Krug, "*Piers Plowman* and the Secrets of Health."

86. Langland, *Vision of Piers Plowman*, XX.81–85.

87. Langland, *Vision of Piers Plowman*, XX.169.

88. Langland, *Vision of Piers Plowman*, XX.174–77.

89. Langland, *Vision of Piers Plowman*, XX.314–15.

90. Langland, *Vision of Piers Plowman*, XX.348.

91. Langland, *Vision of Piers Plowman*, XX.372–73.

92. *Early English Versions of the* Gesta Romanorum, ed. Herrtage, 317, orthography modernized here and in subsequent citations. A more extended reading of this exemplum, with somewhat different emphasis, appears in Orlemanski, "Literary Genre, Medieval Studies, and the Prosthesis of Disability."

93. Bakhtin, *The Dialogic Imagination*, 84.

94. *Early English Versions of the* Gesta Romanorum, ed. Herrtage, 318.

95. *Early English Versions of the* Gesta Romanorum, ed. Herrtage, 318.

96. *Early English Versions of the* Gesta Romanorum, ed. Herrtage, 318.

97. Salter, *Popular Reading in English*, 98–99. Also see Bright, "Anglo-Latin Collections."

98. *Early English Versions of the* Gesta Romanorum, ed. Herrtage, 319.

99. The tales of the *Gesta Romanorum* derive from "oriental apologues, classical literature, saints' lives, chronicles, medieval romance, Aesopic fables, and folklore" (Bright, "Anglo-Latin Collections," 401).

100. Manly and Rickert, *Text of the Canterbury Tales*, 1:207–18.

101. *Early English Versions of the* Gesta Romanorum, ed. Herrtage, 67.

102. *Early English Versions of the* Gesta Romanorum, ed. Herrtage, 67–68.

103. *Early English Versions of the* Gesta Romanorum, ed. Herrtage, 68.

104. *Early English Versions of the* Gesta Romanorum, ed. Herrtage, 68.

105. *Early English Versions of the* Gesta Romanorum, ed. Herrtage, 69.

106. *Early English Versions of the* Gesta Romanorum, ed. Herrtage, 69.

107. *MED*, s.v. "dōm" (n.) 1a, 2, 4b.

108. *Early English Versions of the* Gesta Romanorum, ed. Herrtage, 69.

109. *Early English Versions of the* Gesta Romanorum, ed. Herrtage, 70.

CHAPTER 5

1. For a detailed account of the relation of the "Knight's Tale" to the *Teseida*, see Boitani, *Chaucer and Boccaccio*, 1–60.

2. Muscatine, "Form, Texture, and Meaning," 929.

3. *Canterbury Tales* I.2987, in *Riverside Chaucer*. Subsequent citations occur in text by line number.

4. For instance, see Burlin, *Chaucerian Fiction*, 95–112, Mann, *Geoffrey Chaucer*, and the works listed in Aers, *Chaucer, Langland*, 228n1.

5. For instance, see Salter, *The Knight's Tale and the Clerk's Tale*, 9–36; Blake, "Order and the Noble Life in Chaucer's *Knight's Tale*?"; Aers, *Chaucer, Langland*, 175–95; and Patterson, *Chaucer and the Subject of History*, 165–230.

6. For a recent exploration of medicine and the "Knight's Tale" from a different angle, see Fumo, "The Pestilential Gaze." Fumo's essay makes many striking observations, though I hesitate to follow her in the claim that the tale instances "conscious participation in the discourse of plague-writing" (123). For another suggestive consideration of plague and the "Knight's Tale," see Smith, "Plague, Panic Space, and the Tragic Medieval Household."

7. See Chapter 3.

8. Schweitzer, "Fate and Freedom in 'The Knight's Tale,'" 13.

9. Patterson, *Chaucer and the Subject of History*, 200.

10. The exception is *expellen*; see *MED*, s.v. "expellen" (v.). To determine first recorded usage, I rely on Cannon's lexicon in *The Making of Chaucer's English* (based on proposed date of composition rather than manuscript date). For subsequent usage, see *MED*, s.v. "ventōsing(e" (ger.), "expulsīf, -īve" (adj.), "animal" (adj.), "lacerte" (n.), and "vein(e" (n.(1)) 1d. My claims about this passage do not depend, however, on Chaucer's usage being the very first.

11. Boccaccio, *Teseida* X.11.3–4; Boccaccio, *Book of Theseus*, 263.

12. Boccaccio, *Teseida* X.12.3–4.

13. Readers will notice that I decline to explain shifts in diction or tone in terms of the mental state of the Knight as narrator. Insofar Chaucer is likely to have completed the "Knight's Tale" prior to its incorporation into the *Canterbury Tales* (a point I return to), I choose not to collapse the tale's narrator into the character of the Knight. The scholarly debate concerning the Knight's role as tale-teller has been mapped in Klitgård, *Chaucer's Narrative Voice in "The Knight's Tale,"* 29–38. My sense that the narrator is best regarded as a principle of unity and agency organizing disparate stylistic, narrative, and perceptual effects, occasionally demarcated with the pronoun *I*, is informed by Spearing, *Medieval Autographies*.

14. Wallis, *Medieval Medicine*, 544.

15. *MED*, s.v. "vertu" (n).

16. Joannitius and Constantine the African, *Isagoge*, 142.

17. Avicenna, excerpt from the *Canon*, 717.

18. Kaye, *A History of Balance*, 6.

19. Kolve, *Chaucer and the Imagery of Narrative*, 122.

20. Kolve, *Chaucer and the Imagery of Narrative*, 122.

21. Kolve, *Chaucer and the Imagery of Narrative*, 122.

22. On this foreshadowing, see Schweitzer, "Fate and Freedom in 'The Knight's Tale'" and Patterson, *Chaucer and the Subject of History*, 204–7.

23. See Lowes, "The Loveres Maladye of Hereos."

24. On this tradition, see Wack, *Lovesickness in the Middle Ages*.

25. Fradenburg, "Sacrificial Desire," 50.

26. As Mark Miller has shown, the narration of Emelye's May morning rites (for instance) have the effect of evacuating her agency and rendering her desires "merely as phenomena in a causal sequence" (*Philosophical Chaucer*, 87).

27. Boccaccio, *Teseida* IX.5–7.

28. It is striking that Boccaccio offers an extensive authorial gloss on the stanzas of the *Teseida* where the Fury appears, a gloss that ruminates on the interlocked processes of fiction-making and narrative's etiological manipulation: "In this part, the author attributes what he imagines as happening to the compromise made between Mars and Venus, each eager to serve the one who had prayed to him. . . . And as can be read in the text, Arcite's horse shied and reared up and fell back on his chest. It is a very certain thing that animals shy at some frightening object that they seem to see, but what they see, or what they think they see, no one knows. So the author imagines that it was Erinys." See Boccaccio, *Book of Theseus*, 257–58. However, Chaucer is not thought to have known Boccaccio's glosses.

29. For more on how medieval thinkers understood pagan belief, see Van Dyke, *Chaucer's Agents*, 108–14 and Minnis, *Chaucer and Pagan Antiquity*, 13–17.

30. Augustine, *The City of God* VI.9, 258–59.

31. See Seznec, *The Survival of the Pagan Gods*.

32. Mann, "Planetary Gods," 93. Also see Mann, "Chance and Destiny."

33. Mann, "Planetary Gods," 93.

34. On the astrological additions, see Curry, *Chaucer and the Mediaeval Sciences*, 119–63.

35. Boitani, *Chaucer and Boccaccio*, 102, emphasis original.

36. Kolve links the gods' portrayal in the "Knight's Tale" to a tradition of astrological treatises on "the 'qualities' of the planets—hot, cold, dry, wet—together with the kinds of human occupation each governs and the kind of event each characteristically brings about," a tradition that eventually resulted in the iconography of *Planetenkinder*, or "children of the planets," so resonant with the paintings described on the temple walls. See Kolve, *Chaucer and the Imagery of Narrative*, 115–21.

37. Orlemanski, "Prosopopoeial Heaviness in Chaucer's *Book of the Duchess*."

38. Boccaccio, *Teseida* X.12.5–13.3; Boccaccio, *Book of Theseus*, 263.

39. As it does, for instance, in the *House of Fame*, when Venus's temple of glass is called a "chirche" (line 473, in *Riverside Chaucer*).

40. *MED*, s.v. "natur(e" (n.) 2b.

41. *MED*, s.v. "natur(e" (n.) 1a.

42. For examples of such death lyrics, see "Signs of Death in Middle English," and "How Death Comes," in *Medieval English Lyrics*, 74–75.

43. *MED*, s.v. "vĭtǎl" (adj.) 1a and b.

44. Wallis, *Medieval Medicine*, 550.

45. Boccaccio, *Teseida* XI.1–3.

46. Muscatine, "Form, Texture, and Meaning," 926.

47. Muscatine, "Form, Texture, and Meaning," 926.

48. Schweitzer, "Fate and Freedom in '*The Knight's Tale*,'" 13.

49. The classic formulation is Muscatine's, "Form, Texture, and Meaning."

50. See Kolve, *Chaucer and the Imagery of Narrative*: "The amphitheater that Theseus builds for the tournament between Palamon and Arcite . . . allows Chaucer to assess, in an unusually comprehensive and exploratory way, the possibilities of creating human order within a world apparently governed by chance" (105).

51. *Boece* I.pr5.71–73 and I.pr2.19–21, in *Riverside Chaucer*.

52. *Boece* III.m9.18–21, in *Riverside Chaucer*.

53. *Boece* IV.p6.163–65, in *Riverside Chaucer*.

54. *Boece* II.m8.17–20, in *Riverside Chaucer*.

55. *Boece* III.p11.159–62, in *Riverside Chaucer*.

56. *Boece* III.p11.155, 198–99, in *Riverside Chaucer*.

57. Patterson, *Chaucer and the Subject of History*, 200.

58. *nature*, lines 2758 and 2759; *corrupteth*, 2746; *corrupcioun*, 2754.

59. Patterson, *Chaucer and the Subject of History*, 75.

60. Muscatine, "Form, Texture, and Meaning," 925.

61. On this irony, see Mieszkowski, "The Reputation of Criseyde."

62. McGerr, *Chaucer's Open Books*, 96.

63. Cooper usefully summarizes the evidence; see Cooper, *Oxford Guides to Chaucer*, 61–62. Also see Bowes, "Three Readings of *The Knight's Tale*," esp. 280. For an especially compelling analysis of "Chaucer's decision to use one of his earlier, self-standing poems as the *Knight's Tale*," see Bahr, *Fragments and Assemblages*, 155–207.

64. *Legend of Good Women* F 420, in *Riverside Chaucer*.

65. Cooper, *Oxford Guides to Chaucer*, 94.

66. As Mark Miller has shown, when Chaucer's Miller is considered as an agential subject, he is one governed by normative disciplines and hierarchical ordering, not one who has escaped them. Miller, *Philosophical Chaucer*, 36–81.

CHAPTER 6

1. An earlier version of the arguments of this chapter appears in Orlemanski, "Desire and Defacement."

2. Though it survives only in sixteenth-century witnesses, the *Testament* was composed in the later fifteenth century; it is evidently referred to, and so was in circulation, by 1492. See Fox, introduction to *The Poems of Robert Henryson*, xciv–c.

3. *Testament of Cresseid*, lines 568 and 613, in Henryson, *The Poems of Robert Henryson*, ed. Fox. Hereafter the poem is cited in the text by line number with orthography modernized. My translations rely on the notes and glossary in Henryson, *The Poems of Robert Henryson*, ed. Fox, as well as the glosses in Henryson, *Robert Henryson: The Complete Works*, ed. Parkinson.

4. The phrase is from Pearsall, "'Quha wait?'" 177.

5. Lynch, "Robert Henryson's 'Doolie Dreame,'" 182.

6. Jana Mathews has charted Henryson's connections to fifteenth-century Scottish judiciary procedure and shown particularly how the *Testament* recasts its mythological figures "in terms of contemporary legal theory and practice" ("Land, Lepers, and the Law in *The Testament of Cresseid*," 50).

7. Henryson, *Robert Henryson*, ed. Parkinson, 208n266.

8. Henryson, *The Poems of Robert Henryson*, ed. Fox, 365n311.

9. MacQueen, *Robert Henryson*, 61.

10. Patterson, "Christian and Pagan," 699, emphasis original.

11. Patterson, "Christian and Pagan," 701.

12. Patterson, "Christian and Pagan," 697.

13. As Felicity Riddy points out, the ascription of moral progress to Cresseid presumes that the different articulations of her suffering are the expressions of a steadily developing moral agent, rather than, as Riddy suggests, a "voice" passing through "different genres that provide discontinuous subject positions" ("'Abject Odious,'" 290).

14. Kruger, "Medical and Moral Authority in the Late Medieval Dream," 51.

15. Henryson, *The Poems of Robert Henryson*, ed. Fox, 341nn11–14.

16. Henryson, *The Poems of Robert Henryson*, ed. Fox, 342n34.

17. Riddy notes of the *Testament*'s opening section that "the male body is to be an issue—perhaps the issue—throughout the poem" ("'Abject Odious,'" 291).

18. Numerous scholars have noted the genre's evocation, and Kathryn Lynch, after cataloging the similarities, goes so far as to call the dream vision the *Testament*'s "functional genre." Lynch, "Robert Henryson's 'Doolie Dreame,'" 178; also see Watson, "Outdoing Chaucer," 102–3 and Kruger, "Medical and Moral Authority in the Late Medieval Dream," 51–63.

19. Kruger, "Medical and Moral Authority in the Late Medieval Dream," 55, 62.

20. *House of Fame*, lines 21–22, in *Riverside Chaucer*.

21. For instance, see Hanna, "Cresseid's Dream and Henryson's *Testament*." Also see Kruger, "Medical and Moral Authority in the Late Medieval Dream" for arguments that trouble Hanna's dismissal of Cresseid's dream on account of its bodily and psychological circumstances.

22. Fox, introduction to Henryson, *Testament of Cresseid*, 53.

23. Pearsall, "Quha wait?" 174.

24. Dunai, "'And Doolie Sessoun' and 'Ane Cairfull Dyte.'"

25. Riddy's reading is close to this: "The problem that the poem is wrestling with is not the problem of femininity but a problem within masculinity: its own uncleanness, which is coded as feminine and rejected as polluting" ("'Abject Odious,'" 292).

26. *Canterbury Tales* I.1917, in *Riverside Chaucer*. Also see the lines about Venus's temple specifically: Theseus "estward hath, upon the gate above, / In worshipe of Venus, goddesse of love, / Doon make an auter and an oratorie" (I.1903–5).

27. See Mann, "Planetary Gods."

28. Pearsall, "'Quha wait?'" 181.

29. *Book of the Duchess*, in *Riverside Chaucer*, ed. Benson, lines 48–51.

30. Donaldson, "Criseide and Her Narrator."

31. *Troilus and Criseyde* V.825, in *Riverside Chaucer*.

32. *Troilus and Criseyde* V.1817, in *Riverside Chaucer*.

33. MacQueen, *Robert Henryson*, 55.

34. See Henryson, *The Poems of Robert Henryson*, ed. Fox, 344n61.

35. Stephenson, "The Acrostic 'Fictio.'"

36. Green, *A Crisis of Truth*, esp. chap. 1, "From Troth to Truth." *DOST*, s.v. "Trew(e, True, *adj*."

37. For instance, the *Roman de Troie* by Benoit de St. Maure, which was a wellspring for later vernacular works, commences with a disquisition on the deceptiveness of Homer, and when

Chaucer discusses the poets of Troy in the *House of Fame*, he records the rumor that "Omer made lyes, / Feynynge in hys poetries" (lines 1476–80, in *Riverside Chaucer*).

38. Also see *Testament of Cresseid*, lines 553, 560, 572, 591, in Henryson, *The Poems of Robert Henryson*, ed. Fox.

39. See Watson, "Outdoing Chaucer."

40. *OED*, s.v. "invention," *n*. I.4; this is the first recorded use. *DOST* records Henryson's usage here as the first record for the meaning "Poetic invention or creativeness; an instance of this" (s.v. "Inventio(u)n," n., 2). *MED* lists only two instances, both from John Lydgate's *Fall of Princes*, for "Rhetorical or poetical invention" (s.v. "invencioun" (n.) 2).

41. Watson, "Outdoing Chaucer," 104.

42. Pearsall, "'Quha wait?'" 174.

43. Henryson, *The Poems of Robert Henryson*, ed. Fox, 346n81.

44. Pearsall, "'Quha wait?'" 174.

45. Mann, "Planetary Gods," 101.

46. Wittig, *The Scottish Tradition in Literature*, 47; Gray, *Robert Henryson*, 192, 169; Mann, "Planetary Gods," 98.

47. *Troilus and Criseyde* V.897–99, in *Riverside Chaucer*.

48. See the discussion of exempla and their narrative poetics in Chapter 4.

49. See Bartholomaeus Anglicus and John Trevisa, *On the Properties of Things*, 479–80 for a representative collection of medieval lore on Saturn, typical of what is represented in Henryson's portrait.

50. For more on the astrological determinants of Cresseid's disease, see Parr, "Cresseid's Leprosy Again." For detailed discussion of the medieval medical accounts of leprosy, see Demaitre, *Leprosy in Premodern Medicine*, 103–23, and Rawcliffe, *Leprosy in Medieval England*, 64–78.

51. Bartholomaeus Anglicus and John Trevisa, *On the Properties of Things*, 493, and see 489–94 for the encyclopedia's complete account of the moon.

52. *Troilus and Criseyde* I.101–5, in *Riverside Chaucer*.

53. *Troilus and Criseyde* V.218–21, in *Riverside Chaucer*.

54. Also see *Testament of Cresseid*, lines 88, 92, 325, 329, 396, 520, 615, in Henryson, *The Poems of Robert Henryson*, ed. Fox.

55. Patch, *The Goddess Fortuna in Medieval Literature*, 96–98.

56. Aswell, "The Role of Fortune in *The Testament of Cresseid*," 482–83.

57. Gray, *Robert Henryson*, 174.

58. Fox's introduction and notes to the poem in both of his editions (*Testament of Cresseid* and *Complete Works*) remain reliable guides. Also see Stearns, "Henryson and the Leper Cresseid" and Parr, "Cresseid's Leprosy Again."

59. Fox, introduction to *Testament of Cresseid*, 26.

60. See the discussion of leprosy's diagnosis in Chapter 2.

61. *Amis and Amiloun*, in *Amis and Amiloun, Robert of Cisyle*, lines 1259–60.

62. *Amis and Amiloun*, in *Amis and Amiloun, Robert of Cisyle*, lines 1543–45.

63. *English Metrical Homilies*, 129–30.

64. For an overview, see Brenner, "Recent Perspectives on Leprosy." For a more extensive version of this argument, see Orlemanski, "Leprosies."

65. Demaitre, "The Description and Diagnosis of Leprosy."

66. Thus, despite Saul Brody's influential claims, Cresseid's leprosy does not necessarily indicate her lust or sexual depravity more than it does other transgressions, nor was leprosy's transmission thought to be predominantly sexual. Brody, *The Disease of Soul*, 173–77. For

arguments against Brody's narrow focus on sexuality, see Grigsby, *Pestilence in Medieval and Early Modern English Literature*, 98–102. One piece of scholarship that has bolstered the "venereal" reading of Cresseid's leprosy (though it does not discuss Henryson's poem directly) is Jacquart and Thomasset, *Sexuality and Medicine in the Middle Ages*, 177–94—but for a critique of its arguments, see Demaitre, "The Description and Diagnosis of Leprosy."

67. Mann, "Planetary Gods," 96.

68. See the discussion of physiognomy in Chapter 2.

69. *Ms. Bodley 959*, ed. Lindberg, 5:154. I quote the verse to reflect its correction in the manuscript, noted by Lindberg. For the later version, see *John Wycliffe Bible 1382*.

70. I give a more complete version of the arguments in this and the following paragraph in Orlemanski, "How to Kiss a Leper."

71. Raymond of Capua, *The Life of Catherine of Siena*, 149.

72. For more examples of leprosy as the incitement to both disgust and love, see Orlemanski, "How to Kiss a Leper"; Farmer, "The Leper in the Master Bedroom"; and Peyroux, "The Leper's Kiss."

73. On the traffic between sacred literature and the poetry of secular love in the Middle Ages, see Dronke, "The Song of Songs and Medieval Love-Lyric"; the texts and commentary in Imbach and Atucha, *Amours plurielles*; and Newman, *Medieval Crossover*.

74. Quoted from Stearns, *Robert Henryson*, 96.

CHAPTER 7

1. "My Compleinte," lines 40–42, in Hoccleve, *"My Compleinte" and Other Poems*, orthography modernized. References to this edition are hereafter cited in text by line number, with P to indicate prologue, C to indicate "My Compleinte," and D to indicate "Dialogue"; orthography is modernized throughout.

2. The *Series* is an editorial title given by E. P. Hammond in *English Verse Between Chaucer and Surrey*. The moralizations of each of the two tales of the *Gesta Romanorum* included in the *Series* are in prose.

3. Burrow, "Autobiographical Poetry," 403; Simpson, "Nobody's Man," 158.

4. Burrow, *Thomas Hoccleve*, 215.

5. Hoccleve "did not come to the Exchequer personally between May 1414 and March 1417 to collect payments due to him." Brown, "The Privy Seal Clerks in the Early Fifteenth Century."

6. On the autobiographical qualities of the poem, see Burrow, "Autobiographical Poetry."

7. Burrow, "Hoccleve's *Series*," 266; Simpson, "Madness and Texts," 16; Knapp, *The Bureaucratic Muse*, 161; Watt, "'I this book shal make,'" 134; Spearing, *Medieval Autographies*, 178.

8. After its two-part autobiographical frame, the *Series* is constituted by three translated works: two tales from the *Gesta Romanorum* and a portion of Henry Suso's *Horologium Sapientiae*. Framing "links," like those in the *Canterbury Tales*, precede each of the two tales from the *Gesta Romanorum*. The collection concludes with a dedication to the Countess of Westmoreland in one (holograph) manuscript, Durham University Library, Cosin MS V iii 9.

9. Spearing, *Textual Subjectivity*, 13, emphasis original.

10. Hoccleve, *Regiment of Princes*, line 217.

11. See Lerer, *Chaucer and His Readers* and Lawton, "Dullness and the Fifteenth Century."

12. Patterson, "What Is Me?" 84, 86, 85.

13. Knapp, *The Bureaucratic Muse*, 166.

14. Simpson, "Madness and Texts," 24.

15. Knapp, *The Bureaucratic Muse*, 175.

16. *MED*, s.v. "fōlĭe" (n.) 3.

17. *MED*, s.v. "tāsten" (v.) 4.

18. Rigg, "Hoccleve's *Complaint* and Isidore of Seville"; Burrow, "Hoccleve's *Complaint* and Isidore of Seville Again."

19. Lawton, "Voice After Arundel," 141–44.

20. Burrow, "Hoccleve's *Complaint* and Isidore of Seville Again," 428.

21. Hoccleve, *Regiment of Princes*, lines 1961–62.

22. Hoccleve, *Regiment of Princes*, line 1963.

23. For instance, see Burrow, "Hoccleve's *Series*," 261 and Knapp, *The Bureaucratic Muse*, 165 and the sources noted there.

24. Chaucerian quotations drawn from *Canterbury Tales* I.1–11, in *Riverside Chaucer*.

25. *Canterbury Tales* I.19–24, in *Riverside Chaucer*.

26. *Canterbury Tales* I.25–26, in *Riverside Chaucer*.

27. For powerful accounts of this effect, see Burrow, "Hoccleve's *Series*," 262–64 and Simpson, "Madness and Texts," 19–20.

28. Burrow, "Hoccleve's *Series*," 262.

29. Doob, *Nebuchadnezzar's Children*, 230.

30. Goldie, "Psychosomatic Illness and Identity," 48.

31. Knapp, *The Bureaucratic Muse*, 179.

32. Burrow, "Autobiographical Poetry," 403.

33. This appears in Ellis's note for lines 638–41 in Hoccleve, *"My Compleinte" and Other Poems*.

34. Watt, *The Making of Thomas Hoccleve's "Series,"* 2.

35. *Troilus and Criseyde* I.1065–71, in *Riverside Chaucer*.

36. Strengthening the likelihood that a Chaucerian reference was intentional on Hoccleve's part is the fact that the *Troilus* is the work by Chaucer most frequently cited by fifteenth-century poets; see Lawton, "Dullness and the Fifteenth Century," 780.

37. *Canterbury Tales* III.662–63, in *Riverside Chaucer*.

38. Quotations drawn from *Canterbury Tales* I.725–36, in *Riverside Chaucer*.

39. "What is this world? What asketh men to have?" (*Canterbury Tales* I.2777, in *Riverside Chaucer*).

40. Winstead, "'I am al othir to yow than yee weene,'" 145.

41. For extensive demonstration, see Watt, *The Making of Thomas Hoccleve's "Series."*

CHAPTER 8

1. Quotes from, respectively, Fanous, "Measuring the Pilgrim's Progress," 171; Windeatt, introduction, 10; Watson, "The Making of *The Book of Margery Kempe*," 425; Ross, "Oral Life, Written Text," 236.

2. For a wide-ranging reflection, see Lawton, *Voice in Later Medieval English Literature*.

3. I refer to Margery Kempe largely by her first name, in agreement with Sarah Salih's reasoning in *Versions of Virginity in Late Medieval England*: "The advantages of using the name 'Kempe' are that it avoids the risk of patronizing familiarity. . . . It is, however, Margery's married

name, and the *Book* makes very clear that she is something other than John Kempe's wife. When the character is addressed by name in the book, it is usually as 'Margery.'. . . Referring to women writers by their Christian names is anyway more usual, and so less patronizing, in a medieval context" (173).

4. For an up-to-date reconsideration of the *Book*'s textual production, see Sobecki, "'The writyng of this tretys.'"

5. Certeau, "Mystic Speech," 90–91. Certeau's analysis treats postmedieval texts, which were written once the term *mysticism* came to name and organize a specific field of discourse in the sixteenth century. Nonetheless, his ideas provide useful heuristics for interpreting late medieval visionary writings.

6. Lochrie, *Margery Kempe and Translations of the Flesh*, 62.

7. Kempe, *Book of Margery Kempe*, ed. Staley, book 1, chap. 77. Henceforth, I cite Staley's edition in the body of the text by book and chapter number.

8. See Robertson, "Medieval Medical Views of Women and Female Spirituality."

9. Beckwith, "A Very Material Mysticism," 37.

10. Freud, *Beyond the Pleasure Principle*.

11. Translation cited from Kempe, *Book of Margery Kempe*, trans. Windeatt, 104. Henceforth, I cite Windeatt's translation (with occasional adjustments), in-text by page number.

12. See Bal, *Narratology*, 142–61.

13. Salih, "Margery's Bodies," 173.

14. Watson, "The Making of *The Book of Margery Kempe*," 404.

15. Windeatt notes the *Book*'s consistent distinction between crying and weeping; see Kempe, *Book of Margery Kempe*, trans. Windeatt, 313n8.

16. For a useful discussion, see Voaden, *God's Words, Women's Voices*, 127n61.

17. However, in chapter 62, the *Book* does cite several authorizing antecedents for her cries. For further discussion, see Ellis, "Margery Kempe's Scribe and the Miraculous Books." Angela of Foligno would offer another possible model for Margery's crying, though there is no evidence that Angela or her *Liber de vere fidelium experientia* was familiar to Margery.

18. Watson, "The Making of *The Book of Margery Kempe*," 416.

19. See Irvine, *The Making of Textual Culture*, 93–94.

20. For "iterative" and "singulative," see Genette, *Narrative Discourse*, 114–17.

21. Voaden (*God's Words, Women's Voices*, 112) links the *Book*'s generic hybridity with the "unruly, unconventional nature of the text": "In general hagiographic texts and books of revelations represented the visionary or saint according to well-established models. . . . The *Book of Margery Kempe*, in marked contrast, does not present a carefully edited seamless structure, conforming to a prototype of hagiography or visionary narrative." Sarah Salih remarks that the *Book* is original "in its combination of apparently incompatible models" (*Versions of Virginity in Late Medieval England*, 187).

22. Salih, *Versions of Virginity in Late Medieval England*, 187.

23. Hollywood, *The Soul as Virgin Wife*, 31.

24. For a general account of the situation sketched here, see Mooney, "Voice, Gender, and the Portrayal of Sanctity." Also see Bynum, "The Female Body and Religious Practice in the Later Middle Ages," in *Fragmentation and Redemption*.

25. John Hirsch defines paramystical phenomena to be "on the boundaries between mysticism and devotion": "For the person caught up in paramystical experience, Christ speaks not only to him, but also through him." See Hirsch, *The Revelations of Margery Kempe*, 19.

26. Elliott, *Proving Woman*, 3.

27. Caciola, *Discerning Spirits*, 2. On the discernment of spirits, also see Voaden, *God's Words, Women's Voices* and Elliott, *Proving Woman*.

28. See Voaden, *God's Words, Women's Voices*, 42 and passim.

29. Testifying to the early recognition of a connection between the *Book of Margery Kempe* and the English *discretio* tradition, Henry Pepwell in 1521 printed the "Pistle of Discrecioun of Stirings," the "Tretis of Discrecyon of Spirites," and excerpts from Hilton alongside selections from Margery's *Book*. See Gardner, introduction to *The Cell of Self-Knowledge*.

30. Beckwith, "Problems of Authority," 192, emphasis original.

31. Salih, "Margery's Bodies," 173.

32. Dillon, "Holy Women and Their Confessors," 134.

33. See Orlemanski, "Margery's 'Noyse' and Distributed Expressivity."

34. For a generative account, see Cohen, *Medieval Identity Machines*, esp. chap. 5, "The Becoming-Liquid of Margery Kempe."

35. Certeau, "Mystic Speech," 91.

36. Salih, "Margery's Bodies," 174.

37. Watson, "The Making of *The Book of Margery Kempe*," 424.

38. Voaden, *God's Words, Women's Voices*, 119.

39. Salih, "Margery's Bodies," 173.

40. Uhlman, "The Comfort of Voice, the Solace of Script," 63.

41. See, for instance, Kempe, *Book of Margery Kempe*, ed. Staley, I.24, I.33, I.61, and I.83.

42. Hope Emily Allen draws attention to a note in the manuscript indicating that this friar may be the Franciscan preacher William Melton. See Kempe, *Book of Margery Kempe*, ed. Meech, 321, note 148/28–29.

43. Elliott, *Proving Woman*, 249.

44. Certeau, "Mystic Speech," 92, emphasis original.

45. Certeau, "Mystic Speech," 93, 92.

46. Lawton, "Voice, Authority, and Blasphemy," 101.

47. Lawton, "Voice, Authority, and Blasphemy," 101.

48. Watson observes that "it would have been for the people of Lynn that the *Book* was initially written, with the help of a priestly scribe qualified to produce an exemplar for future copyists in the town's dialect" ("The Making of *The Book of Margery Kempe*," 425).

49. Salih, *Versions of Virginity in Late Medieval England*, 180.

50. Evans, "The Book of Margery Kempe," 509.

51. Erskine, "Margery Kempe and Her Models," 82.

52. Johnson, "Trope of the Scribe," 837.

53. Riddy, "Text and Self in *The Book of Margery Kempe*," 442.

54. Kempe, *Book of Margery Kempe*, ed. Meech, vii.

55. I have found the strongest version of this argument to be that of Watson, "The Making of *The Book of Margery Kempe*." Lynn Staley (formerly, Lynn Staley Johnson) has influentially argued that the scribe may be just a rhetorical device used by the author Margery Kempe to bolster the *Book*'s credibility: "I would like to be able to say that the scribe never existed, that Margery Kempe created him, but I can say that in terms of the shape and function of the *Book*, its author needed a scribe, even a succession of scribes as witnesses and mediators who could authorize the text." See Johnson, "Trope of the Scribe," 837; also see Staley, *Margery Kempe's Dissenting Fictions*.

56. See Hirsch, "Author and Scribe in the *Book of Margery Kempe*" and Spearing, "Margery Kempe."

57. Riddy, "Text and Self in *The Book of Margery Kempe*," 435. Also see Evans, "The Book of Margery Kempe" and Sobecki, "'The writyng of this tretys.'"

58. Sarah Salih writes, "While I would not argue that the *Book* is an accurate historical record, I think it is important to acknowledge that it claims to be" (*Versions of Virginity in Late Medieval England*, 171). I take the phrase "literacy event" from Riddy, "Text and Self in *The Book of Margery Kempe*," 438.

59. Critten, *Author, Scribe, and Book in Late Medieval English Literature*, 83.

CODA

1. For an overview, see Bynum, "Why All the Fuss About the Body?" and Porter, "History of the Body Reconsidered." For an essay collection important to Middle English studies, see Kay and Rubin, *Framing Medieval Bodies*. For a more recent engagement, see Akbari and Ross, *The Ends of the Body*.

2. Hartnell, "Wording the Wound Man."

3. See especially Kerwin, *Beyond the Body*.

Works Cited

Abrahams, P. "The Mercator-Scenes in the Mediaeval French Passion-Plays." *Medium Aevum* 3 (1934): 112–23.

Aers, David. *Chaucer, Langland and the Creative Imagination.* London: Routledge and Kegan Paul, 1980.

Agrimi, J., and C. Crisciani. "Per una ricerca su *experimentum-experimenta*: Riflessione epistemologica e tradizione medica (secoli XIII–XV)." In *Presenza del lessico Greco e Latino nelle lingue contemporanee*, ed. P. Janni and I. Mazzini, 9–49. Macerata: Università degli studi di Macerata, 1990.

Aiken, Pauline. "The Summoner's Malady." *Studies in Philology* 33 (1936): 40–44.

Akbari, Suzanne Conklin, and Jill Ross, eds. *The Ends of the Body: Identity and Community in Medieval Culture.* Toronto: University of Toronto Press, 2013.

Amis and Amiloun, Robert of Cisyle, and Sir Amadace. Ed. Edward E. Foster. Kalamazoo, MI: Medieval Institute Publications, 2007.

Amundsen, Darrel W. "The Medieval Catholic Tradition." In *Caring and Curing: Health and Medicine in the Western Religious Traditions*, ed. Ronald L. Numbers and Darrel W. Amundsen, 65–107. New York: Macmillan, 1986.

Ancrene Wisse: A Corrected Edition of the Text in Cambridge, Corpus Christi College, MS 402, with Variants from Other Manuscripts. Vol. 1. Ed. Bella Millett, EETS o.s. 325. Oxford: Oxford University Press, 2005.

Anglo-Norman Medicine. 2 vols. Ed. Tony Hunt. Woodbridge: D. S. Brewer, 1994–97.

Antonius of Florence. Excerpt from *Summa Theologica.* Trans. Faith Wallis. In *Medieval Medicine: A Reader*, ed. and trans. Faith Wallis, 437–45. Toronto: University of Toronto Press, 2010.

Arderne, John. *Treatises of Fistula in Ano, Hæmorrhoids, and Clysters.* Ed. D'Arcy Power, EETS o.s. 139. London: Kegan Paul, Trench, Trübner, and Co., 1910.

Aristotle. *Analytica posteriora.* Trans. William of Moerbeke (revising James of Venice). *Aristoteles Latinus Database 3.* Turnhout: Brepols, 2017.

———. *Aristotle's Metaphysics.* Ed and trans. W. D. Ross. Oxford: Clarendon Press, 1953.

———. *Metaphysica: Libri I–X; XII–XIII.2 (translationis "mediae" recensio).* Trans. William of Moerbeke. *Aristoteles Latinus Database 3.* Turnhout: Brepols, 2017.

Arnau of Vilanova. *Repetitio super aphorismo Hippocratus "Vita brevis."* Ed. Michael R. McVaugh. In *Arnaldi de Villanova Opera medica omnia.* Vol. 14. Barcelona: Universitat de Barcelona, 2014.

Arrizabalaga, Jon. "Facing the Black Death: Perceptions and Reactions of University Medical Practitioners." In *Practical Medicine from Salerno to the Black Death*, ed. Luis García-Ballester,

Roger French, Jon Arrizabalaga, and Andrew Cunningham, 237–88. Cambridge: Cambridge University Press, 1994.

Astell, Ann W. "Memorial Technai, St. Thomas the Twin, and British Library Additional MS 220." In *The Arma Christi in Medieval and Early Modern Material Culture*, ed. Lisa H. Cooper and Andrea Denny-Brown, 171–202. Aldershot: Ashgate, 2014.

Aswell, E. Duncan. "The Role of Fortune in *The Testament of Cresseid*." *Philological Quarterly* 46 (1967): 471–87.

Augustine. *The City of God Against the Pagans*. Ed. and trans. R. W. Dyson. Cambridge: Cambridge University Press, 1998.

———. *De doctrina christiana*. In *Patrologia Latina*. Vol. 34.

———. Sermon 277. *Sermons (273–305A) on the Saints*. Volume III/8 of *The Works of Saint Augustine* (4th release). Electronic ed. Charlottesville, VA: InteLex Corporation, 2014.

Avicenna (Ibn Sina). Excerpt from the *Canon*. Trans. O. Cameron Gruner and Michael McVaugh. In *A Source Book in Medieval Science*, ed. Edward Grant, 715–20. Cambridge, MA: Harvard University Press, 1974.

Bacon, Roger. *De retardatione accidentium senectutis, cum aliis opusculis de rebus medicinalibus*. Ed. A. G. Little and E. Withington. Oxford: Clarendon Press, 1928.

———. *De signis*. Ed. and trans. K. M. Fredborg, Lauge Nielsen, and Jan Pinborg. In "An Unedited Part of Roger Bacon's 'Opus maius': 'De signis.'" *Traditio* 34 (1978): 75–136.

———. "The Errors of the Doctors According to Friar Roger Bacon of the Minor Order." Trans. Mary Catherine Welborn. *Isis* 18 (1932): 26–62.

———. *Opera hactenus inedita Rogeri Baconi*. Vol. 5. Ed. Robert Steele. Oxonii: E typographeo Clarendoniano, 1920.

Bahr, Arthur. *Fragments and Assemblages: Forming Compilations of Medieval London*. Chicago: University of Chicago Press, 2013.

Bakhtin, M. M. *The Dialogic Imagination: Four Essays*. Trans. Caryl Emerson and Michael Holquist. Austin: University of Texas Press, 1981.

Bal, Mieke. *Narratology: Introduction to the Theory of Narrative*. 2nd ed. Toronto: University of Toronto Press, 1997.

Bartholomaeus Anglicus and John Trevisa. *On the Properties of Things: John Trevisa's Translation of Bartholomaeus Anglicus De Proprietatibus Rerum: A Critical Text*. 3 vols. Ed. M. C. Seymour. Oxford: Clarendon Press, 1975.

Beck, R. Theodore. *The Cutting Edge: Early History of the Surgeons of London*. London: Lund Humphries, 1974.

Beckwith, Sarah. "Problems of Authority in Late Medieval English Mysticism: Language, Agency, and Authority in *The Book of Margery Kempe*." *Exemplaria* 4 (1992): 171–99.

———. "Ritual, Church and Theatre: Medieval Dramas of the Sacramental Body." In *Culture and History, 1350–1600: Essays on English Communities, Identities and Writing*, ed. David Aers, 65–89. Detroit: Wayne State University Press, 1992.

———. "A Very Material Mysticism: The Medieval Mysticism of Margery Kempe." In *Medieval Literature: History, Criticism, and Ideology*, ed. David Aers, 34–57. Brighton: Harvester Press, 1986.

Bernard of Gordon. *Practica seu lilium medicinae*. Italy, 1486. *Gallica*. http://gallica.bnf.fr/ark:/12148/bpt6k58673s.

Beullens, Pieter. "Burgundio of Pisa." In *Medieval Science, Technology, and Medicine: An Encyclopedia*, ed. Thomas F. Glick, Steven J. Livesey, and Faith Wallis, 104–5. New York: Routledge, 2005.

Bishop, Louise M. *Words, Stones, and Herbs: The Healing Word in Medieval and Early Modern England*. Syracuse, NY: Syracuse University Press, 2007.

Blake, Kathleen A. "Order and the Noble Life in Chaucer's *Knight's Tale?*" *Modern Language Quarterly* 34 (1973): 3–19.

Boccaccio, Giovanni. *The Book of Theseus/Teseida delle nozzed'Emilia*. Trans. Bernadette Marie McCoy. New York: Medieval Text Association, 1974.

———. *Teseida: Edizione Critica*. Ed. Salvatore Battaglia. Florence: G. C. Sansoni, 1938.

Boitani, Piero. *Chaucer and Boccaccio*. Oxford: Society for the Study of Mediaeval Languages and Literature, 1977.

Bonser, Wilfrid. *The Medical Background of Anglo-Saxon England: A Study in History, Psychology, and Folklore*. London: Wellcome Historical Medical Library, 1963.

Bower, Hannah. "Similes We Cure By: The Poetics of Late Medieval Medical Texts." *New Medieval Literatures* 18 (2018): 183–210.

Bowes, John M. "Three Readings of *The Knight's Tale*: Sir John Clanvowe, Geoffrey Chaucer, and James I of Scotland." *Journal of Medieval and Early Modern Studies* 34 (2004): 279–307.

Bremond, Claude, Jacques Le Goff, and Jean-Claude Schmitt. *L'"Exemplum."* Turnhout: Brepols, 1982.

Brenner, Elma. "Recent Perspectives on Leprosy in Medieval Western Europe." *History Compass* 8, no. 5 (2010): 388–406.

Bright, Philippa. "Anglo-Latin Collections of the *Gesta Romanorum* and Their Role in the Cure of Souls." In *What Nature Does Not Teach: Didactic Literature in the Medieval and Early-Modern Periods*, ed. Juanita Feros Ruys, 401–24. Turnhout: Brepols, 2008.

Brody, Saul Nathaniel. *The Disease of the Soul: Leprosy in Medieval Literature*. Ithaca, NY: Cornell University Press, 1974.

Brown, A. L. "The Privy Seal Clerks in the Early Fifteenth Century." In *The Study of Medieval Records: Essays in Honour of Kathleen Major*, ed. D. A. Bullough and R. L. Storey, 260–81. Oxford: Oxford University Press, 1971.

Burlin, Robert B. *Chaucerian Fiction*. Princeton, NJ: Princeton University Press, 1977.

Burnett, Charles. "Gerard of Cremona." In *Medieval Science, Technology, and Medicine: An Encyclopedia*, ed. Thomas F. Glick, Steven J. Livesey, and Faith Wallis, 191–92. New York: Routledge, 2005.

Burrow, John A. "Autobiographical Poetry in the Middle Ages: The Case of Thomas Hoccleve." *Proceedings of the British Academy* 68 (1982): 389–412.

———. "Hoccleve's *Complaint* and Isidore of Seville Again." *Speculum* 73 (1998): 424–28.

———. "Hoccleve's *Series*: Experience and Books." In *Fifteenth-Century Studies: Recent Essays*, ed. Robert F. Yeager, 259–73. Hamden: Archon Books, 1984.

———. *Thomas Hoccleve*. Aldershot: Ashgate, 1994.

Bylebyl, Jerome J. "The Medical Meaning of *Physica*." *Osiris* 6 (1990): 16–41.

Bynum, Caroline Walker. *Fragmentation and Redemption: Essays on Gender and the Human Body in Medieval Religion*. New York: Zone Books, 1991.

———. *Holy Feast and Holy Fast: The Religious Significance of Food to Medieval Women*. Berkeley: University of California Press, 1987.

———. *The Resurrection of the Body in Western Christianity: 200–1336*. New York: Columbia University Press, 1995.

———. "Why All the Fuss About the Body? A Medievalist's Perspective." *Critical Inquiry* 22 (1995): 1–33.

Caciola, Nancy. *Discerning Spirits: Divine and Demonic Possession in the Middle Ages.* Ithaca, NY: Cornell University Press, 2003.

Cadden, Joan. *The Meanings of Sex Difference in the Middle Ages: Medicine, Science, and Culture.* New York: Cambridge University Press, 1993.

Calendar of Plea and Memoranda Rolls Preserved Among the Archives of the Corporation of the City of London at the Guildhall AD. 1413–1437. Vol. 4. Ed. A. H. Thomas. Cambridge: Cambridge University Press, 1943.

Cameron, M. L. *Anglo-Saxon Medicine.* Cambridge: Cambridge University Press, 1993.

Cannon, Christopher. *The Making of Chaucer's English: A Study of Words.* Cambridge: Cambridge University Press, 1998.

Cant, P. A. "Thesaurus Pauperum: An Edition of B.M., M.S. Sloane 3489, a Fifteenth Century Medical Miscellany, with Introduction, Notes and Glossary." PhD diss., University of London, 1973.

Carey, Hilary M. "What Is the Folded Almanac? The Form and Function of a Key Manuscript Source for Astro-Medical Practice in Later Medieval England." *Social History of Medicine* 16 (2003): 481–509.

Carlino, Andrea. "Petrarch and the Early Modern Critics of Medicine." *Journal of Medieval and Early Modern Studies* 35, no. 3 (2005): 559–82.

Carmichael, Ann G. "Universal and Particular: The Language of Plague, 1348–1500." *Medical History: Supplement* 27 (2008): 17–52.

Certeau, Michel de. "Mystic Speech." In *Heterologies: Discourse on the Other*, trans. Brian Massumi, 80–100, 244–50. Theory and History of Literature 17. Minneapolis: University of Minnesota Press, 1986.

Chambers, E. K. *The English Folk-Play.* Oxford: Clarendon Press, 1933.

Chaucer, Geoffrey. *The Riverside Chaucer.* Ed. Larry D. Benson. 3rd ed. Boston: Houghton Mifflin, 1987.

Chrétien de Troyes. *Cligès.* Ed. Charles Méla and Olivier Collet. Paris: Le Livre de Poche, 1994.

———. *Cligès.* Trans. Burton Raffel. New Haven: Yale University Press, 1997.

Cicero, Marco Tullius. *De inventione; De optimo genere oratorum; Topica.* Trans. H. M. Hubbell. Cambridge, MA: Harvard University Press, 1949.

Citrome, Jeremy. *The Surgeon in Medieval English Literature.* New York: Palgrave, 2006.

Cohen, Jeffrey Jerome. *Medieval Identity Machines.* Minneapolis: University of Minnesota Press, 2003.

Comrie, John D. *History of Scottish Medicine.* 2nd ed. 2 vols. London: Baillière, Tindall & Cox, 1932.

Cooper, Helen F. *Oxford Guides to Chaucer: The Canterbury Tales.* 2nd ed. Oxford: Oxford University Press, 1996.

Cooper, Lisa H. "The Poetics of Practicality." In *Oxford Twenty-First Century Approaches to Literature: Middle English*, ed. Paul Strohm, 491–505. Oxford: Oxford University Press, 2007.

Critten, Rory G. *Author, Scribe, and Book in Late Medieval English Literature.* Cambridge: D. S. Brewer, 2018.

Croxton Play of the Sacrament. Ed. John T. Sebastian. Kalamazoo, MI: Medieval Institute Publications, 2012.

Currie, George. "Narrative Representation of Causes." *Journal of Aesthetics and Art Criticism* 64 (2006): 309–16.

Curry, Walter Clyde. *Chaucer and the Mediaeval Sciences.* New York: Oxford University Press, 1926.

Decrees of the Ecumenical Councils. 2 vols. Ed. Norman P. Tanner. London: Sheed & Ward, 1990.

Demaitre, Luke. "The Description and Diagnosis of Leprosy by Fourteenth-Century Physicians." *Bulletin of the History of Medicine* 59 (1985): 327–44.

———. *Leprosy in Premodern Medicine: A Malady of the Whole Body.* Baltimore: Johns Hopkins University Press, 2009.

———. *Medieval Medicine: The Art of Healing, from Head to Toe.* Santa Barbara, CA: Praeger, 2013.

Dillon, Janette. "Holy Women and Their Confessors or Confessors and Their Holy Women? Margery Kempe and Continental Tradition." In *Prophets Abroad: The Reception of Continental Holy Women in Late Medieval England*, ed. Rosalynn Voaden, 115–40. Cambridge: D. S. Brewer, 1996.

Dives and Pauper. Vol. 1. Pt. 1. Ed. Priscilla Heath Barnum, EETS o.s. 275. London: Oxford University Press, 1976.

Donaldson, E. Talbot. "Criseide and Her Narrator." In *Speaking of Chaucer*, 65–83. New York: Norton, 1970.

Doob, Penelope B. R. *Nebuchadnezzar's Children: Conventions of Madness in Middle English Literature.* New Haven, CT: Yale University Press, 1974.

Dronke, Peter. "The Song of Songs and Medieval Love-Lyric." In *The Bible and Medieval Culture*, ed. W. Lourdaux and D. Verhelst, 237–62. Leuven: Leuven University Press, 1979.

Dunai, Amber. "'And Doolie Sessoun' and 'Ane Cairfull Dyte': Cresseid and the Narrator in Henryson's *Testament of Cresseid*." *Chaucer Review* 50 (2015): 420–41.

Early English Versions of the Gesta Romanorum. Ed. Sidney Herrtage, EETS e.s. 33. London: N. Trubner, 1987.

Edwards, A. S. G. "Lydgate Manuscripts: Some Directions for Future Research." In *Manuscripts and Readers in Fifteenth-Century England: The Literary Implications of Manuscript Study*, ed. Derek Pearsall, 15–26. Woodbridge: D. S. Brewer, 1983.

Elliott, Dyan. *Proving Woman: Female Spirituality and Inquisitional Culture in the Later Middle Ages.* Princeton, NJ: Princeton University Press, 2004.

Ellis, Roger. "Margery Kempe's Scribe and the Miraculous Books." In *Langland, the Mystics, and the Medieval English Religious Tradition: Essays in Honour of S. S. Hussey*, ed. Helen Phillips, 161–75. Cambridge: D. S. Brewer, 1990.

English Metrical Homilies. Ed. John Small. Edinburgh: William Patterson, 1862.

Erskine, John A. "Margery Kempe and Her Models: The Role of the Authorial Voice." *Mystics Quarterly* 15, no. 2 (1989): 75–85.

Evans, Ruth. "The Book of Margery Kempe." In *A Companion to Medieval English Literature and Culture c. 1350–c. 1500*, ed. Peter Brown, 507–21. Malden, MA: Blackwell, 2007.

Fanous, Samuel. "Measuring the Pilgrim's Progress: Internal Emphases in *The Book of Margery Kempe*." In *Writing Religious Women: Female Spiritual and Textual Practices in Late Medieval England*, ed. Denis Renevey and Christiania Whitehead, 157–78. Toronto: University of Toronto Press, 2000.

Farmer, Sharon. "The Leper in the Master Bedroom: Thinking Through a Thirteenth-Century Exemplum." In *Framing the Family: Narrative and Representation in the Medieval and Early Modern Periods*, ed. Rosalynn Voaden and Diane Wolfthal, 79–100. Tempe: Arizona Center for Medieval and Renaissance Studies, 2005.

Finucane, Ronald C. *Miracles and Pilgrims: Popular Beliefs in Medieval England.* New York: St. Martin's Press, 1995.

Forster, E. M. *Aspects of the Novel.* New York: Harcourt, 1927.

Förster, Max. "Kleinere mittelenglische Texte." *Anglia* 42 (1918): 176–92.

Fox, Denton. "Henryson's 'Sum Practysis of Medecyne.'" *Studies in Philology* 69 (1972): 453–60.

———. Introduction to Robert Henryson, *The Poems of Robert Henryson*, ed. Denton Fox, xiii–cxxiii. Oxford: Clarendon Press, 1981.

———. Introduction to Robert Henryson, *Testament of Cresseid*, ed. Denton Fox, 1–58. London: Nelson, 1968.

Fradenburg, Louise O. "Sacrificial Desire in Chaucer's *Knight's Tale*." *Journal of Medieval and Early Modern Studies* 27 (1997): 47–75.

Freud, Sigmund. *Beyond the Pleasure Principle*. 1920. Ed. and trans. James Strachey. New York: Norton, 1989.

Fumo, Jamie C. "The Pestilential Gaze: From Epidemiology to Erotomania in *The Knight's Tale*." *Studies in the Age of Chaucer* 35 (2013): 85–136.

Garbáty, Thomas J. "The Summoner's Occupational Disease." *Medical History* 7 (1963): 348–58.

Gardner, Edmund G. Introduction to *The Cell of Self-Knowledge: Seven Early English Mystical Treatises*, ed. Edmund G. Gardner, xi–xxvii. New York: Cooper Square Publishers, 1966.

Garrett, Robert Max. "Middle English Rimed Medical Treatise." *Anglia* 34 (1911): 163–93.

Gascoigne, Thomas. *Loci e Libro veritatum: Passages Selected from Gascoigne's Theological Dictionary Illustrating the Condition of Church and State*. Oxford: Clarendon Press, 1881.

Gasse, Roseanne. "The Practice of Medicine in *Piers Plowman*." *Chaucer Review* 39 (2004): 177–97.

Genette, Gérard. *Narrative Discourse: An Essay in Method*. Trans. Jane E. Lewin. Ithaca, NY: Cornell University Press, 1980.

Getz, Faye Marie. "Charity, Translation, and the Language of Medical Learning in Medieval England." *Bulletin of the History Medicine* 64 (1990): 1–17.

———. "The Faculty of Medicine Before 1500." In *The History of the University of Oxford: Late Medieval Oxford*. Vol. 2, ed. J. I. Catto and Ralph Evans, 373–405. Oxford: Clarendon Press, 1992.

———. "Medical Education in Later Medieval England." In *The History of Medical Education in Britain*, ed. V. Nutton and R. Porter, 76–93. Amsterdam: Rodopi, 1995.

———. *Medicine in the English Middle Ages*. Princeton, NJ: Princeton University Press, 1988.

Gillespie, Vincent. "The Study of Classical Authors, from the Twelfth Century to c. 1450." In *The Cambridge History of Literary Criticism*, vol. 2, *The Middle Ages*, ed. Alastair Minnis and Ian Johnson, 142–236. Cambridge: Cambridge University Press, 2005.

Godden, Richard, and Jonathan Hsy. "Analytical Survey: Encountering Disability in the Middle Ages." *New Medieval Literatures* 15 (2013): 313–39.

Goldie, Matthew Boyd. "Psychosomatic Illness and Identity in London, 1416–1421: Hoccleve's Complaint and Dialogue with a Friend." *Exemplaria* 11 (1999): 23–52.

Goldstein, R. James. "Writing in Scotland, 1058–1560." In *The Cambridge History of Medieval English Literature: Writing in Britain, 1066–1547*, ed. David Wallace, 229–54. Cambridge: Cambridge University Press, 1999.

Gray, Douglas. *Robert Henryson*. Leiden: Brill, 1979.

Green, Monica H. "Bodily Essences: Bodies as Categories of Difference." In *A Cultural History of the Human Body in the Middle Ages*, ed. Linda Kalof, 149–72, 264–68. Oxford: Berg, 2010.

———. "The Diversity of Human Kind." In *A Cultural History of the Human Body in the Middle Ages*, ed. Linda Kalof, 173–90, 268–71. Oxford: Berg, 2010.

———. "The Possibilities of Literacy and the Limits of Reading: Women and the Gendering of Medical Literacy." In *Women's Healthcare in the Medieval West*, ed. Monica Green, 1–71. Aldershot, Hampshire: Ashgate, 2000.

———. "Salerno on the Thames: The Genesis of Anglo-Norman Medical Literature." In *Language and Culture in Medieval Britain: The French of England, c. 1100–c. 1500*, ed. Jocelyn Wogan-Browne, 220–32. Woodbridge: York Medieval, 2013.

———. "Women's Medical Practice and Health Care in Medieval Europe." In *Sisters and Workers in the Middle Ages*, ed. J. Bennett et al., 39–78. Chicago: University of Chicago Press, 1989.

Green, Richard Firth. *A Crisis of Truth: Literature and Law in Ricardian England*. Philadelphia: University of Pennsylvania Press, 1999.

Grigsby, Bryon Lee. *Pestilence in Medieval and Early Modern English Literature*. New York: Routledge, 2004.

Grothé, Richard. "Le Ms. Wellcome 564: Deux Traites de Chirurgie en Moyen-Anglais." PhD diss., Université de Montréal, 1984.

Guy de Chauliac. *The Cyrurgie of Guy de Chauliac*, vol. 1, Text. Ed. Margaret S. Ogden, EETS o.s. 265. London: Oxford University Press, 1971.

Ham, Edward B. "The Rutebeuf Guide for Medieval Salescraft." *Studies in Philology* 47 (1950): 20–34.

Hammond, E. P. *English Verse Between Chaucer and Surrey*. Durham, NC: Duke University Press, 1927.

Hanna, Ralph III. "Cresseid's Dream and Henryson's *Testament*." In *Chaucer and Middle English Studies, in Honor of Rossell Hope Robbins*, ed. Beryl Rowland, 288–97. London: Allen and Unwin, 1974.

Harley, M. P. "The Middle English Contents of a Fifteenth-Century Medical Book." *Mediaevalia* 8 (1982): 171–88.

Hartnell, Jack. "Wording the Wound Man." *British Art Studies* 6 (2017). http://dx.doi.org/10.17658/issn.2058-5462/issue-06/jhartnell.

Heng, Geraldine. "The Invention of Race in the European Middle Ages II: Locations of Medieval Race." *Literature Compass* 8 (2011): 332–50.

Henri de Mondeville. *Die Chirurgie des Heinrich von Mondeville*. Ed. Julius Pagel. Berlin: Hirschwald, 1892.

Henry, Duke of Lancaster. *The Book of Holy Medicines*. Trans. Catherine Batt. Tempe: Arizona Center for Medieval and Renaissance Studies, 2014.

———. *Le Livre de Seyntz Medicines*. Ed. E. J. Arnould. Anglo-Norman Texts II. Oxford: Basil Blackwell, 1940.

Henryson, Robert. *The Poems of Robert Henryson*. Ed. Denton Fox. Oxford: Clarendon Press, 1981.

———. *The Poems of Robert Henryson*. Ed. Robert L. Kindrick. Kalamazoo, MI: Medieval Institute Publications, 1997.

———. *Robert Henryson: The Complete Works*. Ed. David J. Parkinson. Kalamazoo, MI: Medieval Institute Publications, 2010.

Hirsch, John C. "Author and Scribe in the *Book of Margery Kempe*." *Medium Aevum* 44 (1975): 145–50.

———. *The Revelations of Margery Kempe: Paramystical Practices in Late Medieval England*. Leiden: Brill, 1989.

Hoccleve, Thomas. *"My Compleinte" and Other Poems: Thomas Hoccleve*. Ed. Roger Ellis. Exeter: University of Exeter Press, 2001.

———. *The Regiment of Princes*. Ed. Charles R. Blyth. Kalamazoo, MI: Medieval Institute Publications, 1999.

Hoeniger, Robert. *Der schwarze Tod in Deutschland: Ein Beitrag zur Geschichte des vierzehnten Jahrhunderts*. Berlin: Grosser, 1882.

Hollywood, Amy. *The Soul as Virgin Wife: Mechthild of Magdeburg, Marguerite Porete, and Meister Eckhart*. Notre Dame, IN: University of Notre Dame Press, 1995.

Holmes, Brooke. *The Symptom and the Subject: The Emergence of the Physical Body in Ancient Greece*. Princeton, NJ: Princeton University Press, 2010.

Horrox, Rosemary, ed. and trans. *The Black Death*. Manchester: Manchester University Press, 1994.

Hsy, Jonathan. "Disability." In *The Cambridge Companion to the Body in Literature*, ed. David Hillman and Ulrika Maude, 24–40. Cambridge: Cambridge University Press, 2015.

Hunt, Tony. *Plant Names of Medieval England*. Cambridge: D. S. Brewer, 1989.

———. "The Poetic Vein: Phlebotomy in Middle English and Anglo-Norman Verse." *English Studies* 77, no. 4 (1996): 311–22.

Imbach, Ruedi, and Iñigo Atucha, ed. and trans. *Amours plurielles. Doctrines médiévales du rapport amoureux de Bernard de Clairvaux à Boccace*. Paris: Éditions du Seuil, 2006.

Irvine, Martin. *The Making of Textual Culture: "Grammatica" and Literary Theory, 350–1100*. Cambridge: Cambridge University Press, 1994.

Isidore of Seville. *The Etymologies of Isidore of Seville*. Trans. Stephen A. Barney et al. Cambridge: Cambridge University Press, 2006.

Jacquart, Danielle. *La Médecine médiévale dans le cadre parisien: XIVe–XVe siècle*. Paris: Fayard, 1998.

———. "Medical Scholasticism." In *Western Medical Thought from Antiquity to the Middle Ages*, ed. Mirko D. Grmek, trans. Antony Shugaar Cambridge, 197–240. Cambridge, MA: Harvard University Press, 1998.

———. "Theory, Everyday Practice, and Three Fifteenth-Century Physicians." *Osiris* 6 (1990): 140–60.

Jacquart, Danielle, and Claude Thomasset. *Sexuality and Medicine in the Middle Ages*. Trans. Matthew Adamson. Princeton, NJ: Princeton University Press, 1988.

Joannitius (Hunayn ibn Ishaq) and Constantine the African. *Isagoge*. Trans. Faith Wallis. In *Medieval Medicine: A Reader*, ed. and trans. Faith Wallis, 139–56. Toronto: University of Toronto Press, 2010.

———. "Johannicius: Isagoge ad Techne Galieni." Ed. Gregor Maurach. *Sudhoffs Archiv* 62, no. 2 (1978): 148–74.

John of Burgundy. "Treatises on Plague." Ed. Lister M. Matheson. In *Sex, Aging, and Death in a Medieval Medical Compendium*, vol. 2, ed. M. Teresa Tavormina, 569–602. Tempe: Arizona Center for Medieval and Renaissance Studies, 2006.

John Wycliffe Bible 1382. In *Textus Receptus Bibles*. http://textusreceptusbibles.com/Wycliffe.

Johnson, Lynn Staley. "The Trope of the Scribe and the Question of Literary Authority in the Works of Julian of Norwich and Margery Kempe." *Speculum* 66 (1991): 820–38.

Jones, Claire. "Discourse Communities and Medical Texts." In *Medical and Scientific Writing in Late Medieval English*, ed. Irma Taavitsainen and Päivi Pahta, 23–36. Cambridge: Cambridge University Press, 2004.

———. "Vernacular Literacy in Late Medieval England: The Example of East Anglian Medical Manuscripts." PhD diss., University of Glasgow, 2000.

Jones, Peter Murray. "Arderne, John (*b.* 1307/8, *d.* in or after 1377)." *ODNB.* Electronic ed.
———. "Argentine, John (*c.* 1443–1508)." *ODNB.* Electronic ed.
———. "Four Middle English Translations of John of Arderne." In *Latin and Vernacular: Studies in Late Medieval Texts and Manuscripts*, ed. Alastair Minnis, 61–89. Cambridge: D. S. Brewer, 1989.
———. "Harley MS 2558: A Fifteenth-Century Medical Commonplace Book." In *Manuscript Sources of Medieval Medicine: A Book of Essays*, ed. Margaret R. Schleissner, 35–54. New York: Garland, 1995.
———. "Information and Science." In *Fifteenth-Century Attitudes: Perceptions of Society in Late Medieval England*, ed. Rosemary Horrox, 97–111. Cambridge: Cambridge University Press, 1994.
———. "Medicine and Science." In *Cambridge History of the Book in Britain*, vol. 3, *1400–1557*, ed. L. Hellinga and J. B. Trapp, 433–48. Cambridge: Cambridge University Press, 2000.
———. "Staying with the Programme: Illustrated Manuscripts of John of Arderne, c. 1380–1550." *English Manuscript Studies, 1100–1700*, no. 10 (2002): 204–27.
———. "The Surgeon as Story-Teller." *Poetica* (2009): 77–91.
———. "Surgical Narrative in Middle English." *ANQ* 18, no. 3 (2005): 3–7.
Jordanus de Turre. "The Symptoms of Lepers." Trans. Michael R. McVaugh. In *A Sourcebook in Medieval Science*, ed. Edward Grant, 754–55. Cambridge, MA: Harvard University Press, 1974.
Kauffman, Corinne E. "Dame Pertelote's Parlous Parle." *Chaucer Review* (1969): 41–48.
Kay, Sarah, and Miri Rubin, eds. *Framing Medieval Bodies*. Manchester: Manchester University Press, 1994.
Kaye, Joel. *A History of Balance, 1250–1375: The Emergence of a New Model of Equilibrium and Its Impact on Thought*. Cambridge: Cambridge University Press, 2014.
Kealey, Edward J. *Medieval Medicus: A Social History of Anglo-Norman Medicine*. Baltimore: Johns Hopkins University Press, 1981.
Keiser, George R. "More Light on the Life and Milieu of Robert Thornton." *Studies in Bibliography* 36 (1983): 111–19.
———. "Robert Thornton's *Liber de Diversis Medicinis*: Text, Vocabulary, and Scribal Confusion." In *Rethinking Middle English: Linguistic and Literary Approaches*, ed. Nikolaus Ritt and Herbert Schendl, 30–41. Frankfurt: Peter Lang, 2005.
———. "Scientific, Medical, and Utilitarian Prose." In *A Companion to Middle English Prose*, ed. A. S. G. Edwards, 231–47. Cambridge: D. S. Brewer, 2004.
———. "Two Medieval Plague Treatises and Their Afterlife in Early Modern England." *Journal of the History of Medicine and Allied Sciences* 58 (2003): 292–324.
———. "Verse Introductions to Middle English Medical Treatises." *English Studies* 84 (2003): 301–17.
———. *Works of Science and Information*. A Manual of the Writings in Middle English, 1050–1500. Vol. 10. New Haven: Connecticut Academy of Arts and Sciences, 1998.
Kempe, Margery. *The Book of Margery Kempe*. Ed. Sanford Brown Meech, with notes by Hope Emily Allen. EETS o.s. 212. London: Oxford University Press, 1940.
———. *The Book of Margery Kempe*. Trans. Barry Windeatt. London: Penguin, 1985.
———. *The Book of Margery Kempe*. Ed. Lynn Staley. Kalamazoo, MI: Medieval Institute Publications, 1996. http://d.lib.rochester.edu/teams/publication/staley-the-book-of-margery-kempe.

Kerwin, William. *Beyond the Body: The Boundaries of Medicine and English Renaissance Drama*. Amherst: University of Massachusetts Press, 2005.

Kibre, Pearl. "The Faculty of Medicine at Paris, Charlatanism, and Unlicensed Medical Practices in the Later Middle Ages." *Bulletin of the History of Medicine* 27 (1953): 1–20.

Kieckhefer, Richard. "The Specific Rationality of Medieval Magic." *American Historical Review* 99 (1994): 813–36.

Klitgård, Ebbe. *Chaucer's Narrative Voice in "The Knight's Tale."* Copenhagen: Museum Tusculanum Press, 1995.

Knapp, Ethan. *The Bureaucratic Muse: Thomas Hoccleve and the Literature of Late Medieval England*. University Park: Pennsylvania State University Press, 2001.

Kolve, V. A. *Chaucer and the Imagery of Narrative: The First Five Canterbury Tales*. Stanford, CA: Stanford University Press, 1984.

Krochalis, Jeanne, and Edward Peters, eds. and trans. *The World of Piers Plowman*. Philadelphia: University of Pennsylvania Press, 1975.

Krug, Rebecca. "*Piers Plowman* and the Secrets of Health." *Chaucer Review* 46 (2011): 166–81.

Kruger, Steven. "Medical and Moral Authority in the Late Medieval Dream." In *The Interpretation of Dreams from Chaucer to Shakespeare*, ed. Peter Brown, 51–83. Oxford: Oxford University Press, 1999.

Lanfranc of Milan. *Lanfrank's "Science of Cirurgie."* Ed. Robert von Fleischhacker, EETS o.s. 102. London: Kegan Paul, Trench, Trübner, and Co., 1894.

Langland, William. *The Vision of Piers Plowman: A Critical Edition of the B-Text Based on Trinity College, Cambridge MS B.15.17*. 2nd ed. Ed. A. V. C. Schmidt. London: J. M. Dent, 1995.

Langum, Virginia. *Medicine and the Seven Deadly Sins in Late Medieval Literature and Culture*. New York: Palgrave Macmillan, 2016.

A Latin Technical Phlebotomy and Its Middle English Translation. Ed. and trans. Linda Ehrsam Voigts and Michael R. McVaugh. Philadelphia: American Philosophical Society, 1984.

Lawton, David. "Dullness and the Fifteenth Century." *ELH* 54 (1987): 761–99.

———. "Sacrilege and Theatricality: The *Croxton Play of the Sacrament*." *Journal of Medieval and Early Modern Studies* 33 (2003): 281–309.

———. "Voice After Arundel." In *After Arundel: Religious Writing in Fifteenth-Century England*, ed. Kantik Ghosh and Vincent Gillespie, 133–52. Turnhout: Brepols, 2011.

———. "Voice, Authority, and Blasphemy in *The Book of Margery Kempe*." In *Margery Kempe: A Book of Essays*, ed. Sandra McEntire, 93–116. New York: Garland, 1992.

———. *Voice in Later Medieval English Literature: Public Interiorities*. Oxford: Oxford University Press, 2017.

Leach, Elizabeth Eva. *Sung Birds: Music, Nature, and Poetry in the Later Middle Ages*. Ithaca, NY: Cornell University Press, 2006.

Leder, Drew. *The Absent Body*. Chicago: University of Chicago Press, 1990.

Lerer, Seth. *Chaucer and His Readers: Imagining the Author in Late Medieval England*. Princeton, NJ: Princeton University Press, 1993.

Lindberg, David C. *The Beginnings of Western Science: The European Scientific Tradition in Philosophical, Religious, and Institutional Context, 600 B.C. to A.D. 1450*. Chicago: University of Chicago Press, 1992.

Livesey, Steven J. "Scientia." In *Medieval Science, Technology, and Medicine: An Encyclopedia*, ed. Thomas F. Glick, Steven J. Livesey, and Faith Wallis, 455–58. New York: Routledge, 2005.

Lochrie, Karma. *Covert Operations: The Medieval Uses of Secrecy*. Philadelphia: University of Pennsylvania Press, 1999.

————. *Margery Kempe and Translations of the Flesh.* Philadelphia: University of Pennsylvania Press, 1991.

Lowes, John Livingston. "The Loveres Maladye of Hereos." *Modern Philology* 11 (1914): 491–546.

Lydgate, John. "The Dietary." In *Codex Ashmole 61: A Compilation of Middle English Verse,* ed. George Shuffelton, 277–79. Kalamazoo, MI: Medieval Institute Publications, 2008.

————. *The Minor Poems of John Lydgate, Vol. II (Secular Poems).* Ed. Henry Noble MacCracken. EETS o.s. 192. London, 1934.

Lynch, Kathryn L. "Robert Henryson's 'Doolie Dreame' and the Late Medieval Dream Vision Tradition." *Journal of English and Germanic Philology* 109 (2010): 177–97.

A Macaronic Sermon Collection from Late Medieval England: Oxford Bodley 649. Ed. and trans. Patrick J. Horner. Toronto: Pontifical Institute of Mediaeval Studies, 2006.

Macdougall, Simone C. "The Surgeon and the Saints: Henri de Mondeville on Divine Healing." *Journal of Medieval History* 26 (2000): 253–67.

MacQueen, John. *Robert Henryson: A Study of the Major Narrative Poems.* Oxford: Clarendon Press, 1967.

Maidstone, Henry. "Miscellanea Relating to the Martyrdom of Archbishop Scrope." In *Historians of the Church of York and Its Archbishops,* ed. James Raine, 2:304–11. London: Longman, 1886.

Manly, John M., and Edith Rickert. *The Text of the Canterbury Tales: Studied on the Basis of All Known Manuscripts.* 8 vols. Chicago: University of Chicago Press, 1940.

Mann, Jill. "Chance and Destiny in *Troilus and Criseyde* and the *Knight's Tale.*" In *The Cambridge Companion to Chaucer,* ed. Piero Boitani and Jill Mann, 93–111. Cambridge: Cambridge University Press, 2004

————. *Chaucer and Medieval Estates Satire: The Literature of Social Classes and the General Prologue to the Canterbury Tales.* Cambridge: Cambridge University Press, 1993.

————. *Geoffrey Chaucer.* Feminist Readings Series. Atlantic Highlands, NJ: Humanities Press International, 1991.

————. "The Planetary Gods in Chaucer and Henryson." In *Chaucer Traditions: Studies in Honour of Derek Brewer,* ed. Ruth Morse and Barry Windeatt, 91–106. Cambridge: Cambridge University Press, 1990.

Mapstone, Sally. "The Scots *Buik of Phisnomy* and Sir Gilbert Hay." In *The Renaissance in Scotland: Studies in Literature, Religion, History, and Culture Offered to John Durkan,* ed. A. A. MacDonald, Michael Lynch, and Ian B. Cowan, 1–44. Leiden: Brill, 1994.

Mathews, Jana. "Land, Lepers, and the Law in *The Testament of Cresseid.*" In *The Letter of the Law: Legal Practice and Literary Production in Medieval England,* ed. Emily Steiner and Candace Barrington, 40–66. Ithaca, NY: Cornell University Press, 2002.

McGerr, Rosemarie P. *Chaucer's Open Books: Resistance to Closure in Medieval Discourse.* Gainesville: University Press of Florida, 1998.

McNiven, Peter. "The Problem of Henry IV's Health, 1405–1413." *English Historical Review* 100 (1985): 747–72.

McVaugh, Michael R. "The 'Experience-Based' Medicine of the Thirteenth Century." *Early Science and Medicine* 14 (2009): 105–30.

————. *Medicine Before the Plague: Practitioners and Their Patients in the Crown of Aragon, 1285–1345.* Cambridge: Cambridge University Press, 1993.

————. "The Nature and Limits of Medical Certitude at Early Fourteenth-Century Montpellier." *Osiris* 6 (1990): 62–84.

————. *The Rational Surgery of the Middle Ages.* Florence: Sismel-Edizioni del Galluzzo, 2006.

McVaugh, Michael R., and Fernando Salmón. Introduction to Arnau of Vilanova, *Repetitio super aphorismo Hippocratus "Vita brevis,"* ed. Michael R. McVaugh, 265–333. In *Arnaldi de Villanova Opera medica omnia.* Vol. 14. Barcelona: Universitat de Barcelona, 2014.

McVaugh, Michael R., and L. García Ballester. "Therapeutic Method in the Later Middle Ages: Arnau de Vilanova on Medical Contingency." *Caduceus* 11 (1995): 73–86.

Medieval English Lyrics: A Critical Anthology. Ed. R. T. Davies. London: Faber and Faber, 1963.

Medieval Woman's Guide to Health: The First English Gynecological Handbook. Ed. Beryl Rowland. Kent, OH: Kent State University Press, 1981.

Merleau-Ponty, Maurice. *Phenomenology of Perception.* 1945. Trans. Colin Smith. London: Routledge & Paul, 1962.

Metzler, Irina. *Disability in Medieval Europe: Physical Impairment in the High Middle Ages, c. 1100–c. 1400.* London: Routledge, 2006.

Mieszkowski, Gretchen. "The Reputation of Criseyde, 1155–1500." *Transactions of the Connecticut Academy of Arts and Sciences* 43 (1971): 71–153.

Miller, Mark. *Philosophical Chaucer: Love, Sex, and Agency in the Canterbury Tales.* Cambridge: Cambridge University Press, 2004.

Mimes français du XIIIe siècle. Ed. Edmond Faral. Paris: H. Champion, 1910.

Mink, Louis O. "Narrative Form as Cognitive Instrument." In *The Writing of History: Literary Form and Historical Understanding,* ed. Robert H. Canary and Henry Kozicki, 129–49. Madison: University of Wisconsin Press, 1978.

Minnis, A. J. *Chaucer and Pagan Antiquity.* Cambridge: D. S. Brewer, 1982.

Mirfield, John. *Johannes de Mirfeld of St Bartholomew's, Smithfield: His Life and Works.* Ed. and trans. Percival Horton-Smith Hartley and Harold Richard Aldridge. Cambridge: Cambridge University Press, 1936.

Mirk, John. *Mirk's Festial: A Collection of Homilies.* Ed. Theodor Erbe, EETS e.s. 96. London: K. Paul, Trench, Trübner, 1905.

Mitchell, J. Allan. *Ethics and Exemplary Narrative in Chaucer and Gower.* Cambridge: D. S. Brewer, 2004.

Mooney, Catherine M. "Voice, Gender, and the Portrayal of Sanctity." In *Gendered Voices: Medieval Saints and Their Interpreters,* ed. Catherine M. Mooney, 1–15. Philadelphia: University of Pennsylvania Press, 1999.

Moorat, S. A. J. *Catalogue of Western Manuscripts on Medicine and Science in the Wellcome Historical Medical Library.* London: Wellcome Institute for the History of Medicine, 1962–73.

Moore, R. I. *The Formation of a Persecuting Society: Power and Deviance in Western Europe, 950–1250.* Oxford: Blackwell, 1987.

Morrissey, Jake Walsh. "'To al indifferent': The Virtues of Lydgate's 'Dietary.'" *Medium Aevum* 84 (2015): 258–78.

Mosher, Joseph A. *The Exemplum in the Early Religious and Didactic Literature of England.* New York: Columbia University Press, 1911.

Ms. Bodley 959: Genesis-Baruch 3.20 in the Earlier Version of the Wycliffite Bible. 5 vols. Ed. Conrad Lindberg. Stockholm: Almqvist & Wiksell, 1959.

Murphy, James J. *Rhetoric in the Middle Ages: A History of Rhetorical Theory from St. Augustine to the Renaissance.* Berkeley: University of California Press, 1974.

Muscatine, Charles. "Form, Texture, and Meaning in Chaucer's *Knight's Tale.*" *PMLA* 65 (1950): 911–29.

Mystères inédits du quinzième siècle. Ed. Achille Jubinal. 2 vols. Paris: Téchener, 1837.

Newman, Barbara. *Medieval Crossover: Reading the Secular Against the Sacred.* Notre Dame, IN: University of Notre Dame Press, 2013

Nutton, Vivian. "The Seeds of Disease: An Explanation of Contagion and Infection from the Greeks to the Renaissance." *Medical History* 27 (1983): 1–34.

O'Boyle, Cornelius. *The Art of Medicine: Medical Teaching at the University of Paris, 1250–1400.* Leiden: Brill, 1998.

———. "Medicine, God, and Aristotle in the Early Universities: Prefatory Prayers in Late Medieval Medical Commentaries." *Bulletin of the History of Medicine* 66 (1992): 185–209.

Olson, Glending. *Literature as Recreation in the Later Middle Ages.* Ithaca, NY: Cornell University Press, 1982.

O'Mara, Veronica, and Suzanne Paul. *A Repertorium of Middle English Prose Sermons.* Turnhout: Brepols, 2007.

Orlemanski, Julie. "Desire and Defacement in *The Testament of Cresseid.*" In *Reading Skin in Medieval Literature and Culture*, ed. Katie L. Walter, 161–81. New York: Palgrave Macmillan, 2013.

———. "How to Kiss a Leper." *postmedieval* 3 (2012): 142–57.

———. "Jargon and the Matter of Medicine in Middle English." *Journal of Medieval and Early Modern Studies* 42 (2012): 395–420.

———. "Leprosies." Forthcoming in the *Ashgate Research Companion to Medieval Disability Studies*, ed. John P. Sexton and Kisha G. Tracy.

———. "Literary Genre, Medieval Studies, and the Prosthesis of Disability." *Textual Practice* 30 (2016): 1253–72.

———. "Margery's 'Noyse' and Distributed Expressivity." In *Voice and Voicelessness in Medieval Europe*, ed. Irit Kleinman, 123–38. New York: Palgrave Macmillan, 2015.

———. "Prosopopoeial Heaviness in Chaucer's *Book of the Duchess.*" In *Chaucer and the Subversion of Form*, ed. Thomas A. Prendergast and Jessica Rosenfeld, 125–46. Cambridge: Cambridge University Press, 2018.

———. "Thornton's Remedies and Practices of Medical Reading." In *Robert Thornton and His Books*, ed. Susanna Fein and Michael Johnston, 235–55. York: York Medieval Press, 2014.

Park, Katharine. *Doctors and Medicine in Early Renaissance Florence.* Princeton, NJ: Princeton University Press, 1985.

———. "Medicine and Society in Medieval Europe." In *Medicine in Society: Historical Essays*, ed. Andrew Wear, 59–90. Cambridge: Cambridge University Press, 1992.

Parr, Johnstone. "Cresseid's Leprosy Again." *Modern Language Notes* 60 (1945): 487–91.

Paston Letters and Papers of the Fifteenth Century. Part 1. Ed. Norman Davis. 1971. EETS s.s. 20. Oxford: Oxford University Press, 2004.

Patch, Howard R. *The Goddess Fortuna in Medieval Literature.* Cambridge, MA: Harvard University Press, 1927.

Patterson, Lee. *Chaucer and the Subject of History.* Madison: University of Wisconsin Press, 1991.

———. "Christian and Pagan in *The Testament of Cresseid.*" *Philological Quarterly* 52 (1973): 696–714.

———. "What Is Me? Hoccleve and the Trials of the Urban Self." 2001. Reprinted in *Acts of Recognition: Essays on Medieval Culture*, 84–119. Notre Dame, IN: University of Notre Dame Press, 2010.

Pearsall, Derek. "'Quha wait gif all that Chauceir wrait was trew?': Henryson's *Testament of Cresseid.*" In *New Perspectives on Middle English Texts: A Festschrift for R. A. Waldron*, ed. Susan Powell and Jeremy J. Smith, 169–82. Cambridge: D. S. Brewer, 2000.

Petrarca, Francesco. *Invectives*. Ed. and trans. David Marsh. Cambridge, MA: Harvard University Press, 2003.

Peyroux, Catherine. "The Leper's Kiss." In *Monks & Nuns, Saints & Outcasts: Religion in Medieval Society*, ed. Sharon Farmer and Barbara H. Rosenwein, 172–88. Ithaca, NY: Cornell University Press, 2000.

Pliny the Elder. *Natural History*. Vol. 7. Trans. W. H. S. Jones. Cambridge, MA: Harvard University Press, 1963.

Pope, Nancy P. "A Middle English Satirical Letter in Brogyntyn MS II.i." *ANQ* 18, no. 3 (2005): 35–39.

Porter, Roy. "History of the Body Reconsidered." In *New Perspectives on Historical Writing*, 2nd ed., ed. Peter Burke, 233–26. University Park: Pennsylvania State University Press, 2001.

Pseudo-Bacon, Roger. "On Tarrying the Accidents of Age (*De retardatione accidentium senectutis*)." Ed. Carol A. Everest and M. Teresa Tavormina. In *Sex, Aging, and Death in a Medieval Medical Compendium: Trinity College Cambridge MS R.14.52, Its Texts, Language, and Scribe*, vol. 1, ed. M. Teresa Tavormina, 133–248. Tempe: Arizona Center for Medieval and Renaissance Studies, 2006.

Pseudo-Cicero. *Rhetorica ad Herennium*. Trans. Harry Caplan. Cambridge, MA: Harvard University Press, 1954.

Quain, Edwin A. "The Medieval *Accessus ad Auctores*." *Traditio* 3 (1945): 215–64.

Rawcliffe, Carole. "The Doctor of Physic." In *Historians on Chaucer: The "General Prologue" to the Canterbury Tales*, ed. Stephen H. Rigby and Alastair Minnis, 297–318. Oxford: Oxford University Press, 2014.

———. *Leprosy in Medieval England*. Woodbridge: Boydell Press, 2006.

———. *Medicine and Society in Later Medieval England*. Stroud: Sutton, 1997.

———. *Urban Bodies: Communal Health in Late Medieval English Towns and Cities*. Woodbridge: Boydell Press, 2013.

Raymond of Capua. *The Life of Catherine of Siena*. Trans. Conleth Kearns. Wilmington: Michael Glazier, 1980.

Reiss, Athene. *The Sunday Christ: Sabbatarianism in English Medieval Wall Painting*. Oxford: Archaeopress, 2000

Renzi, Salvatore de, ed. *Collectio Salernitana*. 5 vols. Naples: Dalla tipografia del Filiatre-Sebezio, 1852–59.

Richards, Peter. *The Medieval Leper and His Northern Heirs*. Cambridge: D. S. Brewer, 1977.

Ricoeur, Paul *Freedom and Nature: The Voluntary and the Involuntary*. 1950. Trans. Erazim V. Kohak. Evanston, IL: Northwestern University Press, 1966.

Riddy, Felicity. "'Abject Odious': Feminine and Masculine in Henryson's *Testament of Cresseid*." In *Chaucer to Spenser: A Critical Reader*, ed. Derek Pearsall, 280–96. Oxford: Blackwell, 1999.

———. "Text and Self in *The Book of Margery Kempe*." In *Voices in Dialogue: Reading Women in the Middle Ages*, ed. Linda Olson and Kathryn Kerby-Fulton, 435–53. Notre Dame, IN: University of Notre Dame Press, 2005.

Rigg, A. G. "Hoccleve's *Complaint* and Isidore of Seville." *Speculum* 45 (1970): 564–74.

Robbins, Rossell Hope. "Medical Manuscripts in Middle English." *Speculum* 45 (1970): 393–415.

———. "Signs of Death in Middle English." *Mediaeval Studies* 32 (1970): 282–98.

Roberts, Phyllis B. "The *Ars Praedicandi* and the Medieval Sermon." In *Preacher, Sermon and Audience in the Middle Ages*, ed. Carolyn Muessig, 41–62. Leiden: Brill, 2004.

Robertson, Elizabeth. "Medieval Medical Views of Women and Female Spirituality in the *Ancrene Wisse* and Julian of Norwich's *Showings*." In *Feminist Approaches to the Body in Medieval Literature*, ed. Linda Lomperis and Sarah Stanbury, 142–67. Philadelphia: University of Pennsylvania Press, 1993.

Robertson, Kellie. *Nature Speaks: Medieval Literature and Aristotelian Philosophy*. Philadelphia: University of Pennsylvania Press, 2017.

Romero-Barranco, Jesus. *The Late Middle English Version of Constantinus Africanus' Venerabilis anatomia in London, Wellcome Library, MS 290 (f. 1r–41v)*. Newcastle-upon-Tyne: Cambridge Scholars Publishing, 2015.

Ross, Robert C. "Oral Life, Written Text." *Yearbook of English Studies* 22 (1992): 226–37.

Rotuli parliamentorum; ut et petitiones, et placita in parliamento tempore Henrici R. V. Vol. 4. Ed. John Strachey et al. London, 1832.

Rymer's Foedera Volume 11. Ed. Thomas Rymer. London: Apud Joannem Neulme, 1739–45. *British History Online*. http://www.british-history.ac.uk/rymer-foedera/vol11/pp618-639.

Salih, Sarah. "Margery's Bodies, Piety, Work and Penance." In *A Companion to the Book of Margery Kempe*, ed. John H. Arnold and Katherine J. Lewis, 161–76. Cambridge: D. S. Brewer, 2004.

———. *Versions of Virginity in Late Medieval England*. Cambridge: D. S. Brewer, 2001.

Salter, Elizabeth. *The Knight's Tale and the Clerk's Tale*. London: Edward Arnold, 1962.

———. *Popular Reading in English, c. 1400–1600*. Manchester: Manchester University Press, 2012.

Scanlon, Larry. *Narrative, Authority, and Power: The Medieval Exemplum and the Chaucerian Tradition*. Cambridge: Cambridge University Press, 1994.

Scarry, Elaine. *The Body in Pain: The Making and Unmaking of the World*. New York: Oxford University Press, 1985.

Schweitzer, Edward C. "Fate and Freedom in 'The Knight's Tale.'" *Studies in the Age of Chaucer* 3 (1981): 13–45.

Scott, Kathleen L. *Later Gothic Manuscripts, 1390–1490*. 2 vols. London: Harvey Miller Publishers, 1996.

———. "Newly Discovered Booklets from a Reconstructed Middle English Manuscript." *English Manuscript Studies* 14 (2008): 112–29.

Secretum Secretorum: Nine English Versions. Ed. Mahmoud Manzalaoui. EETS o.s. 276. Oxford: Oxford University Press, 1977.

Secular Lyrics of the XIV and XV Centuries. 2nd ed. Ed. Rossell Hope Robbins. Oxford: Clarendon Press, 1955.

Seznec, Jean. *The Survival of the Pagan Gods: The Mythological Tradition and Its Place in Renaissance Humanism and Art*. Trans. Barbara F. Sessions. Princeton, NJ: Princeton University Press, 1953.

Sigerist, Henry E. "Bedside Manners in the Middle Ages: The Treatise de Cautelis Medicorum Attributed to Arnald of Villanova." *Quarterly Bulletin of the Northwestern University Medical School* 20, no. 1 (1946): 136–43.

Silva, Chelsea. "Opening the Medieval Folded Almanac." *Exemplaria* 30, no. 1 (2018): 49–65.

Simpson, James. "Madness and Texts: Hoccleve's *Series*." In *Chaucer and Fifteenth-Century Poetry*, ed. Julia Boffey and Janet Cowen, 15–29. London: King's College London, 1991.

———. "Nobody's Man: Thomas Hoccleve's *Regiment of Princes*." In *London and Europe in the Later Middle Ages*, ed. Julia Boffey and Pamela King, 149–80. London: University of London, 1995.

Siraisi, Nancy G. "How to Write a Latin Book of Surgery: Organizing Principles and Authorial Devices in Guglielmo da Saliceto and Dino del Garbo." In *Practical Medicine from Salerno to the Black Death*, ed. Luis García Ballester, Roger French, Jon Arrizabalaga, and Andrew Cunningham, 88–109. New York: Cambridge University Press, 1994.

———. *Medieval and Early Renaissance Medicine: An Introduction to Knowledge and Practice*. Chicago: University of Chicago Press, 1990.

Slack, Paul. *The Impact of Plague in Tudor and Stuart England*. London: Routledge and Kegan Paul, 1985.

Smith, D. Vance. "Plague, Panic Space, and the Tragic Medieval Household." *South Atlantic Quarterly* 98 (1999): 367–414.

Sobecki, Sebastian. "'The writyng of this tretys': Margery Kempe's Son and the Authorship of Her Book." *Studies in the Age of Chaucer* 37 (2015): 257–83.

Spearing, A. C. "Margery Kempe." In *A Companion to Middle English Prose*, ed. A. S. G. Edwards, 83–97. Cambridge: D. S. Brewer, 2004.

———. *Medieval Autographies: The "I" of the Text*. Conway Lectures in Medieval Studies. Notre Dame, IN: University of Notre Dame Press, 2012

———. *Textual Subjectivity*. Oxford: Oxford University Press, 2005.

Stadolnik, Joe. "Gower's Bedside Manner." *New Medieval Literatures* 17 (2017): 150–74.

Staley, Lynn. *Margery Kempe's Dissenting Fictions*. University Park: Pennsylvania State University Press, 1994.

Stearns, Marshall W. "Henryson and the Leper Cresseid." *Modern Language Notes* 59 (1944): 265–69.

———. *Robert Henryson*. New York: AMC Press, 1966.

Steiner, Emily. "Authority." In *Middle English*, ed. Paul Strohm, 142–59. Oxford: Oxford University Press, 2007.

Stephenson, William. "The Acrostic 'Fictio' in Robert Henryson's *The Testament of Cresseid* (Lines 58–63)." *Chaucer Review* 29 (1994): 163–65.

Taavitsainen, Irma, and Päivi Pahta. "Vernacularisation and Medical Writing in Its Sociohistorical Context." In *Medical and Scientific Writing in Late Medieval English*, ed. Irma Taavitsainen and Päivi Pahta, 1–18. Cambridge: Cambridge University Press, 2004.

Tabuteau, Bruno. "Historical Research Developments on Leprosy in France and Western Europe." In *The Medieval Hospital and Medical Practice*, ed. B. S. Bowers, 41–56. Aldershot: Ashgate, 2007.

Tavormina, M. Teresa. "The Middle English 'Letter of Ipocras.'" *English Studies* 88 (2007): 632–52.

———. "Three Middle English Verse Uroscopies." *English Studies* 91 (2010): 591–622.

Thorndike, Lynn, and Pearl Kibre. *A Catalogue of Incipits of Mediaeval Scientific Writings in Latin*. Rev. ed. Cambridge: Mediaeval Academy of America, 1963.

Three Prose Versions of the Secreta Secretorum. Ed. Robert Steele. EETS e.s. 74. London: K. Paul, Trench, Trübner & Co., 1898.

Tiffany, Daniel. *Infidel Poetics: Riddles, Nightlife, Substance*. Chicago: University of Chicago Press, 2009.

Touati, François-Olivier. "Contagion and Leprosy: Myth, Ideas and Evolution in Medieval Minds and Societies." In *Contagion: Perspectives from Pre-Modern Societies*, ed. L. Conrad and D. Wujastyk, 179–201. Aldershot: Ashgate, 2000.

———. *Maladie et société au moyen âge*. Brussels: De Boeck Université, 1998.

Trotula: A Medieval Compendium of Women's Medicine. Ed. and trans. Monica H. Green. Philadelphia: University of Pennsylvania Press, 2001.

Tubach, Frederic C. "Exempla in the Decline." *Traditio* 18 (1962): 407–17.

———. *Index Exemplorum: A Handbook of Medieval Religious.* FF Communications 204. Helsinki: Suomalainen Tiedeakatemia, 1969.

Turner, Marion. "Illness Narratives in the Later Middle Ages: Arderne, Chaucer, and Hoccleve." *Journal of Medieval and Early Modern Studies* 46 (2016): 61–87.

Uhlman, Diana R. "The Comfort of Voice, the Solace of Script: Orality and Literacy in *The Book of Margery Kempe*." *Studies in Philology* 91 (1994): 50–69.

Ussery, Huling E. *Chaucer's Physician: Medicine and Literature in Fourteenth-Century England.* New Orleans: Tulane University, 1971.

van 't Land, Karine. "Internal Yet Extrinsic: Conceptions of Bodily Space and Their Relation to Causality in Late Medieval University Medicine." In *Medicine and Space: Body, Surroundings and Borders in Antiquity and the Middle Ages*, ed. Patricia A. Baker, Han Nijdam, and Karine van 't Land, 85–116. Leiden: Brill, 2011.

van D'Elden, Stephanie Cain. "The Salerno Effect: The Image of Salerno in Courtly Literature." In *L'Imaginaire Courtois et Son Double*, ed. Giovanna Angeli et Luciano Formisano, 503–15. Naples: Edizioni scientifiche italiane, 1991.

Van Dyke, Carolynn. *Chaucer's Agents: Cause and Representation in Chaucerian Narrative.* Madison, NJ: Fairleigh Dickinson University Press, 2005.

Voaden, Rosalynn. *God's Words, Women's Voices: The Discernment of Spirits in the Writings of Late Medieval Women Visionaries.* York: York Medieval Press, 1999.

Voigts, Linda Ehrsam. "Fifteenth-Century English Banns Advertising the Services of an Itinerant Doctor." In *Between Text and Patient: The Medical Enterprise in Medieval and Early Modern Europe*, ed. Florence Eliza Glaze and Brian K. Nance, 245–77. Florence: SISMEL, 2011.

———. "Herbs and Herbal Healing Satirized in Middle English Texts." In *Herbs and Healers from the Ancient Mediterranean Through the Medieval West: Essays in Honour of John M. Riddle*, ed. Ann Van Arsdall and Timothy Graham, 217–30. Farnham: Ashgate, 2012.

———. "Multitudes of Middle English Medical Manuscripts, or the Englishing of Science and Medicine." In *Manuscript Sources of Medieval Medicine*, 183–95. New York: Garland, 1995.

———. "Scientific and Medical Books." In *Book Production and Publishing in Britain, 1375–1475*, ed. Jeremy Griffiths and Derek Pearsall, 345–402. Cambridge: Cambridge University Press, 1989.

———. "The 'Sloane Group': Related Scientific and Medical Manuscripts from the Fifteenth Century in the Sloane Collection." *British Library Journal* 16 (1990): 26–57.

———. "What's the Word? Bilingualism in Late Medieval England." *Speculum* 71 (1996): 813–26.

Voigts, Linda Ehrsam, and Patricia Deery Kurtz. *Scientific and Medical Writings in Old and Middle English: An Electronic Reference.* CD-ROM. Ann Arbor: University of Michigan Press, 2001.

———. *Voigts-Kurtz Search Program.* University of Missouri–Kansas City. http://cctr1.umkc.edu /cgi-bin/search, accessible via https://medievalacademy.site-ym.com/?page=Books#etk.

von Moos, Peter. "The Use of Exempla in the *Policraticus* of John of Salisbury." In *The World of John of Salisbury*, ed. Michael Wilks, 207–64. Oxford: Basil Blackwell for the Ecclesiastical History Society, 1979.

von Nolcken, Christina. "Gascoigne [Gascoygne], Thomas (1404–1458)." *ODNB.* Electronic ed.

Wack, Mary. *Lovesickness in the Middle Ages: The Viaticum and Its Commentaries.* Philadelphia: University of Pennsylvania Press, 1990.

Wallis, Faith, ed. and trans. *Medieval Medicine: A Reader.* Toronto: University of Toronto Press, 2010.

Walsh, Martin M. "Rubin and Mercator: Grotesque Comedy in the German Easter Play." *Comparative Drama* 36 (2002): 187–202.

Watson, Nicholas. "The Making of *The Book of Margery Kempe*." In *Voices in Dialogue: Reading Women in the Middle Ages*, ed. Linda Olson and Kathryn Kerby-Fulton, 395–434. Notre Dame, IN: University of Notre Dame Press, 2005.

———. "Outdoing Chaucer: Lydgate's *Troy Book* and Henryson's *Testament of Cresseid* as Competitive Imitations of *Troilus and Criseyde*." In *Shifts and Transpositions in Medieval Narrative: A Festschrift for Dr. Elspeth Kennedy*, ed. Karen Pratt, 89–108. Cambridge: D. S. Brewer, 1994.

Watt, David. "'I this book shal make': Thomas Hoccleve's Self-Publication and Book Production." *Leeds Studies in English* 34 (2003): 133–60.

———. *The Making of Thomas Hoccleve's "Series."* Liverpool: Liverpool University Press, 2013.

Whearty, Bridget. "The Leper on the Road to Canterbury." *Mediaevalia* 36/37 (2015/2016): 223–61.

Williams, Steven J. *The Secret of Secrets: The Scholarly Career of a Pseudo-Aristotelian Text in the Latin Middle Ages*. Ann Arbor: University of Michigan Press, 2003.

Windeatt, Barry. Introduction to Margery Kempe. In *The Book of Margery Kempe*, trans. Barry Windeatt, 9–28. London: Penguin, 1985.

Winstead, Karen A. "'I am al othir to yow than yee weene': Hoccleve, Women, and the *Series*." *Philological Quarterly* 72 (1993): 143–55.

Wittig, Kurt. *The Scottish Tradition in Literature*. Edinburgh: Oliver and Boyd, 1958.

Wright, Stephen K. "What's So 'English' About Medieval English Drama? An East Anglican Miracle Play and Its Continental Counterpart." In *To Make His English Sweete upon His Tonge*, ed. Marcin Krygier and Liliana Sikorska, 71–92. Frankfurt: Peter Lang, 2007.

Yunck, John A. "Satire." In *A Companion to Piers Plowman*, ed. John A. Alford, 135–54. Berkeley: University of California Press, 1988.

Ziegler, Joseph. *Medicine and Religion c. 1300: The Case of Arnau de Vilanova*. Oxford: Clarendon Press, 1998.

Index

Acknowledgments

Looking back over this book's coming to be, I am happy to see just how entangled its sentences are with others' generosity and brilliance. *Symptomatic Subjects* began with insights sparked by James Simpson, Nicholas Watson, Katharine Park, and Marjorie Garber. James was long ago responsible for my abrupt decision to become a medievalist, and conversations with him and Nicholas helped me cut a path for myself through medieval studies. Katy Park opened the historiography of medieval medicine and made me believe I could find my way to contributing. My time at Harvard University was lit by many friendships. Maia McAleavey and Marcella Frydman Manoharan buoyed me up through the grim bits and celebrated everything else; they continue to be among my dearest friends. Debating with Daniel Shore remains a favorite intellectual pastime. Many happy occasions were shared with Matthew Barrett, Jason Manoharan, Timothy Michael, Stephen Hequembourg, Hannah Sullivan, and Ian Martin. The "Hegel Reading Group" (which became the Mahindra Humanities Center Seminar on Dialectical Thinking) was my essential intellectual community at Harvard; I thank Gordon Teskey, Jamey Graham, William Baldwin, Martin Moraw, and Robert S. Lehman for sustaining it. The English Department's Medieval Colloquium was also a wellspring of scholarly conviviality, especially Ingrid Nelson and Alexis Becker. The early part of my time in Cambridge, Massachusetts, was made much brighter by the company of Blake Doughty.

The completion of *Symptomatic Subjects* was made possible by institutional support. The Mellon ACLS Fellowship, the Mahindra Humanities Center at Harvard Postdoctoral Fellowship, and the Huntington Library Mellon Fellowship all provided me with time to think and work. During my year at the Humanities Center, Annie McClanahan was my fierce and constant comrade. While at the Huntington Library, I was welcomed to California by Rebecca Davis, Jennifer Jahner, and Andrea Denny-Brown, and I became fast friends with Jessica Davies and Stefanie Sobelle. A Frank Knox Memorial

Traveling Fellowship allowed me to spend a year abroad in England, where I was delighted to befriend Virginia Langum and Annie Ring. The first complete draft of this manuscript was finished at the dining-room table of Tasha Graff, a wonder of patience and grace. This past year I've had the pleasure of completing revisions while at the Institute for Advanced Study in Princeton; my thanks to the librarians for their tireless procurement of books and to Patrick Geary and to Joan Scott each for a generous welcome. While I was an undergraduate at the University of Georgia, long before this project was under way, the English Department made studying literature intoxicating, and I am thankful to it as well as to the Foundation Fellowship for their support. The University of Pennsylvania Press, especially as personified in Jerry Singerman, has made publishing a pleasure, and I am especially grateful to the press's two readers, Kellie Robertson and Bruce Holsinger, whose at once exacting and encouraging reports made the final manuscript much better. One para-institution, the BABEL Working Group, has helped transform medieval studies into a more joyous, promiscuous, and equitable field, and this book tries to do justice to its expansiveness. Eileen A. Joy was the spark for it, and over the years BABEL has put me in touch with a catalogue of wonderful people, including Myra Seaman, Liza Blake, J. Allan Mitchell, Lara Farina, Karl Steel, Jonathan Hsy, Suzanne Conklin Akbari, Ruth Evans, Jeffery Jerome Cohen, Daniel Remein, Roland Betancourt, Holly Crocker, and the inimitable Arthur Russell, among many others. Marion Turner stands out as well for her generosity. All of these individuals and these forms of institutional provision have helped me see *Symptomatic Subjects* through and thrive along the way; I thank them.

The English Department at Boston College was a felicitous environment for setting forth on faculty life, and I particularly thank Robert Stanton and Mary Crane for their kind wisdom. That first year at BC coincided with the events of Occupy Boston, and so, as I remember it, my education in new things unfolded between Chestnut Hill and Dewey Square. It makes me smile that I met Ian Cornelius there before realizing we were both medievalists. More recently the University of Chicago has been an excellent intellectual home. Mark Miller is an extraordinary colleague, whose conversation and care have made this book stronger. Daisy Delogu, Aden Kumler, and Lucy Pick make the study of the Middle Ages vibrant in Hyde Park, as do brilliant graduate students like Carly Boxer, Hannah Christensen, Jack Dragu, Luke Fidler, Andres Millan, Jo Nixon, Matthew Vanderpoel, and Jacqueline Victor. Gratitude is also due to the Midwest Middle English Reading Group and especially the vibrant Liza Strakhov. The English Department at the University of Chicago has constantly supported my work while pushing it further; I particularly thank Lauren Berlant, Frances Ferguson, and Lisa Ruddick. The members of the Chicago-area Junior Faculty Working Group, and the city's cohort of young scholars more broadly, have all strengthened this book, and time and again I've found myself savoring dialogue with Adrienne Brown, Alexis Chema, Andi Diamond, David Diamond, Harris Feinsod, Leah Feldman, Andrew Ferguson, Rachel Galvin, Edgar Garcia, Timothy M. Harrison, Anna Kornbluh, Andrew Leong, Benjamin Morgan, Nassar Mufti, John Muse, Kim O'Neil, Zachary Samalin, David Carroll Simon, Christopher Taylor, and Sonali Thakkar. And the very best thing about Chicago is Peter Coviello, whose talents for joy, for argument, for fast-flashing intelligence, and for unplumbable kindness have made everything brighter, this book included. My thanks and love and futureward dreaming are with him. Finally, I dedicate *Symptomatic Subjects* to my family, especially to Gene and Madylene Walsh, to Dennis and Debbie Orlemanski, and to Katie Orlemanski Mayfield. I often feel our happiness beneath other happiness, a bedrock for flourishing.

Milton Keynes UK
Ingram Content Group UK Ltd.
UKHW042032081123
432218UK00004B/45/J